# Health Communication for Social Justice

This textbook combines whole person and social justice perspectives to educate students on the role of communication in promoting inclusive and person-centered healthcare practices.

This book explores health inequities experienced by disadvantaged and marginalized populations and outlines the actions students can take to address these challenges. The book demonstrates how physical, mental, and emotional health is connected to equitable understandings of individual, community, and environmental health. It considers how social, interpersonal, and systemic factors such as personal relationships, language, literacy, religion, technology, and the environment affect health equity. To present strategies and invite action to support the goals of the whole person, social justice activist approach, the book provides contemporary examples, interviews with communication scholars, and case studies that examine local communities and the everyday contexts of health meaning making.

This textbook serves as a core or supplemental text for graduate and upper-level undergraduate courses in health communication.

Online resources include PowerPoint slides and an instructor manual containing sample syllabi, assignments, and test questions. They are available online at www.routledge.com/9781032081038.

**Vinita Agarwal** is Professor of Communication at Salisbury University, USA. She is the founder of Whole Person Health Consulting, LLC, and the author of *Medical Humanism, Chronic Illness, and the Body in Pain* (2020). Her work has appeared in journals, including *Health Communication, Journal of Advanced Nursing,* and *Journal of American College Health,* and the *International Encyclopedia of Health Communication.*

Routledge Social Justice Communication Activism Series
Lawrence R. Frey and Patricia S. Parker, Series Editors

For additional information on this series please visit https://www.routledge.com/Routledge-Social-Justice-Communication-Activism-Series/book-series/RSJCAS, and for information on other Routledge titles visit www.routledge.com.

# Health Communication for Social Justice

## A Whole Person Activist Approach

Vinita Agarwal

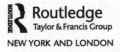
Routledge
Taylor & Francis Group

NEW YORK AND LONDON

Designed cover image: Valerii Minhirov/© Getty Images

First published 2024
by Routledge
605 Third Avenue, New York, NY 10158

and by Routledge
4 Park Square, Milton Park, Abingdon, Oxon, OX14 4RN

Routledge is an imprint of the Taylor & Francis Group, an informa business

ISBN: 978-1-032-10262-7 (hbk)
ISBN: 978-1-032-08103-8 (pbk)
ISBN: 978-1-003-21447-2 (ebk)

DOI: 10.4324/9781003214472

Typeset in Times New Roman
by SPi Technologies India Pvt Ltd (Straive)

Access the Support Material: www.routledge.com/9781032081038

To my family, Sangeet, Arjun, and Appa, for their unconditional love.

# Contents

# Foreword

I am very pleased this exciting new book, *Health Communication for Social Justice: A Whole Person Activist Approach*, is now part of the growing and vibrant body of health communication literature. The book makes important contributions to expanding understanding of the relevance and intricacy of health communication in modern life. The whole person healthcare approach (that is highlighted in the book) clearly describes the multiple interdependent communication factors that are at work in the delivery of care and promotion of health, including how powerful underlying cultural norms influence health beliefs, expectations, and actions that are unique to each person. The book shows that we each are products of the different intersectional cultural communication experiences that have continually shaped and continue to reshape the ways that we make sense of and react to health and illness.

To help people productively adapt to the serious health challenges they experience, this book helps us understand how individual unique cultural perspectives demand culturally sensitive and responsive health communication. This underscores the need to gather information from those who are confronting health problems to learn about their most memorable and influential personal (and observational) experiences with health and illness that shape their responses to health challenges. The book also illustrates the need to communicate strategically in the delivery of healthcare to elicit information about the variety of health issues that individuals are most concerned about so we can help them address these concerns with appropriate care and health promotion activities. The book suggests that the best healthcare communication is person-centered, speaking to each person's individual health history and sharing information to engage each person (and often members of their social networks) in participating in healthcare and health promotion activities.

The important information presented in this book is directly relevant to everyone who confronts personal health challenges (which basically includes all of us!) to help promote individual health and well-being. It is relevant to everyone who delivers healthcare services and advice (which includes more than just trained healthcare professionals since the vast majority of healthcare services are provided outside of formal healthcare facilities by personal connections, by our family members, friends, and colleagues). It is relevant to healthcare team members who need to share relevant information with each other to promote collaboration for making the best possible health decisions. It is relevant to health educators who provide needed guidance to healthcare providers and consumers about health risks and response strategies. The information in this book is also relevant to health system policymakers to guide their important decisions about establishing and refining effective guidelines for delivering care and promoting health.

It is my hope that many people will use the powerful information in this book to help them strategically use communication to promote their own health and enable them to help others achieve their health goals too!

**Gary L. Kreps, PhD**
George Mason University

# Preface

## Health Communication for Social Justice: A Whole Person Activist Approach

### Focus and Scope

Talking about health communication in everyday contexts has never been more important. From determining the credibility of the daily barrage of health information and suggestions that people receive from media sources and campaigns conducted by organizations, to knowing how to engage in social interactions that ensure equitable and accessible opportunities for health, health communication embeds every facet of people's lives. In whole person healthcare (hereafter, WPHC), people are seen as individuals who are embedded in social relations, leading to healthcare that is grounded in their unique values, needs, and goals. WPHC invites us to consider the facets of an individual's circumstances that impact healthcare conceptualization, delivery, and outcomes from a social justice (SJ) lens. These include the individual's family, community, and other relationships and resources; the environment and how it shapes their lived contexts and those of the species that share our planet; provision of clinical follow-up on their health needs; their religious and spiritual beliefs and how these are addressed in healthcare settings; wellness education and treatment support; and coordination of care to reduce Medicare or Medicaid expenses, urgent care, and emergency department visits and hospitalization outcomes and costs. WPHC accounts for the individuals' diet, exercise, and healthy relationships as the foundation of well-being, ensuring food security, mobility, high-touch care, and virtual health coach visits. WPHC, thus, considers the many individual, institutional, policy, environmental, global, religious, and social factors that affect people's health.

The textbook will delve into each of these facets in detail. It will provide an insightful, comprehensive, and action-oriented look at how each facet shapes WPHC and how we as individuals, caregivers, community members, and critical healthcare consumers and producers, can intervene to make WPHC equitable, inclusive, and accessible for all. The textbook is unique in centering multiple forms of intersectionalities through the social determinants of health (SDoH) perspective with respect to whole person and social justice activism (SJA). Chapters include ample instances and discussion of intersectionalities (e.g., race and gender and ability status) both in pedagogical features and chapter content. Social movements, and the political, ideological, and social-historical contexts underlying these topics are central to describing WPHC and its SJA intersections.

## Main Themes and Objectives

*Health Communication for Social Justice: A Whole Person Activist Approach* helps students to:

- Know and attend to the many types/forms of health (e.g., physical, mental, and spiritual) and health contexts and interactions (e.g., interpersonal, group, organizational, institutional, societal, and global) when a whole person approach is adopted.
- View health through a SJ lens to identify and address health inequalities/disparities (e.g., access) that affect members of oppressed communities.
- Identify the different healthcare models in use and their comparative strengths in WPHC.
- Understand how we communicate and think about health shapes our health outcomes in relationship with others.
- Understand how individual health is intricately connected with social, global, religious and spiritual, and environmental health.
- Examine health communication in everyday life from diverse perspectives.
- Understand how evolving communication technologies can contribute to achieving holistic, socially just healthcare.
- Engage in communicative action to achieve the goals of the whole person, SJ approach to health.

## Organization and Rationale

The textbook is organized around three sections:

I. **Conceptualizing Health**: This section introduces *how we theorize health*. The three central themes of the textbook are *whole person* and *SJA* framework within a *social constructionist* approach to health. Thus, the three chapters that discuss frameworks for these themes are placed in this section.

II. **Constructing Health**: The second section emphasizes the *constructed nature of health and health-related meaning making*. This emphasizes how the WPHC SJA is based on health-related meaning making in *situated, historical, political, social, and economic contexts*. The chapters on *evolving understandings of health, healthcare relationships, healthcare systems*, and *health literacy* are placed here.

III. **Contextualizing Health**: This focuses on the *contexts in which health practices are enacted and health communication occurs*. The contexts in which health-related meaning making occurs and in which health practices are enacted shape our conceptualization and construction of health. These factors provide a point of entry to discuss SJ principles (e.g., equity, access, and fairness). The chapters on *health and the environment; technology and health; health, religion, and spirituality*; and *global health* are placed here.

## Significance

Finally, the significance of enduring structural change is knit through the chapters in numerous discursive and organizational ways through the *pedagogical features* and *chapter content*. Each chapter includes ample provocative and intervention-oriented material with the following features: chapter organization; communication scholar(s) interviews work that connects their research to a whole person, social justice context; textboxes and table(s) with theories, definitions placed in engaged, applied contexts, resources, and SJA prompts and activities; discussion questions and thought scenarios for student reflection; present challenges and future directions exercise for students; and reference list of sources cited in chapters, along with helpful sources in each textbox. Together, the textbook provides the conceptual foundations and action-oriented lens to achieve a whole person vision of health.

# Acknowledgments

I would like to thank my publishing team at Routledge, especially Alexandra de Brauw, commissioning editor, and Sean Daly, editorial assistant, for their invaluable guidance; series coeditor Dr. Larry Frey, for the invitation to write the textbook; Fulton School of Liberal Arts dean, Maarten Pereboom, for his support of the effort; and my students, who inspire and guide the way we will tread the path of justice and health for those who need it most in the present and the future.

# Selected Abbreviations

| | |
|---|---|
| **AI** | Artificial intelligence |
| **ACA** | Affordable Care Act |
| **ADA** | Americans with Disabilities Act |
| **AHRQ** | Agency for Healthcare Research and Quality |
| **AMA** | American Medical Association |
| **BM** | Biomedical model |
| **BSM** | Biopsychosocial model |
| **CAM** | Complementary and Alternative Medicine |
| **CBC** | Community-based care |
| **CBPA** | Community-based participatory approach |
| **CBPR** | Community-based participatory research |
| **CDC** | Centers for Disease Control and Prevention |
| **CHC** | Community health center |
| **CIM** | Complementary and Integrative Medicine |
| **CMS** | Centers for Medicaid and Medicare |
| **COPD** | Chronic obstructive pulmonary disease |
| **CPE** | Clinical pastoral education |
| **CVD** | Cardiovascular disease |
| **DC** | Diagnostic care |
| **EHR** | Electronic health record |
| **EM** | Ecological model |
| **ER** | Emergency room |
| **FCC** | Federal Communications Commission |
| **FCH** | Family cancer history |
| **FDA** | US Food and Drug Administration |
| **FHH** | Family health history |
| **GHSA** | Global Health Security Agency |
| **HH** | Health humanities |
| **HHC** | Home healthcare |
| **HHS** | US Department of Health and Human Services |
| **HINTS** | Health Information National Trends Survey |
| **HM** | Holistic model |
| **HRSA** | Health Resources Services Administration |
| **IM** | Integrative medicine |
| **IOM** | Institute of Medicine |

| IPC | Interprofessional communication |
| IPCC | Intergovernmental Panel on Climate Change |
| LMIC | Low- and middle-income countries |
| NCD | Noncommunicable diseases |
| NCI | National Cancer Institute |
| NLM | National Library of Medicine |
| NNLM | Network of the National Library of Medicine |
| NP | Nurse practitioner |
| NTD | Neglected tropical diseases |
| PA | Physician assistant |
| PC | Primary care |
| PCC | Patient-centered communication |
| PCP | Primary care providers |
| PHI | Personal health information |
| RC | Rehabilitative care |
| RHM | Rhetoric of health and medicine |
| SC | Secondary care |
| SCoH | Social construction of health |
| SDoH | Social determinants of health |
| SDG | Sustainable Development Goals |
| SJ | Social justice |
| SJA | Social justice activism |
| SM | Social mobilization |
| SUD | Substance abuse disorders |
| TC | Tertiary care |
| UN | United Nations |
| WHO | World Health Organization |
| WPHC | Whole person healthcare |

# Section I

# Conceptualizing Health

# A Whole Person Framework of Health

## Chapter Learning Outcomes

Upon completing **Chapter 1, A Whole Person Framework of Health**, the student should be able to apply **whole person health communication** (WPHC) **social justice activism** (SJA) principles to:

1. Explain the tenets of a WPHC framework from the perspective of the individual, the healthcare provider, and healthcare systems.
2. Explain how health can be understood from a social constructionist perspective and seen as relational, interdependent, and reflexive.
3. Understand how the WPHC includes complementary and integrative medicine (CIM) approaches in the conceptualization and delivery of care.
4. Identify how the social determinants of health (SDoH) contribute to health outcomes for individuals from diverse backgrounds.
5. Explain how the WPHC framework supports an inclusive and rights-based approach to health.

## Consider the following contexts:

Social isolation, understood as a lack of social connections and interactions (see, e.g., House, 2001), can have significant effects on an individual's health and well-being. The US Surgeon General's Advisory underscores the urgency of attending to the public health crisis of loneliness, isolation, and lack of connection in America (The US Surgeon General, 2023). The report highlights the implications of social media use on adolescents' social, educational, psychological, and neurological development. Social media usage does not occur in isolation; rather, it involves the larger domain of stakeholders ranging from local and national public policy, health professionals, systems, and relationships; researchers and educators; workplaces; community-based organizations, technology, media, and entertainment industries, parents caregivers; and individuals. Young adults with high social media usage, measured as time and frequency of use, for instance, demonstrate higher degrees of social isolation (Primack et al., 2017). On the other hand, because many socially isolated people use social media, social media platforms offer a useful venue for

DOI: 10.4324/9781003214472-2

intervention. Social media platforms, including Facebook, X (formerly known as Twitter), YouTube, LinkedIn, Instagram, and Snapchat, whose usage is prevalent among young adults, offer an opportunity to mediate social isolation and aggravate it.

Social isolation among vulnerable populations such as older adults can increase the risk of experiencing chronic health conditions that include cardiovascular disease, type 2 diabetes, chronic stress, depression, and anxiety (Lubben, 2017; Nicholson, 2012; Tomaka et al., 2006). The negative effects of social isolation on older adults' physical, mental, and emotional health are especially severe for those who have limited mobility, do not engage in daily physical activity engagement, and/or are managing multiple chronic health conditions. Moreover, the deleterious effects of such forms of social isolation accumulate over a lifetime (American Psychological Association, 2021; Taylor et al., 2019). Social isolation, thus, is a public health issue. The American Association of Retired Persons (AARP) Foundation (2016) reported that social isolation is a growing epidemic in the United States affecting more than eight million older adults. Social isolation can lead to loneliness, or a negative feeling of being alone or separated (National Institute on Aging, 2021). However, people with many social contacts can also feel lonely and socially isolated, and those with few social contacts can feel socially connected (Cacioppo et al., 2009, 2011). Hence, whether people feel socially isolated or socially connected is not about the number of social contacts but about how people see and feel about their relationships with those in their social network.

Research indicates that African Americans, compared to non-Hispanic Whites, are less likely to live alone. However, factors such as race-related stress, stemming from older African Americans' distrust of healthcare providers, can contribute to an increase in their social isolation, putting them at increased risk of myriad negative health outcomes (Cornwell et al., 2008).

Social isolation is a complex mental health issue. For those who are vulnerable, thoughtful engagement on social media can enhance self-worth, connections, and well-being. Such usage can help address the public health crisis stemming from bullying, prejudice, and exclusion that can aggravate mental health challenges, societal violence, and the potential for self-harm.

## Chapter Organization

**Chapter 1, A Whole Person Framework of Health**, is organized as follows: **First**, the chapter conceptualizes the WPHC approach, focusing on how health is an individual and collective concern, and teases out the distinctions between health, illness, and disease. It situates the WPHC framework with the value-based ethic of care in relationship with CIM, coordination of care, and preventative care as a socially constructed concept. **Second**, the chapter connects WPHC as centrally connected with the tenets of **social justice** (hereafter, **SJ**) by explaining how the SDoH contribute to inclusive health outcomes and the relational and socially constructed nature of health. **Third**, the chapter considers the WPHC as an inclusive approach with a rights-based approach to health framework. **Fourth**, the chapter concludes with a discussion of how WPHC's "health-for-all" philosophy is an SJ-rights-based approach to health. Along the way, the chapter will **present applied WPHC contexts** and **SJA discussion prompts**

and activities ranging from mental and physical health challenges faced by individuals who identify as LGBTQIA+ to the WPHC model in clinical settings, healthy neighborhoods, substance abuse disorders, and SDoH-related racial disparities in cardiovascular diseases. The communication **scholar interview** with Dr. Gary L. Kreps, foundational scholar of health communication, presents his research and advocacy in the domain of the WPHC approach to health. Students are invited to engage in **actionable ways** with the SJA dimensions of each WPHC context to intervene, advocate, promote, or increase awareness of the concepts with each activity. The chapter concludes with the **present challenges and future directions exercise** on going out into the field and involving community members to identify barriers and organize collectively for crafting communicative avenues for change.

## Conceptualizing WPHC

The COVID-19 pandemic led to the implementation of social isolation policies to limit the spread of the virus. Virtually everyone, from very young children to older adults, struggled with adapting to the unprecedented quarantining and social distancing measures. For instance, Berg-Weger and Morley (2020) found that during the pandemic, older adults experienced an acute sense of social isolation and loneliness, resulting in increased depression, anxiety, and financial challenges. However, they also discovered an unexpected positive aspect of the pandemic: people of all ages who experienced social isolation increased their awareness of its negative effects on their health. Because of that increased awareness, Berg-Weger and Morley argued that people are now aware of the need to address the effect of social isolation on health for members of vulnerable populations, such as older adults.

## The WPHC Approach

### Health as an Individual and Collective Concern

Good health is integral to people's well-being and quality of life. Any time that people's health is negatively affected, it has an immediate and indirect impact on their daily well-being. It is, therefore, important to understand how people make meaning of health, sickness, well-being, and malaise, as well as the distinction between illness and disease. Moreover, health-related concerns are not just limited to the individuals who experience them; as the COVID-19 pandemic has demonstrated, individuals' health is intimately and powerfully connected with the health of their family members and friends, the communities and society in which they live, and the planet. Health, thus, is both an individual and a collective issue.

### Health, Illness, and Disease

The WPHC approach views health not just as a physical condition but as a combination of physical, mental, social, relational, spiritual, and other aspects that a "whole" person experiences. Health is defined by the World Health Organization (WHO) as "a state of complete physical, mental, and social well-being and not merely the absence of disease or infirmity" (2021b). That definition is in line with medical philosophers who have argued that health is more than the absence of disease. Rather, this definition of health emphasizes the ability to assimilate the experience of disease and illness in an individual vision of health. An illness emphasizes people's perceptions of a health condition they (or others) experience, such as pain, discomfort, or fatigue. (Boyd, 2000). A disease is understood as an objectively measured deviation from a biological norm. In contrast to an illness, which people manage themselves at home, a disease often requires medical intervention and treatment in clinical settings. In making sense of disease, illness, and health, therefore, people rely upon value judgments to determine their meaning in individual contexts. The WPHC considers the patient as an individual with a body, emotions, thoughts, beliefs, hopes, and desires.

## Defining the WPHC Framework of Health

This section provides a brief look at WPHC through a systemic and individual lens. It situates the WPHC framework in alignment with the biomedical approach to health and describes the concerns of value-based care. **Chapter 2, Models for Representing Health and Disease** will provide a more detailed look at the biomedical model of care along with the biopsychosocial model of health, integrative care model, and holistic care model. **Chapter 6, Healthcare Systems** will discuss the premise of value-based care in greater detail.

### WPHC

The WPHC is concerned with the health of the "whole person," which includes physical, emotional, mental, spiritual, and psychosocial facets, along with the context in which individuals construct the meanings of health. In WPHC, the contextual dimensions of people's lives can range from the health of their interpersonal and group relationships and physical environments in which they live to the health of their communities and society, writ large. Conceptualization and delivery of WPHC, therefore, must address the many health dimensions of people's lives.

### WPHC in Comparison with Biomedical Approach

The biomedical approach understands disease one organ system at a time, with health and disease considered to be two separate states (Langevin, 2020). WPHC references care for the whole person rather than focusing on a single diagnosis or health condition. WPHC is, thus, patient-centered and uses diverse healthcare resources to deliver all aspects of care in a whole

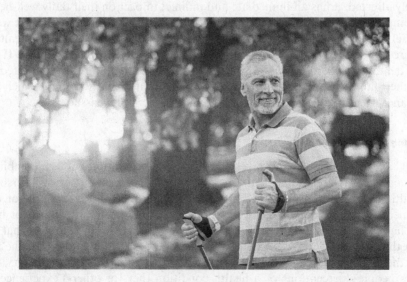

*Figure 1.1* Whole person health includes physical, mental, spiritual, and psychosocial facets.

person context. In clinical contexts, WPHC is seen as being multidimensional, emphasizing coordination of care, recognizing the physicians' humanity, highlighting the therapeutic relationship between the patient and the provider (Agarwal, 2018a, 2018b, 2019), recognizing healthcare recipients' personhood, viewing health as more than an absence of disease, and employing a range of CIM treatment modalities (Thomas et al., 2018).

## WPHC and the Shift to Value-Based Care

WPHC centers value-based care by prioritizing coordination of care at multiple levels. The levels of care can range from primary care (e.g., the primary care physician), secondary care, tertiary care, and quaternary care (see **Chapter 6, Healthcare Systems**, for the different levels of care) and range from the primary care physician to specialists, community-based care, and CIM approaches. WPHC seeks to ensure that individuals receive comprehensive and integrative care in a cost-effective manner. By emphasizing coordination of care, WPHC seeks to address the complexity of an individual's health needs important for clinical and self-management in multimorbid disease domains like chronic conditions in a manner that leads to optimum health outcomes. Chronic conditions like hypertension, diabetes, osteoarthritis, and chronic obstructive pulmonary disease (COPD) are often characterized by multimorbidity and require coordination of care across primary care services, specialist care, medication use, hospital admissions, and community-based care (Ellner & Phillips, 2017). For instance, individuals with type 2 diabetes will also often have comorbidities including hypertension, obesity, hypothyroidism, and dyslipidemia. Multimorbidity is characterized by the presence of two or more chronic conditions in an individual at the same time.

## THE SHIFT TO VALUE-BASED CARE

The systemic shift to value-based care sees healthcare recipients as individuals whose health status should be interpreted as a confluence of the socioeconomic circumstances that may make them vulnerable to specific health risks. Value-based care emphasizes the need to address population health in an optimal, cost-effective manner, particularly for high-risk groups. Communication, coordination, and collaboration are considered the three key components of WPHC. Value-based care is discussed in greater detail in **Chapter 6, Healthcare Systems**. To deliver value-based care, WPHC institutions strive to integrate behavioral health services into every healthcare recipient's experience and to treat both their physical and behavioral health needs. Behavioral health services are often delivered in community-based settings and include mental health treatments, addiction counseling, and preventative care. In WPHC, healthcare delivery is also integrated into community settings to span the continuum from inpatient operations to outpatient operations and community outreach.

## CHALLENGE TO WPHC

One challenge that WPHC faces at the systemic level is that not all the care components (e.g., CIM approaches) are covered by healthcare insurance. That lack of health coverage poses a challenge for members of marginalized and vulnerable populations to access preventative and health promotion services. Unlike biopsychosocial care, that lack of insurance coverage also poses challenges for the providers who utilize an integrative care model to provide better patient care.

*Review **Textbox 1.1** for a look at the key conceptual terms and their meanings.*

---

### Textbox 1.1   A Whole Person Framework of Health

#### WPHC Context

The five domains below reference key conceptual domains in the WPHC framework and their meanings.

WPHC is care that is:

- **Multidimensional**
  Health comprises the physical, mental, social, relational, environmental, and spiritual aspects that make up a whole person.
- **Subjective**
  Health outcomes go beyond the physical body to understand how our feelings, emotions, thoughts, and beliefs play into our perceptions of being healthy.
- **Person-centered**
  Health is person-centered, seeking to meet individuals' physical, emotional, cognitive, sexual, occupational, social, and existential needs.
- **Value-based**
  Looks at patients as individuals whose health status should be interpreted as a confluence of the socioeconomic circumstances that may make them vulnerable to health risks.
- **Integrative**
  Hospitals and health systems focus on integrating behavioral health services into every aspect of patient care, as well as coordinating and connecting with community resources.

#### SJA Discussion Prompt

Individuals who identify as LGBTQIA+ populations are at risk of poorer mental and physical health as compared with individuals from heterosexual and cisgender populations. These poorer health outcomes are often related to barriers in the healthcare system that perpetuate these health inequities. Healthcare factors such as a distrust of the healthcare system and discriminatory experiences by healthcare providers can exacerbate these concerns. The concerns are also exacerbated by the intersection of race and ethnicity, geographic region, and socioeconomic factors. Some of the domains of health disparities evidenced in the LGBTQIA+ populations include a higher rate of mental health concerns, substance abuse, risky sexual behaviors, self-harm, and suicide.

Consider the WPHC concepts of healthcare as multidimensional, subjective, person-centered, value-based, and integrative.

1. What advice will you give nurse practitioners and healthcare providers from the perspective of the WPHC framework of health to ensure their communication with LGBTQIA+ is inclusive and culturally sensitive?
2. Design one recommendation to help healthcare providers engage in gender-affirming communication that encourages recognition of the barriers and challenges faced by individuals from this population.

### Resource

Medina-Martínez, J., Saus-Ortega, C., Sánchez-Lorente, M. M., Sosa-Palanca, E., Garciá-Martínez, P., & Mármol-López, M. I. (2021). Health inequities in LGBT people and nursing interventions to reduce them: A systematic review. *International Journal of Environmental and Public Health, 18*(22), Article 11801. https://doi.org/10.3390/ijerph182211801

## WPHC and Integrative Medicine

The integrative medicine (IM) model promotes health by emphasizing the balance between the body, mind, and spirit through evidence-based complementary and alternative medicine (CAM) approaches and conventional medicine. WPHC approaches are employed by providers working in IM healthcare settings, which focus on value-based healthcare and offer holistic treatment for people's long-term physical and mental health. IM combines WPHC value-based and CIM approaches to address the multiple dimensions of whole person care, including people's bodies, minds, emotions, and spirits. The goal of WPHC is to apply scientific and technological advances in healthcare to address the mental and spiritual aspects of well-being that play an important part in health-related meaning making and outcomes.

Review *Textbox 1.2 Scholar Interview* with *Dr. Gary Kreps, one of the earliest founders of the field of Health Communication, and a recognized scholar-advocate of the WPHC framework.*

---

### TEXTBOX 1.2   Scholar Interview

**Dr. Gary L. Kreps**
University Distinguished Professor and Director of the Center for Health and Risk Communication, George Mason University

1.  What does the "whole person healthcare" (WPHC) approach mean to you? How is WPHC relevant in the current sociopolitical context?
    The WPHC approach illustrates how multiple powerful factors influence health promotion, healthcare, and health outcomes. The approach examines the ways that many different societal and cultural communication factors influence health, such as the unique ways that individuals and collectives create meanings to make sense of health and illness, such as the ways that communication can influence our emotions, beliefs, levels of understanding, anxiety, uncertainty, confidence, comfort, and faith related to health and healthcare. Symbolic aspects of health guide the ways we respond to health problems. We are directly influenced by the health communicative practices that we engage in. For example, the use of validating health communication from significant others (including healthcare providers, family members, romantic partners, friends, and community leaders) concerning health issues can provide us with the needed support, encouragement, and direction to help us address challenging health risks we may face. While the lack of supportive and validating health communication can often discourage people from disclosing their health concerns, actively seeking needed care, and engaging in health-promoting activities. WPHC illustrates that the influences of health communication in different social contexts,

cultural groups, personal relationships, and organizations can have strong influences on important health outcomes. This suggests that health communication research and practice must address the variety of key sociopolitical and ecological health communication factors that are directly related to promoting health and well-being.

2. Your work has advocated for communication to promote justice in the healthcare system. What advice would you offer those who would like to apply the WPHC approach to advocate for social justice?

The WPHC approach suggests the need to carefully examine how access to relevant health information and support within unique social systems can influence health outcomes. To promote justice in the healthcare system we need to develop communication programs, policies, practices, and technologies that fit the unique needs, expectations, and perspectives of different individuals and groups. The WPHC approach also suggests the need for conducting community-based collaborative research and intervention efforts that work closely with members of different at-risk communities to address serious health issues and risks they face.

3. How can health communication professionals employ the ethos of the WPHC approach to advocate for equitable health outcomes for minorities and marginalized populations?

Health communication professionals interested in promoting equitable health outcomes for marginalized populations can use the WPHC approach to guide their multimethodological community-based research efforts to help identify the unique interrelated factors that lead to poor health outcomes for different individuals and groups. Data from such research can guide the design and implementation of culturally sensitive communication interventions, programs, policies, and technologies to address health disparities.

4. In your point of view, what is one particularly good example of a community-based application of the WPHC approach that promotes social justice?

The INSIGHTS (International Studies to Investigate Global Health Information Trends) research consortium program that I coordinate uses the WPHC approach to promote social justice, by collecting revealing data in multiple countries about serious gaps in health information access and use faced by different population segments. The data from this research can be used to guide the development of evidence-based, social justice communication intervention strategies to provide at-risk populations with needed information and support, both within each country and across countries.

### Coordination of Care in WPHC

The WPHC approach is patient-centered and emphasizes the allocation and coordination of multiple resources such as behavioral, physical, and social support in the care of the whole person. Coordination of care involves the seamless sharing of patient information and health status across all healthcare provider domains involved in patient care with the goal of achieving optimal health outcomes and cost efficiencies. The WPHC approach sees individuals' medical information as being an important, but incomplete, part of their health story. Along with clinical care, the WPHC also considers intersections of care such as how an individual may get to the physician's office and access care.

### The Individual's Health Story

Aspects of individuals' complete health picture will include their lived contexts, such as where they live. For example, the health picture will consider where they live (i.e., whether they live in a disadvantaged neighborhood, e.g., one with poor access to healthy food sources or health services), their race, their socioeconomic status, their ethnicity, the language they speak, their religious values and beliefs, housing stability, food insecurity, and cultural practices. By thinking of health and disease as two ends of a continuum and not two distinct and isolated concepts, the WPHC approach shifts attention from the clinical disease symptoms to encompassing people's lifestyle and belief-related health behaviors, such as, for instance, their poor diet, sedentary lifestyle, chronic stress, and poor sleep. Thus, WPHC is whole person centered in its conceptualization of health, illness, and disease.

### Supporting a Preventative Approach

Addressing lifestyle and belief-related health behaviors can prevent chronic health conditions, such as diabetes, cardiovascular disease, degenerative joint disease, and depression. In turn, recognizing health and disease as being on a continuum can lead to achieving better health outcomes by taking a preventative approach and addressing these behaviors at an early stage to prevent the occurrence of multiple diseases down the line. A range of behavioral health statistics, from mental illness to substance use disorders, are essential for effective, integrated care.

### Creating a Continuum of Care

In WPHC, healthcare systems integrate behavioral health services into every aspect of people's healthcare, as well as coordinate and connect health recipients with community resources that can help them. This coordination and connection of care supports the goal to create a continuum of care that reflects integration at each point on the road to accomplishment of overall good health (American Hospital Association [AHA], 2021). The type of integrated healthcare that the WPHC approach offers is needed in myriad healthcare contexts, from cardiac rehabilitation to breast cancer survivorship care. WPHC approaches may include community-based whole-health systems, such as Ayurveda and Traditional Chinese Medicine (TCM), and integrated complementary and conventional, biomedical, and biopsychosocial approaches.

Review *Table 1.1 The Whole Person Model of Care in Clinical Settings*.

*The information under the column "Clinical Contexts" provides an illustrative example of one clinical context for patient care.*

*The information under the column "WPHC Component: Healthcare Settings" provides examples of WPHC components of care in healthcare settings.*

*The information under the column "WPHC Component: Community-Based Settings" provides examples of WPHC components of care applicable to that clinical setting.*

*The information under the column "WPHC Component: CIM Settings" provides examples of CIM modalities as applicable to a WPHC framework of care in that clinical setting. Respond to the SJA prompt that follows.*

Table 1.1 Whole Person Model of Care in Clinical Settings

| Clinical Contexts | WPHC Component: Healthcare Settings | WPHC Component: Community-Based Settings | WPHC Component: CIM Settings |
|---|---|---|---|
| Oncology | Care coordination includes:<br><br>• Physicians<br>• Nutrition therapists<br>• Psychotherapists<br>• Clinical social workers<br>• Genetic counselors<br>• Pharmaceutical experts | • Personalized care by a team of professionals<br>• Convenient access to ancillary support services (e.g., financial counselors) | Combined with evidence-based CIM therapies to care for the whole person through:<br><br>• Exercise<br>• Nutrition<br>• Yoga<br>• Acupuncture for pain management<br>• Mental health<br>• Chemotherapy side effects<br>• Post-surgical recovery support |
| Chronic Pain | Multidisciplinary rehabilitation including:<br><br>• Patient counseling<br>• Health coaching<br>• Psychiatric care<br>• Behavioral health therapy<br>• Functional medicine combining illness coping and pain management. | Community-based education that includes:<br><br>• Exercise self-management programs<br>• Social network support<br>• Patient expertise and preferences<br>• Patient empowerment | Includes CIM approaches such as:<br><br>• TCM Acupuncture<br>• Yoga therapist<br>• Tai chi |
| Substance Abuse | Addresses people's multiple needs tailored to their age, gender, ethnicity, and culture, including:<br><br>• Medical Psychological<br>• Social<br>• Vocational<br>• Legal<br>• Cognitive behavioral therapies<br>• Medication management<br>• Detoxification<br>• Individual, family, and group therapy<br>• Personal training and cardiovascular exercise | Care coordination programs that:<br><br>• Provide appropriate levels of funding support.<br>• Assess need for mental health and substance abuse disorder treatment and services.<br>• Make referrals to programs to match treatment and service needs to facilitate substance abuse disorder prevention, treatment, and recovery. | Include CIM therapies such as:<br><br>• Animal assistance<br>• Arts programs<br>• Sports<br>• Spiritual instruction<br>• Acupuncture<br>• Meditation |

## SJA Prompt

For each of the three illustrative clinical contexts provided in Table 1.1, oncology, chronic pain, and substance abuse, consider the contribution of an individual's lived contexts such as neighborhoods, education, or financial stability (these will be captured by the SDoH, discussed in a later section) toward successfully achieving the goals of WPHC:

1.  Identify one key attribute of the individual's lived context that seems specifically relevant to each clinical context.

    a.  Is it easy to identify just one?
    b.  Would you need to include more than one facet of the individual's lived context?

2.  What factors went into your decision to include that one key attribute and not another?

## WPHC and the Transactional Healthcare Model

### WPHC as Distinct from the Transactional Model

The WPHC approach differs from the transactional healthcare model, which sees disease in isolation from the whole person. Shifting from a transactional model to a value-based WPHC approach has affected chronic condition management in vulnerable populations, where many whole-health factors affect individuals' ability to achieve and maintain optimal health and well-being.

For example, in a transactional model, people who have diabetes need to coordinate interaction with their primary care physician (PCP), optometrist, and podiatrist individually. If the PCP performed blood tests, those results would not automatically be shared with those other healthcare providers. Moreover, those healthcare providers would not discuss certain topics that are the province of the other healthcare providers; for instance, the PCP would not discuss with their patient that person's mental health.

### WPHC in Comparison with the Transactional Model

The WPHC approach coordinates people's healthcare with respect to all their healthcare providers and the behavioral health and social services they are receiving. For example, a person experiencing a chronic health condition might see a dentist, who may identify an underlying pathology and share their report with the person's PCP, enabling timely preventative treatment. Using WPHC, people who are at high risk of experiencing chronic health issues with high comorbidity, thus, receive more sustainable health outcomes and, ultimately, effective healthcare.

## SDoH in WPHC

One way to identify the many intersecting factors that contribute to an individual's health is by using the SDoH framework. SDoH, according to The Centers for Disease Prevention and Control (CDC, 2021), are the "conditions in the places where people live, learn, work, and play that affect a wide range of health and quality-of-life risks and outcomes." The WHO (2021a) noted that SDoH capture the way the "distribution of money, power, and resources at global, national, and local levels" impact individual health outcomes. SDoH relate to the myriad aspects that comprise an individual's life, ranging from personal safety and mobility to violence prevention, urban health, and healthy aging as they affect individual health, and reflect social inequities experienced at local, national, and global levels. In this manner, they cross different sectors such as education, infrastructure, environment, and places of employment. Thus, addressing SDoH to achieve WPHC is a multisectoral endeavor that requires cooperation across healthcare agencies and a sustained focus on the interrelated factors that shape people's living conditions.

### Domains of SDoHs

Healthy People 2030 is a national public health initiative that seeks to highlight public health priorities that need attention in the coming decade. Healthy People 2030 identifies five key areas of SDoHs: "(a) healthcare access and quality, (b) education access and quality, (c) social and community context, (d) economic stability, and (e) the neighborhood and built environment." These domains are described as follows:

*Healthcare Access and Quality*

This domain describes the "connection between people's access to and understanding of health services and their own health" (Health.gov, 2023) Factors affecting that **connection** include whether and the extent to which people have healthcare insurance, available primary care, and their health literacy (the ability to understand and to use information about their health conditions to make informed decisions).

*Education Access and Quality*

This domain refers to the "connection of education to health and well-being," and is assessed regarding enrollment in high school or in an institution of higher education, language literacy, and early childhood education and development.

*Social and Community Context*

This domain describes the "connection between characteristics of the contexts within which people live, learn, work, and play, and their health and well-being." That area includes, among other things, the cohesiveness of people's relationships and the geographical community, their participation in civic life, workplace conditions, and whether they have been incarcerated.

*Economic Stability*

This domain connects "the financial resources people have—income, cost of living, and socio-economic status—and their health" (CDC, 2023).

*Neighborhood and Built Environment*

This domain describes the relationship "between where a person lives—housing, neighborhood, and environment—and their health and well-being" (Health.gov, 2023).

*Review* **Textbox 1.3 Healthy Neighborhoods***. As you consider the different facets of a healthy neighborhood and their impact on residents' health, imagine what a whole person approach to designing a healthy neighborhood would look like.*

*How would it approach a neighborhood that supports a health-relevant social, built, and land use environment? What systemic interventions might be required to design a neighborhood that minimizes geographical and spatial bases of health inequities caused by the built environment?*

---

**Textbox 1.3  Healthy Neighborhoods**

**WPHC Context**

Where we live is important to our health. Our neighborhoods are defined not only by the houses we live in and their physical features such as the presence of walkways and green spaces but also by the sense of community they cultivate. Safe and aesthetically pleasing neighborhoods are characterized by plenty of green spaces, access to clean drinking water, good schools, healthy food sources, low air pollution, and high social connectedness. Healthy neighborhoods have the potential to support positive health outcomes by lowering stress and improving mental and physical health by providing greater opportunities for physical exercise and healthy eating, among other mechanisms. Structural policies such as those promoting mixed-income neighborhoods can reduce residential segregation by social class and promote greater health equity by reducing differential access to preferential resources and services by disadvantaged populations (Roux, 2016).

## SJA Prompt

A neighborhood is not a single, unitary entity. It is composed of several interrelated components, some of which are described in the WPHC context. Imagine an ideal neighborhood that supports the WPHC approach for all individuals in the community. As you brainstorm what a picture of a healthy neighborhood should look like, consider the effect of interrelatedness of neighborhood factors on the health of its residents and respond to the prompts that follow:

1. What would a neighborhood that provides a healthy environment for its residents look like?
2. What are some elements that a healthy neighborhood *must* have?
3. What are some elements that the neighborhood *could* have should resources permit?
4. How will the neighborhood meet the whole person health needs of people of all ages?

## Resource

Roux, A. V. D. (2016). Neighborhoods and health: What do we know? What should we know? *American Journal of Public Health, 106*(3), 430–431. https://doi.org/10.2105/AJPH.2016.303064

### The SDoHs in the WPHC Approach

The WPHC approach considers the five key SDoHs and the need to collect, acquire, validate, analyze, and integrate the data about the many areas that comprise SDoHs. For instance, identifying an individual's housing status as part of the clinical record is now considered to be essential for understanding their health status. These new forms of data privilege non-medical root causes of people's health issues, such as the stability of their housing situation, utilization of transitional or public housing, and/or the conditions characterizing an individual's living conditions in their homes (e.g., amount of unhealthy noise, dust, and environmental pollutants). Collecting medical data beyond individuals' biological markers can support how the healthcare experience is tailored to their daily lived conditions in whole person ways. For instance, understanding a person's housing status, education level, and languages spoken can be helpful in conceptualizing care that is effective in the patient's context. The SDoH perspective emphasizes an effort to understand why health inequities exist and aims to reduce them.

## The Relational and Socially Constructed Nature of Health

One of the benefits of good health is that people are self-sufficient and do not have to depend on others to take care of them.

### The Objectivist View

The objectivist view of the healthy individual draws upon theories of human physiological functioning and normative beliefs about human behavior, actions, and well-being, which is helpful in defining health and disease in the clinical domain. An objectivist approach considers health as being centered on the individual, removed from the factors that shape their environmental and sociocultural context. In the objectivist view, departures from the typical way in which people's bodies function help to determine malfunctions, and their corresponding assessments of health and well-being. Such an approach helps health communication and public health professionals design individual- and population-level treatments and interventions based on health risks and outcomes. For example, to confront smoking-related illnesses and sexually transmitted diseases, public health interventions and health communication campaigns target individual health beliefs and motivations to drive behavior change.

### Limitations of the Objectivist View

Important understandings of health can be garnered through biomedical knowledge of human physiology. However, conceptualizing health as determined solely by objective biopsychosocial indicators has shortcomings. As explained next, by considering health from a relational and inclusive perspective and as an intersection of the many facets of an individual's physiological, biological, environmental, social, psychological, emotional, spiritual, and system-level factors, the constructivist approach to health is a central premise of the WPHC framework.

Review **Textbox 1.4** for an understanding of the WPHC context of substance abuse disorders and attempt the SJA prompt.

---

### Textbox 1.4   Substance Abuse Disorders and Health Communication Contexts

**WPHC Context**

Substance abuse disorder (SUD) is a major health challenge in the United States. SUDs often co-occur with mental health disorders (e.g., depression, bipolar disorders, attention-deficit hyperactivity disorder, antisocial personality disorder, and psychotic illness). Health communication professionals play a vital role in shaping how people make sense of health issues, challenges, barriers, and behaviors.

**SJA Prompt**

Give an example of one communication initiative for each of the following health communication contexts:

- Campaigns
- Public relations
- Media
- Workplace

---

For example, an example of a campaign for the health communication context under the first column titled, "Campaigns," the *Truth Initiative* conducted a "Truth about Opioids" campaign in 2019. You would, thus, examine the campaign to respond to the following prompts.

1. Take one of the messages from that campaign and explain how it illustrates the whole person healthcare approach to SUD.
2. Does that message focus on a SJ concern, and, if so, how?
3. What actions does that message suggest?
4. Alternatively, is there some action you would recommend for addressing the SUD concern?

### Resource

*Truth Initiative*. (2019, May 6). The truth about opioids campaign wins Emmy award. Retrieved April 26, 2021, from https://truthinitiative.org/press/press-release/truth-about-opioids-campaign-wins-emmy-award

### The Constructivist Approach

The constructivist approach starts with the premise that health and disease reflect human biases. For instance, an objectivist approach will consider the healthy body norm as one that seeks to achieve a body weight in accordance with certain biomedical criteria and markers. In this instance, those over the desirable expectation of healthy body weight will appear as out of normative range. Thus, an objectivist approach will design health interventions to detect, intervene, and treat a condition and will drive behavior based on the motivation of weight loss through the association of body fat with health risks. For the objectivist, the research on blood pressure or life expectancy shapes the stigma associated with body weight, fat, and obesity. It assumes that being obese is not normal and places the onus for losing weight through interventions on the individual. A weight-inclusive constructivist approach, on the other hand, would claim that providing people with nonstigmatizing healthcare increases their ability to maintain a healthy body and achieve a state of well-being in relationship with their weight. A constructivist approach to healthy weight management will emphasize achieving the optimum weight for an individual based on health behaviors and nutrition approaches that fit into their lifestyle and values.

### WPHC and a Social Constructionist Approach to Health

Social constructionism is a theoretical orientation that scholars employ to understand how people make sense of a phenomenon, such as health, illness, and disease.

### UNDERSTANDING SOCIAL CONSTRUCTIONISM

Social constructionism argues that people make meaning of health through creating a shared understanding of how health conditions are experienced at an individual level, how meaning making occurs both individually and collectively, and how diseases are evaluated and treated.

Social constructionism will emphasize shared meaning making of health and disease as a sociocultural phenomenon rooted in understandings of illness, disease, medical knowledge, and treatment.

STRENGTHS OF A SOCIAL CONSTRUCTIONIST APPROACH

The social constructionist approach to health (social construction of health [SCoH]) is a useful lens for illuminating how people make meaning through interaction and dialogue and how these meanings shape our understanding of health and disease conditions. Illness and disease can carry a range of subjective meanings for different individuals, cultures, socioeconomic contexts, and time, and is not universal in their evaluation, assessment, or treatment approaches. The SCoH is central to the WPHC framework because it considers the whole person as shaped by the socio-historical, cultural, and individual influences on health-related meaning making, evaluation, assessment, treatment, and outcomes.

Health communication research employing SCoH reinforces an inclusive, integrative, and shared understanding of health in multiple domains. This research with populations who are disadvantaged shows how the SCoH accounts for the multiple intersecting factors that shape an individual's health and well-being status and outcomes.

*Applications of SCoH in WPHC Contexts*

Many communication scholars have conducted research using the SCoH perspective by people experiencing stigmatizing or under-researched health issues and negative media constructions. Rafferty and Sullivan (2017), for instance, studied how parents of children diagnosed with complex chronic conditions advocate for their children. They interviewed 35 parents of children diagnosed with chronic conditions. Their study found that parental advocacy was socially constructed through communicative behaviors in relationships with medical professionals, family members, and school educators. As another example, Gill and Babrow (2007) used problematic integration theory to examine challenges that women face in coping with their uncertainty about and the ambivalence they felt about having breast cancer. In line with the SCoH emphasis on cultural understandings of health, the findings showed that the coping approaches constructed through an interpretive analysis of all breast cancer articles appearing in top-circulating US women's magazines between 1997 and 2002 were somewhat imperfect. Coping was illustrated through simplification, information-seeking/provision, affect management, trusting intuition, sustaining hope, and metaphoric reframing.

Frohlich (2016) studied how people with inflammatory bowel disease (IBD) use social media networks to make sense of living with IBD and their struggles with coping with the stigmatizing views that people have of those with IBD as being unattractive. Her study takes a SCoH approach by eschewing objective and standardized definitions of IBD and attractiveness. The findings showed that those she interviewed who had IBD used social media technologies to redefine the subjective meanings of living with IBD by using different terms when speaking with others. Interviewees' redefinitions negotiated stigmatization that stemmed from surgery and its scarring effects on their bodies and adverse effects on their weight. The findings showed how the self-identity of those with a stigmatizing disease is (re)created by members of social media IBD groups about people's physical attractiveness, as when people posted photos of themselves that were "liked" by members of the community, it reconstructed the meaning of "physical beauty."

Focusing on how meanings are subjective and continually in the process of negotiation in SCoH, Omillion-Hodges et al. (2019) researched the meanings young adults ascribe to the word "death." They analyzed young adults' word choices used to describe death and how they constructed meaning from these descriptions. Their study sought to gain insight into the communicative aspects associated with death and dying by understanding how the youths co-constructed the meaning of death in conversations. The researchers employed the communication management of meaning theory (CMM; see, e.g., Pearce & Cronen, 1980), which posits that meaning is constructed through six levels that build upon and are embedded in each other: (a) the content (e.g., verbal and nonverbal cues); (b) the performance of cues (e.g., speech acts); (c) contracts, or rules that guide interactions; (d) episodes, sequences of speech acts; (e) identity, or life scripts, which reflects individuals' sense of self as created through lived experience; and (f) cultural archetype. Their study showed that when youth talked about death, sociocultural beliefs related to values such as religion, spirituality, and expression of emotion, should be taken into no account. In this manner, in line with SCoH, meaning is not fixed but varies with context, content, and channel, among other factors.

Matsaganis and Golden (2015) examined reproductive healthcare disparities among African American women in a small, disadvantaged urban community located in the north-eastern United States. Their study was guided by communication infrastructure theory (CIT), which looks at the multilevel storytelling network (STN) of micro-, meso-, and macrolevel actors that is set in its communication action context (CAC). Community residents are microlevel actors, whereas community-based organizations (community-oriented media) are mesolevel actors, with large institutions and media organizations being macrolevel actors. According to CIT, communication among STN agents is enabled and constrained by the CAC in interaction with the environment, such as organizational resources, transportation, and health-related resources.

Matsaganis and Golden (2015) studied how the women's urban environment and their social construction of that environment interacted to produce a "field of action." The researchers found that women with lower income and racial and ethnic minorities bore a disproportionate burden of negative reproductive health outcomes, ranging from disparities in maternal and newborn health outcomes and sexually transmitted infections (STIs) to reproductive tract infections and lack of access to and utilization of reproductive health services. Their study showed how the availability of healthcare resources, transportation services, communication resources, and personal privacy illustrate the dependencies among the STN and CAC factors, and the specific field of health action for the African American women in the community. They recommended that for healthcare interventions to be successful, they need to address the factors in an interdependent manner. For instance, they pointed out that an intervention, such as a taxi voucher program, must address people's transportation challenges alongside the barriers due to privacy concerns for the intervention to be completely successful. This study highlights how the interplay of individual and collective factors, a tenet of SCoH, shapes the understanding of effective interventions in achieving healthcare goals.

## Reflexivity and Interdependence in Healthcare Approaches

### Reflexivity in WPHC

Reflexivity references the aware, critical, and informed process of drawing on information or complex attributes of a phenomenon to make sense of and/or decisions with respect to that phenomenon. Reflexivity involves people thoughtfully and critically examining their beliefs, values, judgments, actions, and practices that they typically take for granted. Reflexivity is a central tenet of the WPHC framework because it encourages a critical and nuanced examination of health that is contextual, open to multiple interpretations, and emphasizes meaning making processes as key elements of health. This section describes how reflexivity can be understood at an individual level, at a contextual level, and in the research process.

*Reflexivity at an Individual Level*

Communication scholars have studied reflexivity regarding how people make sense of health information. For instance, Mendes et al. (2017) studied "reflexive actors" who strive to make well-informed decisions about their health by actively seeking information and rationally considering its pros and cons. Specifically, they studied young adults' health information-seeking practices. The findings revealed that healthy young adults saw health professionals as reliable sources of health information advice, whereas they perceived online health information as unreliable. Mendes et al. defined reflexivity as an assimilation of complex and multilayered information through a thoughtful evaluation of its credibility, reliability, and trust to engage in informed decision-making.

*Review **Textbox 1.5**. Respond to the SJA discussion prompt that follows.*

---

### Textbox 1.5 Reflexivity in SDoH-related Disparities in Cardiovascular Diseases: Media Messages

#### WPHC Context

Cardiovascular diseases (CVDs) are the leading cause of morbidity and mortality globally. People of color bear a disproportionate burden of CVD-related morbidity and mortality and poor disease outcomes. The evidence linking race and racism with negative CVD outcomes is increasingly becoming clear (Javed et al., 2022). Not surprisingly, this evidence indicates how the five key SDoHs (healthcare access and quality, education access and quality, social and community context, economic stability, and the neighborhood and built environment) shape barriers to CVD health and increase health disparities in this domain.

For instance, racial differences in socioeconomic determinants (e.g., in wealth and income) are associated with poor CVD health and quality of life. Black and Hispanic employees are 48% to 52% more likely to experience insecurity and be exposed to increased psychosocial occupational stressors stemming from low job control, long commutes, and high work-related demands (Schultz et al., 2018). Psychosocial occupational stressors are, in turn, strong predictors of CVD risk factors, including diabetes and hypertension. Increasing awareness of CVD risk factors is one way of addressing health-related disparities in the CVD domain. Media messages can play a powerful role in supporting the goals of WPHC in this regard.

#### SJA Prompt

Conduct an online search for recent promotional messages about CVD health (e.g., advertisements, campaigns, product marketing, brands, and/or organizational messages).

1. How inclusive are they of people of various races, ethnicities, ages, gender identities, and sexual orientations?

2. Which populations do they predominantly seem to address, and which are left out?
3. Take one of those messages and modify it to include one of the populations that is underrepresented.
4. How will you ensure you are being reflexive about your biases in designing the message?

### Resources

Javed, J., Maqsood, M. H., Yahya, T., Amin, Z., Valero-Elizondo, J., Andrieni, J. … Nasir, K. (2022). Race, racism, and cardiovascular health: Applying a social determinants of health framework to racial/ethnic disparities in cardiovascular disease. *Circulation, 15*(1). https://doi.org/10.1161/CIRCOUTCOMES.121.007917

Schultz, W. M., Kelli, H. M., Lisko, J. C., Varghese, T., Shen, J. … Sperling, L. S. (2018). Socioeconomic status and cardiovascular outcomes: challenges and interventions. *Circulation, 137*(20), 2166–2178. https://doi.org/10.1161/CIRCULATIONAHA.117.029652

*Reflexivity in the Contextual Level*

#### REFLEXIVITY IN THE CONTEXT OF MEDIA REPRESENTATIONS OF HEALTH

Health communication researchers also have examined reflexivity about how media representations of health and people experiencing health issues represent health topics. For instance, in examining the swine flu in Australia, Holland and Blood (2013) focused on reflexivity as a means of critically engaging with media, evaluating the government's response, and enacting vigilance and behavior change by those who medical authorities deemed to be "at risk." Holland and Blood, thus, interrogated how people construct categories of who is deemed to be at risk and how those categories are informed by people's own value systems and taken-for-granted norms that subsume hierarchical relationships.

*Reflexivity in Health Communication Research*

#### RESEARCHER REFLEXIVITY

Communication scholars also have studied how researchers, themselves, engage in reflexivity. For instance, Russell (2019) examined how health communication researchers engage reflexivity in their embodied interactions with research participants to negotiate complex issues involving trust, vulnerability, and risk. Dutta (e.g., 2010, 2018) has centered reflexivity in their employment of the culture-centered approach (CCA) when examining health disparities for subaltern voices (see **Chapter 11, Global Health**, for more on the CCA). Reflexivity in the research process encourages researchers to interrogate how their identity and positionality shape the research process, interactions, and findings.

#### REFLEXIVITY IN THE RESEARCH PROCESS

Reflexivity also means that researchers consider their own thought process and its construction as it bears upon the focus of their research. For instance, Dutta and de Souza (2008) examined the sociopolitical context in which health scholars design health communication campaigns. They attended to tensions that health communication campaign designers experience between the past and the present, the global and the local, and the modern and postmodern. Employing a critical cultural approach that examines the assumptions behind beliefs and norms, the researchers highlighted how campaign designers think through and become aware of the role of media, culture, health responsibility, structural conditions, and politics of knowledge. They took structure-level factors into account to understand how individuals who are socially disadvantaged are constructed as vulnerable vs. empowered and as having agency or as lacking agency. Their research reinforces how reflexivity has powerful implications for the agency of those whose voices are being represented by others. By encouraging individual ownership and critical examination of the beliefs and knowledge domains that contribute to the SCoH norms and conditions, reflexivity is central to fulfilling the goals of the WPHC approach.

### Interdependence in WPHC

Interdependence directs people's awareness of their connections with others, social contexts, organizations, and with the environment. Interdependence considers mutual dependence, shared power, and cooperation in relationships. One theory that has been used often to understand interdependence in health contexts is the actor-partner interdependence model (APIM; Kenny et al., 2006). This theory considers the intrapersonal and interpersonal contexts of health behavior. Intrapersonal contexts refer to those facets of relationships that occur within a person, whereas interpersonal interactions refer to those that occur between people. In an interpersonal context, Matsuda (2017) used that model to examine how couples influenced one another regarding the connection between sexual communication and relationship power, general communication, and views on family planning. Magsamen-Conrad et al. (2019) applied the APIM to understand the response patterns of support, reciprocity, emotional reaction, and avoidance for romantic couples managing cancer. Interdependence helps to understand contexts of health disruption, such as those caused by cancer (Magsamen-Conrad et al., 2019). Communication of concerns and disclosure of fear and thoughts helps to manage illness, which, in turn, decreases the amount of distress and burden that the partner experiences (Stanton et al., 2002; Venetis et al., 2014). Interdependence has also been examined in spousal communication and sense-making after a miscarriage about its impact on spouses' well-being, perspective-taking, and relational satisfaction (Horstman & Holman, 2018).

Reflexivity and interdependence thus are important to WPHC, as they address key aspects of relational, emotional, and social health and well-being. As the next section shows, they also are key to health equity.

*Textbox 1.6 provides a select list of WPHC concepts with their definitions for this chapter. Attempt the SJA discussion prompt that follows.*

---

**Textbox 1.6   Selected WPHC Concepts with Definitions**

- **Health**: a state of complete physical, mental, and social well-being and not merely the absence of disease or infirmity.
- **Well-being**: includes the presence of positive emotions and moods (e.g., contentment and happiness), absence of negative emotions (e.g., depression and anxiety), satisfaction with life, fulfillment, and positive function. Well-being can be described as people judging their life positively and feeling good (CDC, 2018, 2021).
- **Disease**: an illness or sickness characterized by specific signs or symptoms.

- **Social isolation**: the absence of social interactions, contacts, and relationships with family, friends, and neighbors, and with "society at large" (Berg & Cassells, 1992).
- **Biomedical knowledge**: pertains to the processes underlying the manifestations of a disease, and incorporates knowledge about domains that include biochemistry, microbiology, and physiology.
- **SDoH**: conditions in the places where people live, learn, work, and play that affect a wide range of health and quality-of-life risks and outcomes.
- **Value-based model of care**: View people as individuals whose health status should be interpreted as a confluence of socioeconomic circumstances that may make them vulnerable to health risks.
- **Complementary, alternative, and IM**: If a practice that is not mainstream is used **together with** conventional medicine, it is "complementary." If a nonmainstream practice is used **in place of** conventional medicine, it is "alternative." Integrative healthcare brings conventional and complementary approaches together in a coordinated way emphasizing a holistic, person-focused approach to healthcare and wellness—often including mental, emotional, functional, spiritual, social, and community aspects— and treating the whole person rather than, for example, one organ system. Integrative healthcare aims for well-coordinated care between various providers and institutions (NCCIH, 2021).
- **IM**: practice of medicine that reaffirms the importance of the relationship between healthcare providers and patients, focuses on the whole person, is informed by evidence, and makes use of all appropriate therapeutic approaches, healthcare professionals, and disciplines to achieve optimal health and healing (American Board of Physician Specialties, 2021)
- **Transactional communication**: communication that is characterized by shared power, mutual influence, attentiveness to both verbal and nonverbal cues, and the value of feedback and diversity (du Pré & Foster, 2015).
- **Objectivist approach**: defines social problems by concrete, scientifically measurable damage conditions cause or objective dangers they pose to human life.
- **Constructivist approach**: defines social problems by the public concern that conditions generate.
- **Social constructionism**: theory of knowledge that holds that characteristics typically thought to be immutable and solely biological (e.g., gender, race, class, ability, and sexuality) are products of human definition and interpretation, shaped by cultural and historical contexts. Social constructionism highlights the ways in which cultural categories(e.g., "men," "women," "Black," and "White") are concepts that are created, changed, and reproduced through historical processes within institutions and culture.
- **Illness**: an anomaly that can manifest to create a condition of being unhealthy, sick, or diseased.
- **Communicative management of meaning**: theorizes communication as a process that allows people to create and manage social reality by describing how communicators engage in meaning making, which is understood as a hierarchical process, about their lived conditions.
- **CIT**: posits that storytelling is central to building and maintaining a community, as well as to effecting social change at the community level (Ball-Rokeach et al., 2001).

- **Reflexivity**: people being aware of their actions and the belief and value systems that guide them in critical and interpretive ways.
- **Interdependence**: processes, actions, or activities that require one individual to work with another.
- **Openness**: a basic personality trait denoting receptivity to new ideas and experiences. It is one of five core personality dimensions that drive behavior in the Five-Factor Model of Personality. People with high, as compared to low, levels of openness are more likely to seek out a variety of experiences, be comfortable with that which is unfamiliar, exhibit high levels of curiosity, and pay attention to their feelings.
- **Vulnerable populations**: Those at greater risk for poor health status and health access who are considered vulnerable, including racial and ethnic minorities; those who are economically disadvantaged; and those with chronic health conditions experience greater risk factors, worse access to care, and increased morbidity and mortality compared to the general population.
- **Agency**: capacity of individuals to act independently and make choices.
- **APIM**: a model of dyadic relationships that integrates a conceptual view of and statistical techniques for measuring interdependence.
- **Inclusive healthcare**: the ethical premise of the health-for-all ethos that recognizes and seeks to eliminate all barriers to people's participation in receiving health.
- **Right to health**: The belief that people have an innate entitlement to good health, with health understood as an inclusive right to the factors needed to help lead a healthy life (e.g., safe drinking water, safe food, adequate nutrition and housing, healthy working and environmental conditions; health-related education and information; and gender equality); freedoms (free from nonconsensual medical treatment, inhuman or degrading treatment, or punishment; equality of opportunity to enjoy the highest attainable level of health; right to prevention, treatment, and control of disease; and access to essential medicines, among others); health services, goods, and facilities provided to all without any discrimination; all services must be available, accessible, acceptable, and of good quality.

## SJA Discussion Prompt

- In what way does this list of concepts and their definitions highlight the concerns of WPHC?
- What SJA themes stand out as most important to you in considering the goals of WPHC?

## Resources

American Board of Physician Specialties. (2021). *Integrative medicine defined*. Retrieved from https://www.abpsus.org/integrative-medicine-defined/

Ball-Rokeach, S. J., Kim, Y.-C., & Matei, S. (2001). Storytelling neighborhood: Paths to belonging in diverse urban environments. *Communication Research*, *27*(4), 392–427. https://doi.org/10.1177/009365001028004003

Berg, R. L., & Cassells, J. S. (Eds.). (1992). *The second fifty years: Promoting health and preventing disability*. National Academies Press. Retrieved from https://www.nap.edu/catalog/1578/the-second-fifty-years-promoting-health-and-preventing-disability

Berg-Weger, M., & Morley, J.E. (2020). Loneliness and social isolation in older adults during the COVID-19 pandemic: Implications for gerontological social work. *Journal of Nutrition, Health, & Aging, 24*(5), 456–458. https://doi.org/ 10.1007/s12603-020-1366-8

Centers for Disease Control and Prevention (CDC). (2021, May 6). *Social determinants of health: Know what affects health*. Retrieved from https://www.cdc.gov/socialdeterminants/index.htm

du Pré, A., & Foster, E. (2015). Transactional communication. In E. Wittenberg, B. R. Ferrell, Goldsmith, J., Smith, T., Glajchen, M., & Handzo, G. F. (Eds.), *Textbook of palliative communication* (pp. 14–21). Oxford University Press. https://doi.org/10.1093/med/9780190201708. 003.0003

Institute on Medicine (IOM). Committee on Monitoring Access to Personal Healthcare Services. (1993). *Access to healthcare in America*. National Academy Press. Retrieved from https://www.nap.edu/catalog/2009/access-to-healthcare-in-america

National Center for Complementary and Integrative Health. (2021, June 24). *Complementary, alternative, or integrative health: What's in a name?* Retrieved from https://www.nccih.nih.gov/health/complementary-alternative-or-integrative-health-whats-in-a-name

## WPHC and the Inclusive and Rights-Based Approach to Health

### WPHC as an Inclusive Approach to Health

Viewing health through the lens of equity, access, and disparity foregrounds its ethical foundations. To be meaningful and relevant, any understanding of health must necessarily speak to the perspectives and needs of all people. An inclusive healthcare system is one that is reflexive in its efforts to be sensitive to all people's needs, provide equitable access, and ensure all people's full participation. Inequities are revealed in systematic patterns of unfair, avoidable, and remediable differences in people's health status based on, for instance, their gender, ethnicity, socioeconomic status, and education.

An inclusive approach to health affects both individuals' health and public health. In looking at weight-loss interventions, for example, Tylka et al. (2014) critiqued the weight-normative approach that relates weight and weight loss to health and well-being. They argued that the focus on a normative expectation of weight is ineffective because many people regain the pounds that they lose and fall into a pattern of using weight-loss interventions, which, when they fail, further aggravate their health and well-being. A biomedical weight-normative approach also stigmatizes weight, further linking it with adverse health and well-being outcomes. Weight-inclusive approaches, in contrast, improve physical (blood pressure), behavioral (binge eating), and psychological indices (e.g., depression), as well as avoid stigmatizing those whose weight does not meet the normative standards imposed. Tylka et al. (2014) noted that the Health-at-Every-Size model upholds nonmaleficence and beneficence.

### Inclusive Approach and Intersectoral Coordination

Research shows that paradoxically, even as health status improves at the population level, social health inequities continue to widen. This disparity has been attributed in part to negligence of factors in sectors like education, transportation, housing, and finance, and treating them as separate from those related to health. Public health policies that focus on intersectoral action consider how social policies across all sectors such as education and housing, contribute to the overall context that shapes an individual's health status and outcomes.

For instance, public health policies directed toward domains like tobacco control may depend on insurance, service delivery, and meaningful health leadership to be effective. Thus, intersectoral coordination is deeply connected with SDoHs.

### Inclusive Approach and Continuum of Care

An inclusive approach to health considers facets of service delivery that focus on disadvantaged populations to assist with the continuum of care where the health inequities are most exacerbated and where healthcare system utilization is most disparate. Continuum of care emphasizes care continuity over time, such as through diagnosis to testing to recovery, sustainable maintenance, and community support. Healthcare policy that examines data by ethnicity, social class, and geographical area can make these disparities visible for hard-to-reach populations and bridge the power gap between healthcare systems and the people they serve. Globally, power differentials exist between many countries. For instance, WHO (2007) noted that only 38% of the population in low-income countries has access to improved sanitation facilities, whereas 100% of the population living in high-income countries has that access. Moreover, more than 60% of children in South Asia and sub-Saharan Africa are deprived of reasonable shelter. The right to health, thus, also includes the right to the underlying determinants of health, freedom from discrimination, participation, and accountability.

Review **Textbox 1.7**. Respond to the SJA discussion prompt that follows.

---

**Textbox 1.7    A Social Justice Inventory for Your Neighborhood**

**WPHC Context**

The premise of inclusive healthcare advocates the removal of individual, social, institutional, and community-level barriers; making accommodations; and providing culturally sensitive and informed care to enable individuals who are socially disadvantaged to effectively access and utilize healthcare for optimal outcomes. It also means that healthcare providers recognize and acknowledge their client's unique experiences, choices, and knowledge in designing their care. Inclusive health is based on the principles of equitable access and full participation while accounting for any barriers posed by the SDoH. An inclusive approach to healthcare is nonstigmatizing and supports the ability of everyone to access health services equally, regardless of their racial and ethnic status, age, gender, sexual identity, and other differences.

**SJA Discussion Prompt**

This exercise will support your understanding of socially disadvantaged populations in your local geographical community based on each of the SDoH criteria (listed in the table that follows).

1. Identify a nonprofit organization in your community that works with the SDoH criteria and fill in the "community" column. For example, a homeless shelter that works with those facing housing should be placed in the "community" column of the "housing status" SDoH row.

---

2. What is one health challenge that members of the vulnerable population in your community face? For example, those in the housing status category may face challenges obtaining oral hygiene and preventative services. Fill in challenges as they fall under the "inclusion," "access," and "equity" columns. Be short, focused, and evidence-based when identifying each element in the following table.

| SDoH | Community | Health Concern | Inclusion | Access | Equity |
|------|-----------|----------------|-----------|--------|--------|
| Race |  |  |  |  |  |
| Gender |  |  |  |  |  |
| Age |  |  |  |  |  |
| Housing status |  |  |  |  |  |
| Neighborhood |  |  |  |  |  |

### WPHC and Right to Health in Healthcare

The premise of right to health is based on a legal understanding of achieving a healthful status. However, it references much more than its legal interpretation by also focusing attention on rights in terms of social ethics (Sen, 2008). Rights viewed from an ethics perspective attend to what a good society must have and provide for its members. As Sen (2008) emphasized, understanding the right to health as a right of all demands action to promote the goal of health for all. Such action goes beyond the provision of personal liberties and political facets, such as the right to vote. It also includes the right to health, understood as the ability of all to achieve the highest possible accomplishment of their personal vision. The right-to-health approach assumes that healthcare is only one component of good health; good health also depends on nutrition, lifestyle, education, gender equality, elimination of inequities, and a free society (Sen, 2008). Thinking of health from a right-for-all perspective is a key WPHC tenet that strengthens the collective social commitment to good health for all members of society in inclusive ways.

### Health as a Human Right

Global advocacy efforts to achieve health for all have focused on strengthening primary healthcare (PHC; see **Chapter 6**, "**Healthcare Systems**," for more on PHCs) with regard to health equity, community participation, and intersectoral action (Rasanathan et al., 2011). PHC originated in the ethos of community-based healthcare offered in low- and middle-income countries in the 1950s and 1960s. These were codified at the Alma Ata conference to include basic, vital healthcare sectors related to national and community development, such as housing, food, education, communication, and agriculture. In both PHC and SDoH approaches, the concern for health equity is closely associated with the view of health as a human right (Commission on Social Determinants of Health, 2007). The view of health as a human right expands the thinking of health fundamentally beyond merely viewing health as being the absence of disease. Thinking about health as a human right changes the way that healthcare systems, policies, and implementation of healthcare are perceived by emphasizing how all aspects of health and well-being as well as an individual's environment and context are a fundamental part of the WPHC. As Rasanathan et al. (2011) pointed out, both the PHC and SDoH emphasize health promotion, disease prevention, and wellness, as well as support people in having access to resources that they need to stay healthy and to protect themselves from health and disease. The shared concern of PHC and SDoH on health equity is based on a broad vision of WPHC, rather than the narrow biomedical view of healthcare as clinical intervention and treatment. The WPHC also assumes the PHC is situated in a relationship of multisectoral and shared efforts toward strengthening the health system.

### WPHC and the Inclusive, Rights-Based Approach to Health

An inclusive, rights-based approach to health references the SDoH and PHC paradigms and identifies disempowerment and marginalization of populations in society as a barrier to achieving health equity (Rasanathan et al., 2011). Both approaches call for an examination of processes and responses that address the inequitable distribution of power. They highlight the role of community empowerment and the importance of health services in responding to community needs and participation in healthcare. Empowered communities are involved in service provision, collaboration, and health policy decision-making. Including the community in healthcare approaches shifts the focus to the impact of community-based factors (e.g., distribution of resources, empowerment, social inclusion and exclusion, relative social status, and community resiliency and support) on people's health (Chandanabhumma et al., 2020). A rights-based approach to health is closely connected with inclusive health. The ethos of the rights-based approach to health includes the political, social, economic, scientific, and cultural actions that can be taken by everyone to ensure good health for all (Sen, 2008). Embedded in the inclusive approach to health is the WPHC assumption that health services improve people's health and well-being, and that those services both prevent disease and the social conditions that lead to disease.

## Conclusion

In conclusion, **Chapter 1**, "**A Whole Person Framework of Health**" introduces the key tenets and principles comprising the WPHC approach. It describes how the WPHC approach can inform how we think about, conceptualize, and deliver healthcare in a manner that is reflexive, inclusive, and adopts value-based care and rights-based inclusive understanding of health. The key constructs of WPHC laid out in Chapter 1 are examined and elaborated upon in the subsequent chapters in the textbook. **Chapter 2**, "**Models for Representing Health and Disease**," will begin by describing the four models of health and disease.

*Review **Textbox 1.8**. How can community involvement support sustainable change in individuals who are socially disadvantaged?*

---

### Textbox 1.8   Present Challenges and Future Directions: Involving the Community

#### WPHC Context

Researchers Betancourt et al. (2003) advocate that health promotion models, to be effective, must embrace not only individual-level but also community-level factors. They should also be accompanied by institutional change. They suggest that structural and sociocultural change can be achieved through strategies such as forming supportive internal and external alliances and increasing awareness of the need for cultural competence interventions. Recruiting more individuals from minority populations in health professions can be one such step. Likewise, Professor Dutta and colleagues discuss the need for community-grounded participatory solutions (2019) to increase community knowledge of health promotion behaviors. In Professor Dutta and colleagues' campaign on cardiovascular disease knowledge awareness, knowledge for change was created by community members and disseminated in local spaces such as health fairs and church meetings by community members.

## SJA Activity

This exercise involves going out into the community and speaking with members, community leaders, and community organizations.

1. Identify any one vulnerable population in your community. This population could be those facing housing instability, food insecurity, or single parents, or it could be low-income neighborhoods with a predominantly minority population.
2. Make an appointment with the county health department to understand the healthcare needs and challenges faced by the minority populations in the community. This preliminary research will give you an introduction to county-level health behaviors and risk factors grouped by population characteristics.
3. Next, try to identify two or three institutional barriers that contribute to these challenges for one specific minority population. Examples of institutional barriers can include insufficient program funding, restrictive policies, and lack of culturally and linguistically appropriate health resources.
4. How can you involve the community members to identify barriers and organize their collective knowledge to create communicative avenues for change? For instance, one communication student planned to address the lack of education among providers in his county on racial/ethnic testing data on health plans and delivery systems by going to the nearby hospitals in his county and speaking with a group of providers and nurses about their knowledge and awareness of racial and ethnic differences in the health issue. Armed with this information, he said he would create pamphlets that include each race group in a table with an indication of different health issues.
5. How can you create sustainable change? What is one opportunity for strengthening one of the resources that the community must help for it to grow stronger in the future?
   a. What other problems and barriers do you anticipate (e.g., loss of transportation)?
   b. How can you work with the community members and organizations to create awareness and support their resources to grow productively in the future?

## Resources

Betancourt, J. R., Green, A. R., Carrillo, J. E., & Ananeh-Firempong, O., II (2003). Defining cultural competence: A practical framework for addressing racial/ethnic disparities in health and health care. *Public Health Reports*, *118*(4), 293–302. https://doi.org/10.1093/phr/118.4.293

Dutta, M. J., Collins, W., Sastry, S., Dillard, S., Anaele, A., Kumar, R., Roberson, C., Robinson, T., & Bonu, T. (2019). A culture-centered community-grounded approach to disseminating health information among African Americans. *Health Communication*, *34*(10), 1075–1084. https://doi.org/10.1080/10410236.2018.1455626

## References

American Hospital Association (AHA). (2021). 2022 Health care talent scan. Retrieved from https://www.aha.org/system/files/media/file/2021/10/AHA-Health-Care-Talent-Scan-2022.pdf

American Psychological Association. (2021). *African American older adults and race-related stress: How aging and healthcare providers can help*. Retrieved from https://www.apa.org/pi/aging/resources/african-american-stress.pdf

American Psychological Association (APA). (2021). The risks of social isolation. Retrieved from https://www.apa.org/monitor/2019/05/ce-corner-isolation

Agarwal, V. (2018a). Reconceptualizing pain through patient-centered care in the complementary and alternative medicine therapeutic relationship. *Journal of Advanced Nursing, 74*(10), 2406–2415. https://doi.org/10.1111/jan.13734

Agarwal, V. (2018b). The provider's body in the therapeutic relationship: How complementary and alternative medicine providers describe their work as healers. *Health Communication, 34*(11), 1350–1358. https://doi.org/10.1080/10410236.2018.1489201

Agarwal, V. (2019). Patient communication of pain in the complementary and alternative medicine therapeutic relationship. *Journal of Patient Experience*, 1–7. https://doi.org/10.1177/2374373519826137

Boyd, K. M. (2000). Disease, sickness, health, healing, and wholeness: Exploring some elusive concepts. *Medical Humanities, 26*(1). http://doi.org/10.1136/mh.26.1.9

Cacioppo, J. T., Fowler, J. H., & Christakis, N. A. (2009). Alone in the crowd: The structure and spread of loneliness in a large social network. *Journal of Personality and Social Psychology, 97*(6), 977–991. https://doi.org/10.1037/a0016076

Cacioppo, J. T., Hawkley, L. C., Norman, G. J., & Berntson, G. G. (2011). Social isolation. *Annals of the New York Academy of Sciences, 1231*(1), 17–22. https://doi.org/10.1111/j.1749-6632.2011.06028.x

CDC. (2018, October 31). *Well-being concepts*. Retrieved from https://www.cdc.gov/hrqol/wellbeing.htm#three

Centers for Disease Prevention and Control (CDC). (2023). Economic stability. Retrieved from https://www.cdc.gov/prepyourhealth/discussionguides/economicstability.htm#:~:text=SDOH%20are%20grouped%20by%20Healthy,socioeconomic%20status%E2%80%94and%20their%20health

Chandanabhumma, P. P., Duran, B. M., Peterson, J. C., Pearson, C. R., Oetzel, J. G., Dutta, M. J., & Wallerstein, N. B. (2020). Space within the scientific discourse for the voice of the other? Expressions of community voice in the scientific discourse of community-based participatory research. *Health Communication, 35*(5), 616–627. https://doi.org/10.1080/10410236.2019.1581409

Commission on Social Determinants of Health. (2007). *Achieving health equity: From root causes to fair outcomes*. http://apps.who.int/iris/bitstream/handle/10665/69670/interim_statement_eng.pdf;jsessinid=CA6E32D29A015FC852DB47AB69983EFC?sequence=1

Cornwell, B., Laumann, E. O., & Schumm, P. L. (2008). The social connectedness of older adults: A national profile. *American Sociological Review, 73*(2), 185–203. https://doi.org/10.1177/000312240807300201

Dutta, M. J. (2010). The critical cultural turn in *Health Communication*: Reflexivity, solidarity, and praxis. *Health Communication, 25*(6–7), 534–539. https://doi.org/10.1080/10410236.2010.497995

Dutta, M. J. (2018). Culture-centered approach in addressing health disparities: Communication infrastructures for subaltern voices. *Communication Methods and Measures, 12*(4), 239–259. https://doi.org/10.1080/19312458.2018.1453057

Dutta, M. J., & de Souza, R. (2008). The past, present, and future of health development campaigns: Reflexivity and the critical-cultural approach. *Health Communication, 23*(4), 326–339. https://doi.org/10.1080/10410230802229704

Frohlich, D. O. (2016). The social construction of inflammatory bowel disease using social media technologies. *Health Communication, 31*(11), 1412–1420. https://doi.org/10.1080/10410236.2015.1077690

Gill, E. A., & Babrow, A. S. (2007). To hope or to know: Coping with uncertainty and ambivalence in women's magazine breast cancer articles. *Journal of Applied Communication Research, 35*(2), 133–155. https://doi.org/10.1080/00909880701263029

Health.gov (2023). Healthy People 2030. Retrieved from https://health.gov/healthypeople

Holland, K., & Blood, W. R. (2013). Public responses and reflexivity during the swine flu pandemic in Australia. *Journalism Studies, 14*(4), 523–538. https://doi.org/10.1080/1461670X.2012.744552

Horstman, H. K., & Holman, A. (2018). Communicated sense-making after miscarriage: A dyadic analysis of spousal communicated perspective-taking, well-being, and parenting role salience. *Health Communication, 33*(10), 1317–1326. https://doi.org/10.1080/10410236.2017.1351852

House, J. S. (2001). Social isolation kills, but how and why? *Psychosomatic Medicine, 63*(2), 272–274. https://doi.org/10.1097/00006842-200103000-00011

Kenny, D. A., Kashy, D. A., & Cook, W. L. (2006). *Dyadic data analysis.* Guilford Press.

Langevin, H. (2020, April 27). *Considering whole person health as we develop NCCIH's next strategic plan.* National Center for Complementary and Integrative Health. Retrieved from https://www.nccih.nih.gov/about/offices/od/director/past-messages/considering-whole-person-health-as-we-develop-nccihs-next-strategic-plan

Lubben, J. (2017). Addressing social isolation as a potent killer! *Public Policy and Aging Report, 27*(4), 136–138. https://doi.org/10.1093/ppar/prx026

Magsamen-Conrad, K., Venetis, M. K., Checton, M. G., & Greene, K. (2019). The role of response perceptions in couples' ongoing cancer-related disclosure. *Health Communication, 34*(9), 999–1009. https://doi.org/10.1080/10410236.2018.1452091

Matsaganis, M. D., & Golden, A. G. (2015). Interventions to address reproductive health disparities among African-American women in a small urban community: The communicative reconstruction of a "field of health action". *Journal of Applied Communication Research, 43*(2), 163–184. https://doi.org/10.1080/00909882.2015.1019546

Matsuda, Y. (2017). Actor–partner interdependence model analysis of sexual communication and relationship/family planning factors among immigrant Latino couples in the United States. *Health Communication, 32*(5), 612–620. https://doi.org/10.1080/10410236.2016.1160317

Mendes, A., Abreu, L., Vilar-Correia, M. R., & Borlido-Santos, J. (2017). "That should be left to doctors, that's what they are there for!"—Exploring the reflexivity and trust of young adults when seeking health information. *Health Communication, 32*(9), 1076–1081. https://doi.org/10.1080/10410236.2016.1199081

National Institute on Aging. (2021, January 14). *Loneliness and social isolation—Tips for staying connected.* Retrieved from https://www.nia.nih.gov/health/loneliness-and-social-isolation-tips-staying-connected

Nicholson, N. R. (2012). A review of social isolation: An important but underassessed condition in older adults. *Journal of Primary Prevention, 33*(2–3), 137–152. https://doi.org/10.1007/s10935-012-0271-2

Omilion-Hodges, L. M., Manning, B. L., & Orbe, M. P. (2019). "Context matters:" An exploration of young adult social constructions of meaning about death and dying. *Health Communication, 34*(2), 139–148. https://doi.org/10.1080/10410236.2017.1384436

Pearce, W. B., & Cronen, V. E. (1980). *Communication, action, and meaning: The creation of social realities.* Praeger.

Primack, B. A., Shensa, A., Sidani, J. E., Whaite, E. O., Yi Line, L., Rosen, D. … Miller, E. (2017). Social media use and perceived social isolation among young adults in the U.S. *American Journal of Preventive Medicine, 53*(1), 1–8. https://doi.org/10.1016/j.amepre.2017.01.010

Rafferty, K. A., & Sullivan, S. L. (2017). "You know the medicine; I know my kid": How parents advocate for their children living with complex chronic conditions. *Health Communication, 32*(9), 1151–1160. https://doi.org/10.1080/10410236.2016.1214221

Rasanathan, K., Montesinos, E. V., Matheson, D., Etienne, C., & Evans, T. (2011). Primary healthcare and the social determinants of health: Essential and complementary approaches for reducing inequities in health. *Journal of Epidemiology and Community Health, 65*(8), 656–660. https://doi.org/10.1136/jech.2009.093914

Russell, L. D. (2019). Encountering the unexpected: Revelations of trust, vulnerability, and embodied ways of knowing. *Health Communication, 34*(11), 1380–1382. https://doi.org/10.1080/10410236.2018.1481493

Sen, A. (2008). Why and how is health a human right? *Lancet, 372*(9655). https://doi.org/10.1016/S0140-6736(08)61784-5

Stanton, A. L., Danoff-Burg, S., & Huggins, M. E. (2002). The first year after breast cancer diagnosis: Hope and coping strategies as predictors of adjustment. *Psycho-Oncology: Journal of the Psychological, Social and Behavioral Dimensions of Cancer, 11*(2), 93–102. https://doi.org/10.1002/pon.574

Taylor, R. J., Chatters, L. M., & Taylor, H. O. (2019). Race and objective social isolation: Older African Americans, Black Caribbeans, and non-Hispanic Whites. *Journals of Gerontology: Series B, 74*(8), 1429–1440. https://doi.org/10.1093/geronb/gby114

The US Surgeon General's Advisory. (2023). *Our epidemic of loneliness and isolation.* Retrieved May 16, 2023, from https://www.hhs.gov/sites/default/files/surgeon-general-social-connection-advisory.pdf

Thomas, H., Mitchell, G., Rich, J., & Best, M. (2018). Definition of whole person care in general practice in the English language literature: A systematic review. *BMJ Open, 8*(12), Article e023758. https://doi./org/10.1136/bmjopen-2018-023758

Tomaka, J., Thompson, S., & Palacios, R. (2006). The relation of social isolation, loneliness, and social support to disease outcomes among the elderly. *Journal of Aging and Health, 18*(3), 359–384. https://doi.org/10.1177/0898264305280993

Tylka, T. L., Annunziato, R. A., Burgard, D., Daníelsdóttir, S., Shuman, E., Davis, C., & Calogero, R. M. (2014). The weight-inclusive versus weight-normative approach to health: Evaluating the evidence for prioritizing well-being overweight loss. *Journal of Obesity*, Article 983495. https://doi.org/10.1155/2014/983495

Venetis, M. K., Magsamen-Conrad, K., Checton, M. G., & Greene, K. (2014). Cancer communication and partner burden: An exploratory study. *Journal of Communication, 64*(1), 82–102. https://doi.org/10.1111/jcom.12069

World Health Organization (WHO, 2007). Water. Retrieved from https://www.afro.who.int/health-topics/water

World Health Organization. (2021a). *Social determinants of health.* Retrieved from https://www.who.int/teams/social-determinants-of-health

World Health Organization. (2021b, April 19). *What is the WHO definition of health?* Retrieved from https://www.who.int/about/who-we-are/frequently-asked-questions

## Additional Resources

### Healthcare Institutions and Plans

Inner-City Fund (ICF). Kaiser the shift from transactional to whole-person care. Retrieved from https://www.icf.com/next/insights/health/new-approach-whole-person-care#

Picker Institute. (n.d.). Care of the whole person. Retrieved from https://www.picker.org/picker-impact-report-2019-2020/#p=6

### Global and US-Based Organizations

World Health Organization. Retrieved from https://www.who.int/news-room/fact-sheets/detail/primary-health-care

Centers for Disease Prevention and Control. (n.d.). *Whole school, whole community, whole child (WSCC) initiative.* Retrieved from https://www.cdc.gov/healthyschools/wscc/

San Francisco Department of Health. *Whole person care.* Retrieved from https://www.sfdph.org/dph/comupg/oprograms/wpc/default.asp

Arizona Healthcare Cost Containment System (AHCCCS). (n.d.). *AHCCS Whole Person care initiative (WPCI).* Retrieved on April 26, 2021, from https://www.azahcccs.gov/AHCCCS/Initiatives/AHCCCSWPCI/

# Models for Representing Health and Disease

## Chapter Learning Outcomes

At the end of **Chapter 2**, **Models for Representing Health and Disease**, students should be able to apply WPHC SJA principles to:

1. Critique the biomedical, biopsychosocial, holistic, and IM models of health with respect to whole person care, equitable relationships, coordination of care, and collaborative decision-making.
2. Explain how health communication as a field is interdisciplinary in its focus and gain an overview of how health communication perspectives attend to issues of health equity, policy communication, public advocacy, cultural competence, and health literacy.
3. Understand how behavior change theories can be applied to individual health behaviors and to building local-clinical stakeholder health partnerships.
4. Explain critical, cultural, and narrative approaches to health and medicine with particular attention to patient-centered care and relationships, eliminating health disparities, achieving health equity, and improving the health of all populations.
5. Consider how relational, humanistic approaches can be designed and implemented to promote the goals of socially just WPHC from the perspective of those who have been historically oppressed, disadvantaged, and marginalized.
6. Engage health communication theories and models to applied contexts in dialogic health communication and digital platforms ranging from entertainment-education and social network storytelling to designing two-way visual communication messages.

## Consider this context:

Otitis media (OM) is a form of inflammation and infection of the middle ear. It is also sometimes known as "runny ears." Damage to the outer or middle ear is one of the most common causes of hearing loss in children. Hearing loss, in turn, is associated

DOI: 10.4324/9781003214472-3

with poor learning, language development and communication, and impaired psychosocial development in children, leading to speech delay, social isolation, and educational disadvantage (WHO, 2004). OM rates are higher where conditions of overcrowded housing, poor nutrition, compromised hygiene, smoke exposure, and limited access to routine care exist. Aboriginal and Torres Strait Islander children have some of the highest rates of OM in the world (DeLacy et al., 2020). In fact, in the remote communities across the Northern Territory of Australia, only one in ten Aboriginal children younger than 3 years has healthy years (Leach et al., 2021).

In Indigenous children, the hearing loss experienced in early childhood can have a devastating impact on their ability to connect with family members, play with friends, and develop academically. They may find education frustrating and difficult. This may cause them to disengage from school, leave early, and ultimately get in trouble with the law. Recent studies in the Northern Territory of Australia find that around 90% of Indigenous prison inmates have significant hearing loss (Center of Research Excellence in Ear and Hearing Health of Aboriginal and Torres Strait Islander Children, 2021).

Hearing impairment, in turn, affects understanding of complex interactions with services and authorities, including hospitals, police, and the criminal justice system. For example, researchers Vanderpoll and Howard carried out testing with 44 Aboriginal inmates within the Darwin Correctional Center and Alice Springs Correctional Centers Center in Australia and found that 94% of Aboriginal inmates had significant hearing loss. This was exemplified in the comments the researchers heard from the inmates related to hearing loss. The researchers note how the hearing loss had resulted in violent altercations with others and the criminal justice system. For example:

> I can't hear what my family says.
> School was hard for me to listen.
> Family always tell me stuff I can't hear.
> Can't hear them police or them court man.
> Hard for me in prison.
> Get in trouble from police can't hear what they're talking.

(2012, p. 4)

Current interventions focus on treating disease with advances in research on vaccines and antibiotics. Vaccines and antibiotics are essential for providing high-quality clinical care for OM. Some researchers, such as DeLacy et al., note that alongside advances in vaccines and antibiotics, a broader public health lens is also necessary. A public health perspective can contribute by addressing underlying social factors that drive the gap in OM rates between Aboriginal and non-Aboriginal children (2020). Yet, DeLacy et al. note that 62% of peer-reviewed articles in their study did not mention the need to address SDoH in their future directions for researching OM. In fact, about 46% of the articles reviewed in their study recommended solely a biomedical model (BM) approach by advocating for research into antibiotic treatment and vaccine development and the need for a greater understanding of OM-associated bacterial carriage.

The biopsychosocial model (BSM) approach goes beyond the BM to emphasize the context by attending to the environment where people live, work, and interact, and the importance of community for the individual. In the case of OM research, only 10% of the articles included recommendations for policy development intended to address SDoH to reduce the high rates of OM in Aboriginal children. By emphasizing community involvement, the BSM can help in providing coordination, access, and delivery of services, enhancing capacity building within communities, and sharing Aboriginal control of research activities and their translation to empower Aboriginal communities to manage OM in a culturally safe way (DeLacy et al., 2020). An integrative model further extends the BSM by incorporating the cultural health practices of the Aboriginal communities. It can, for instance, include evidence-based research on CAM modalities, such as massage, acupuncture, and chiropractic, among others, to integrate them into patient care.

A WPHC approach incorporating cultural-, individual- and community-based values can more comprehensively address Aboriginal understandings of health, which include taking the body, mind, spirit, land, environment, community and family relationships, and social structures into account. Such an approach will also be socially just and conceptualize health outcomes that are based on the principles of health equity, access, and culturally tailored healthcare.

## Chapter Organization

**Chapter 2, Models for Representing Health and Disease** is organized as follows: **First**, the chapter covers the historical and conceptual domains of four models: BM, BSM, holistic model (HM), and IM, and provides a critique of each. **Second**, the chapter provides an overview of dominant health communication theories and models, situating health communication as an interdisciplinary field. **Third**, the chapter covers health communication behavior change theories and applies them to considerations such as those involved in message design. **Fourth**, the chapter covers critical, critical cultural, social constructionist, and narrative approaches to health, providing an overview of their principles, dominant theoretical foci, and relational orientation. **Fifth**, the rhetorical and humanistic approaches to health and medicine section provides an overview of the methods, theoretical orientation, and foci among these approaches. Discussion exercises foregrounding the WPHC SJA approach provide students an opportunity to engage their principles in applied contexts ranging from reproductive health as a rights-based issue, palliative care and psychosocial approaches, to social media platforms and chronic condition self-management, entertainment-education and social network storytelling, and the notion of health competence. The scholar interview with Dr. Kenneth Gergen, a foundational scholar of the social constructionist paradigm, illustrates his view of the paradigm. Students gain an overview of the settings of health communication theory and practice and the evolution of the definition of health communication over the decades.

## Biomedical, Biopsychosocial, Holistic, and Integrative Models of Health and Disease

### The Biomedical Model (BM)

#### A Brief History

Until the nineteenth century, illness and disease, and health and wellness were mysterious phenomena. Explanations of illness and disease began to be formulated with advances in cell theory, germ theory of disease, and bacteriology. Rudolf Virchow was the first to introduce the idea that every pathology arises from a damaged cell. His work paved the way for the BM's future advances in biomolecular foundations, such as those seeking to understand the onset of cancer from a malfunction of host cells. In this way, in BM, disease and illness were identified as originating with malfunction at the simplest structural and functional level of organisms (i.e., the cell), and their treatment was associated with corresponding pharmaceutical interventions.

#### Assumptions of the BM

However, the BM does more than emphasize the diagnosis and treatment of diseases through pharmaceutical approaches. It also posits a change in the way illness and health are conceptualized in popular culture and medicine. The BM assumes all diseases have a biological cause, usually understood as a deviation from the norm or a biological abnormality. For example, infection is explained by the invasion of parasites, a metabolic disorder with a genetic mutation, and a disability with neuronal damage. Correspondingly, the BM assumes that diseases can be treated by biological treatment that targets the underlying biological dysfunction (e.g., du Pre, 2002). The goal of treatment research is to discover the exact therapeutic agents that can specifically target the disease process without harming the organism (Moncrieff, 2008).

*Review* **Textbox 2.1** *for a look at racial inequities in obstetrical care for Black and Hispanic women in the United States. Respond to the SJA prompt that follows.*

---

### Textbox 2.1   "Just Birth": Biomedical and Holistic Medicine

#### WPHC Context

Historically, there have been higher rates of cesarean deliveries for low-risk births among Black and Hispanic women in the United States. This trend reflects racial inequities as they play out in obstetrical care. It has been argued that the vaginal birth after cesarean (VBAC) procedure is racially biased because it naturalizes racial differences, compromises patient autonomy through medicalization of racial differences, and undermines informed consent. West's study of the VBAC procedure illustrates the tension between the description of VBAC as a medical procedure by the BM profession on the one hand and its definition as "just birth" by birth advocates on the other hand (2020). The groups that advocate for VBAC as a medical procedure expand the use of the term "risk" to include factors outside the hospital and by positioning pregnant women as patients whose rights to VBAC may be superseded by an expert authority, such as a physician, an insurance company, or a judge.

As a field, obstetrics involves care given during preconception, pregnancy, childbirth, and the period immediately following delivery. Obstetric risk factors include obesity, diabetes, epilepsy, high blood pressure, heart or blood disorders, and thyroid disease, among others. Underlying the disparity between higher numbers of low-risk cesareans among women of color, SJA argue, are medical definitions of what constitutes obstetric risk factors. These factors, it has been argued, are historically defined through the lens of slavery, oppression, and racism, and as biological markers of difference between human populations and unfairly constrained birth choice for women of color.

On the other hand, the groups that advocate for VBAC as a rights-based issue form a counter-public (i.e., one that is defined by [its] tension with a larger public' that "maintains, at some level, conscious or not, an awareness of its subordinate status"; Warner, 2005, p. 56). The counter-public groups describe birth in the language of a normal, physiologic process that is a natural part of a woman's reproductive life.

## SJA Prompt

Bioethicists argue that structural inequities and inequities in healthcare treatments often place women of color and historically oppressed populations at a clinical disadvantage in postcesarean recovery.

1. How can the WPHC approach help reconceptualize considerations to aid clinicians and patients in critical reflection on race-conscious medicine (racism as an SDoH) vs. race-based medicine (race as SDoH) as a key determinant of illness and health?
2. What are some ways explicit and implicit ways that racism may structure obstetric risks, quality of postoperative care, and clinicians' willingness to respect women's care preferences?

## Resources

Rubashkin, N. (2022, March). Why equitable access to vaginal birth requires abolition of race-based medicine. *AMA Journal of Ethics*, 24(3), E233–E238. https://doi.org/10.1001/amaethics. 2022.233

Warner, M. (2005). *Publics and counterpublics*. Zone Books.

West, J. E. (2020). "Just birth": Childbirth advocacy and the rhetoric of feminist health justice. *Women's Studies in Communication*, 43(2), 131–156. https://doi.org/10.1080/07491409.2020.17 37289

*Critiques of the BM*

One critique of the BM is that it does not consider the context, such as the social, psychological, or behavioral facets of the illness to be significant (Engel, 1977). The BM assumes that diseases can be understood and treated by addressing their deviations from the biological (somatic, biochemical, or neurophysiological) parts, taking each in isolation, or reductively. It takes a mechanistic view of biology and analyzes the parts as separate parts. It assumes that disease is independent of social behavior, behavioral aberrations, and psychological factors. Medicalization of health and disease refers to the tendency to treat existential and life events as biomedical issues. For instance, instead of characterizing a trait as shyness, the BM might categorize it as social anxiety.

Communication researchers have examined the doctor-patient relationship using the BM lens. For instance, communication research on communication skills training programs and how communication affects patient satisfaction and compliance in clinical settings is often structured from a BM perspective. Following the BM, the research on the doctor-patient relationship follows a paternalistic, consumerist model. Communication researcher de Souza (2012) explored how 31 participants living with the human immunodeficiency virus (HIV) in urban India respond to the values, assumptions, and dictates of the BM of medicine to make sense of their health and illness. She looks at how the ideologies and practices of biomedicine were appropriated by individuals living with HIV and how they reconciled contradictions between their chronic disease and the dichotomy of health and illness. She foregrounds culture, understood as the medium within which experiences are contextualized to provide an interpretive context (Goffman, 1974) to understand the feelings and processes of medical- and healthcare contexts. De Souza's participants reinforced BM understandings of health and illness by describing themselves as sick based on the biomedical markers of physical symptoms, prescription medication, and laboratory reports. She describes how the participants expanded the meaning of health to include psychological well-being, lack of worry about finances, children, prognosis uncertainty, and even death. Her study calls for

> a sensitive practice of health which allows for cultural and medical truths to coexist, because it understands the power of medicine to prevent and treat certain disease and the power of culture to provide a framework to encompass the limitations of biomedicine.
>
> (p. 183)

*Review **Textbox 2.2** to apply SJA principles to health information shared on social media platforms in a dialogic manner.*

---

**Textbox 2.2   Social Media Platforms and Dialogic Health Communication**

**WPHC Context**

**Social media platforms** such as X (formerly Twitter) allow healthcare organizations such as the CDC to engage with other organizations and target publics directly. **Social media**

facilitate two-way communication. Guidry et al. (2020) found that often public health organizations and practitioners use social networks like X to share information and make health issues and services visible through one-way efforts. However, these studies also find that the organizations do not use them to create dialogue with their target publics.

### SJA Discussion Prompts

Apply one of the theoretical perspectives and models covered thus far in this chapter to craft a **visual communication** that shares a health promotion message with a target audience of your choice. Your health promotion message could concern a significant domain such as CVD, cancer, diabetes, mental health, sexual health, or HIV/AIDS.

- What message format (images, infographics, or videos) would be most effective and why?
- How might you seek to evoke emotion in your selected audience's response to the message?
  - Would emotional arousal be an ethical and appropriate strategy?
  - When might it not be preferable?
- How should nonprofit and government organizations employ social network communication to achieve optimum health outcomes?
- Should all social network communication essentially be dialogic and two-way?
  - Under what conditions would two-way communication be preferable to one-way communication and vice versa?

### Resource

Guidry, J. P. D., Meganck, S. L., Lovari, A., Messner, M., Medina-Messner, V., Sherman, S., & Adams, J. (2020). Tweeting about #diseases and #publichealth: Communicating global health issues across nations. *Health Communication*, *35*(9), 1137–1145. https://doi.org/10.1080/104102 36.2019.1620089

### The Biopsychosocial Model (BSM)

The BSM recognizes the humanistic and patient-centered side of medicine. It includes the social and psychological domains alongside the biological domain in informing medical decision-making. The BSM draws upon the general system theory, which posits a structural and functional interconnection between all entities (Engel, 1977). It recognizes that acknowledging this interconnection helps not only in the medical care of patients by treating their disease but that their psychological and social needs would also be included in the care and treatment process. In the BSM, the human being is understood as comprising the biological levels (described as "below") and the psychological and social levels (described as "above") to comprise a singular biopsychosocial entity. Moreover, the model states that each level operates as a unique system. For example, the tissues and organs will operate at the biological level, perception and experience at the psychological level, and attribution of meaning at the social level. To understand the patient, the integration of these systems to develop their biopsychosocial story is necessary.

*Review **Textbox 2.3**. In what ways can the WPHC approach help address the challenges in integrating the concerns of palliative care and BM approaches in a patient-centered manner? Consider the SJA prompt that follows to apply the holistic care model to this WPHC context.*

---

### Textbox 2.3   "The Death Doctor": Palliative Care and Psychosocial Approach to Medicine

#### WPHC Context

Palliative care involves fulfilling the physical, psychosocial, emotional, practical, and spiritual needs of individuals at the end of life or in tandem with curative treatment. In the traditional BM, curative treatment is privileged with an emphasis on saving lives. As researchers Omillion-Hodges et al. found in their study, a palliative care physician noted that this difference might be because "most physicians treat diseases, not people" thus, "it was impossible to communicate comprehensively about end-of-life care or options if you don't know what to do in the absence of a treatment plan" (p. 1276).

For the medical specialists approaching this context from a biomedical perspective, death was viewed as a failure for physician, patient, and family members" as opposed to the palliative care community that "views death as a natural process" and "embrace as an accepted part of life." Medical colleagues in the biomedical community "strive to prevent it by prolonging a patient's life, because in the case that they do not, they have not achieved their goal or that of the patient" (p. 1278).

In Omillion-Hodges et al.'s study, the tensions between advocates of palliative care and the BM perspective were illustrated vividly by an example shared by a palliative care physician. Jim, a palliative care physician faced obstruction and discomfort in the physician's dining room and public hallways of the hospital. One day, he found his unit was decorated in the style of a Halloween graveyard: "plastic tombstones, urns, cobwebs, [even] a scythe with a black cloak propped" against his office door. Jim was upset by the lack of understanding of the specialty [and] fear of death among other physicians" (p. 1276).

#### SJA Prompt

A WPHC approach to palliative care addresses physical, emotional, spiritual, psychological, and environmental contexts of care for patients in the context of their relationships and life goals.

1. Palliative care is recognized under the human right to health. It focuses on relief from pain, meaningfulness and quality of life, and spiritual aspects to care. Try your hand at constructing three communicative messages that emphasize the partnership between a palliative care nurse and patient in the negotiation of care that is meaningful for the patient, their family, and the provider.
2. What communicative attributes would highlight caring and compassionate teamwork from a WPHC perspective?
3. How can palliative care communication be designed to be inclusive and culturally sensitive?

**Resource**

Omillion-Hodges, L. M., & Swords, N. M. (2017). The grim reaper, hounds of hell, and Dr. Death: The role of storytelling for palliative care in competing medical meaning systems. *Health Communication, 32*(10), 1272–1283. https://doi.org/10.1080/10410236.2016.1219928

*Critiques of the BSM*

The BSM has been critiqued for being too generic and vague. Other models, such as the phenomenological model, which views the patient as an embodied person within a lived context, have sought to address its shortcomings by emphasizing a complete understanding of patients. Yet others have proposed the infomedical model to emphasize the aspects of information to be gathered. However, the BSM at present continues to be the dominant model in making the practice of medicine more scientific.

As an instance of BSM, Robinson and Nussbaum, two communication researchers, look at elder health through the lens of social support and its religious dimension through church attendance. They examine the place of religion in the BSM of medicine and physician-patient communication about religion (for more on religion and health (Robinson & Nussbaum, 2004), see **Chapter 10, Health, Religion, and Spirituality**). Their study attends to the domain between physical and mental health, social support, and aging. They find that religious events, such as weekly mass, prayer groups, and Bible school provide a sense of belonging, fellowship, and cohesiveness that contributes to instrumental and emotional resources (Koenig & Larson, 1998). The authors highlight how physicians are reluctant to initiate inquiries into patients' religious behaviors. Their study presents physician limitations to facilitate and reinforce such behaviors ethically and pragmatically (du Pre, 2002). Textbox 2.7 presents a slightly different perspective by focusing on health competence. How do you feel the notion of health competence can contribute to the BSM in furthering ownership of health?

### The Holistic Model (HM)

The HM considers multidimensional aspects of wellness including the intellectual, social, spiritual, physical, mental, and emotional. It is best exemplified by the 1947 WHO definition: "[A] state of complete physical, mental, and social wellbeing and not merely the absence of disease or infirmity." It is considered a patient-centered model that applies CAM approaches. CAM therapies fall under the description of HM, which means they consider the whole person, including physical, mental, emotional, and spiritual aspects (IOM, 2005). CAM approaches include a broad range of healing philosophies, approaches, and therapies like acupuncture, herbs, homeopathy, therapeutic massage, and TCM.

CAM therapies may be used alone (HM), as an alternative to conventional therapies (CAM model), or in addition to conventional, mainstream therapies (CIM model). In 1984, the WHO proposed a dynamic approach to health that presented it as a process or a force. In 1986, the Ottawa Charter for Health Promotion defined health from the HM perspective as

the extent to which an individual or a group is able to realize aspirations and satisfy needs, and to change or cope with the environment. Health is a resource for everyday life, not the objective of living; it is a positive concept, emphasizing social and personal resources as well as physical capacities.

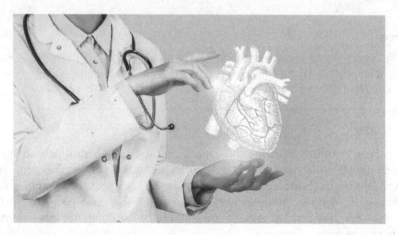

*Figure 2.1* HM Considers the Whole Person.

Other related approaches arising from the holistic and wellness models view health in terms of resiliency, defined as "the capability of individuals, families, groups, and communities to cope successfully in the face of significant adversity or risk" (Vingilis & Sarkella, 1997). A second related approach is the ecological approach, defined as "a state in which humans and other living creatures with which they interact can coexist indefinitely" (Last, 1995). Yet others (e.g., Aboriginal conception of health mentioned at the beginning of the chapter) are even broader and include spiritual dimensions.

*Critiques of the HM*

The practice of medicine is based on a commitment to improve the quality of healthcare alongside a duty of beneficence, i.e., a duty to do good, such as by acting in the best interests of the patients (IOM, 2005). One of the critiques faced by HM is that many of its constructs are hard to measure because of their subjective nature (and thus, may inadvertently do harm). Second, the HM also gives patients more leeway in judging their own health. A third critique is the lack of evidence-based research supporting the application of CAM modalities in healthcare. Structurally, the Federation of State Medical Boards assists the state medical boards in ensuring that licensees utilize CAM in a clinically responsible and ethically appropriate manner within the boundaries of professional practice and accepted standard of care.

Communication researchers Evelyn Ho and Carma Bylund studied acupuncture discourse (as an example of CAM and HM) in an acupuncture clinic that had one licensed acupuncturist and about six interns (Ho & Bylund, 2008). They describe the practitioner-client relationship in the acupuncture-related field site through the lens of holism as a model of health. For instance, the authors highlight how essential Chinese medical theories of *qi*, energetic organs, and *yin* and *yang* are difficult to translate into English and thus, to apply in BM and BSM. Their study participants are amused by the scientific acceptability of FDA-approved drugs despite their many contraindications. For instance, Kate, a participant in their study, notes that a drug for treating nausea that has complications like constipation, diarrhea, low back pain, and stroke is not considered holistic in philosophical terms, as it does not treat the whole person. Although holistic practitioners often employ the paternalistic model in their study, they note that the models of interaction (paternalistic, collaborative) are dynamic and may shift in the patient-provider interaction.

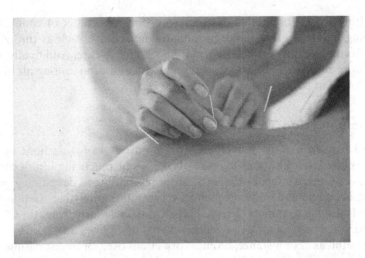

*Figure 2.2* A Patient Undergoing Acupuncture.

### The Integrative Medicine (IM) Model

The IM model (IOM, 2009) states that to be patient-centered, the practice of medicine should include medical training, CAM therapies, and technology. In this way, medicine can treat the complex human being made up of body, mind, emotions, and spirit. IM reaffirms the importance of the relationship between practitioner and patient, focuses on the whole person, is informed by evidence, and makes use of all appropriate therapeutic and lifestyle approaches, healthcare professionals, and disciplines to achieve optimal health and healing (Academic Consortium for Integrative Medicine and Health, 2021). IM practitioners believe that simply treating the body is not good medicine and that having a positive purpose in life is as important an indicator of good health as good BM clinical indicators. IM advocates attending to the social and physical environment as being as important as having, for instance, a low low-density lipoprotein reading (LDL; or "bad" cholesterol; Guarneri, 2007).

IM has several aims that embody its core values in practice and encapsulate its principles. These are described as follows:

The first aim of IM is patient-centeredness, with an emphasis on dialogue and shared control, the ability to give patients the help they want and need, when they want and need it. The second aim of IM is the individualization of care. IM practitioners believe that care should be tailored to each individual, such as through using technological- and genome-related advances. The third aim of IM is to include the patient's family, loved ones, and community in their care. The fourth aim is to maximize healing influences in the healthcare environment through design that reduces patient, family, and staff stress, prevents errors and nosocomial infections (or healthcare-associated infections that are contracted in the process of receiving care), and increases positive influences on health status. Its fifth aim is to maximize healing influences outside the care system, such as supporting provider learning and patient empowerment through healing practices that treat or minimize the impact of illness or disability. Its sixth aim is to rely on evidence-based care, such as recognizing approaches to learning that are less known and validated than experimental designs and randomized trials. Its seventh aim is to use all relevant capacities. For instance, in primary care (PC), exploring all possible avenues of support would include expanding the view of the capacity of all human beings and utilizing insights from the patient's family and community about the person's condition to enhance the provider's knowledge. Its eighth aim underscores the importance of connection, whereby potential helping influences that build on human connections, such as through integrating health navigators and health coaches, information systems in care. And finally, the ninth aim of IM emphasizes an attitude of cooperation and collaboration among all individuals and institutions involved in patient care (IOM, 2009).

## Health Communication Theories and Models

The COVID-19 pandemic took individuals, institutions, and organizations by surprise and resulted in unexpected modifications to established ways of practicing health communication. Health communication is a crucial social process for responding to devastating pandemics that demand timely, accurate, and culturally sensitive communication that meaningfully informs coordinated and effective responses (Kreps, 2021). On the scholarly front, the COVID-19 pandemic increased collaboration among scientists across disciplines and borders to help find a solution to the outbreak. For instance, prompt corrections over journalist misinterpretations of supposed pangolin origins to the SARS-CoV-2 outbreak were invaluable in facilitating counter-narratives from the scientific community. This was seen during instances of controversial scientific communication, such as in interpreting public health policies and their alignment with "herd immunity" during the early days of the pandemic (Pollett & Rivers, 2020). On the programmatic front, Kreps employed the systems principle of requisite variety and community-based sensemaking from Weick's model of organizing to develop strategic communication responses to pandemics. He points out that pandemics demand novel responsive programs and policies that emphasize sharing of relevant health information, promoting sensemaking, and encouraging coordination that can empower effective responses by enhancing understanding of health threats, enabling development of evidence-based strategies for responding to threats, and providing guidance for averting and addressing future pandemics.

*Review **Textbox 2.4**. Consider crafting a definition of health communication that addresses the principles of WPHC SJA to meet the evolving health challenges for the next decade, keeping in mind the challenges and opportunities offered by artificial intelligence (AI).*

---

**Textbox 2.4   Selected Definitions of Health Communication Through the Decades**

- Gary Kreps and Barbara Thornton (1992):
  Health communication is concerned with the way we seek, process, and share health information.

- Ratzan et al. (1994):
  The art and technique of informing, influencing, and motivating individuals, institutional, and public audiences about important health issues. Its scope includes disease prevention, health promotion, healthcare policy, and business, as well as enhancement of the quality of life and health of individuals within the community (p. 362).

- Rogers (1995):
  Health communication is any type of human communication whose content is concerned with health.

- CDC (2021), the National Cancer Institute, and the US Department of Health and Human Services:

The study and use of communication strategies to inform and influence individual and community decisions that enhance health.

- IOM Report (2003):
An ecological model assumes that health and well-being are affected by interaction among determinants, including biology, behavior, and the environment. Interaction unfolds over the life course of individuals, families, and communities, and evidence is emerging that societal-level factors are critical to understanding and improving the health of the public.

- Thompson, T.L. (2000):
Health communication coalesces around identifying the boundaries and scope of a condition, person, profession, or situation associated with health or healthcare, giving meaning to health status by "naming and defining its cause" (Thompson, 2000, p. 3).

## SJA Prompt

Historically, the content of health information that has been communicated to different audiences has evolved from the description of communicable diseases during Hippocrates' time in the 4th century BC to descriptions of scurvy among sailors by James Lind in the 18th century, and Margaret Sanger, who advocated for public education on birth control and safe sex in the early twentieth century.

As we move to the post-COVID-19 pandemic experience and other challenges that have defined the twenty-first century:

1. How would you revise the definition of health communication?
   a. What elements would it include that may be missing in present definitions?
   b. What understandings of WPHC would you emphasize?
2. How will you ensure your definition of health communication is socially just?
   a. How will its objectives be inclusive?
   b. How might they support the goals of health ownership and access to information, and create conditions for empowerment?
3. What steps might you advocate for health communication to emphasize the need for alertness to health misinformation in the age of communication dominated by content that is communicated through digital platforms and increasingly produced by AI?

## Resources

CDC. (2021, December 9). *Health communication gateway*. https://www.cdc.gov/healthcommunication/index.html

IOM (US) Committee on Educating Public Health Professionals for the 21st Century. (2003). In K. Gebbie, L. Rosenstock, & L. M. Hernandez (Eds.). *Who will keep the public healthy? Educating public health professionals for the 21st century*. National Academies Press. https://www.ncbi.nlm.nih.gov/books/NBK221192/

Kreps, G. L., & Thornton, B. C. (1992). *Health communication theory & practice*. Waveland Press.

Ratzan, S. C., Stearns, N. S., Payne, J. G., Amato, P. P., Liebergott, J. W., & Madoff, M. A. (1994). Education for the health communication professional: A collaborative curricular partnership. *American Behavioral Scientist*, *38*(2), 361–380. https://doi.org/10.1177/0002764294038002015

Rogers, E. M. (1995). *Diffusion of innovations* (4th ed.). Free Press.

Thompson, T. L. (2000). The nature and language of illness explanations. In B. B. Whaley (Ed.), *Explaining illness: Research, theory, and strategies* (pp. 3–40). Lawrence Erlbaum Associates.

## An Overview of Health Communication

Health communication lies at the intersection of the two disciplines of health and communication. As health communication scholar and expert Gary Kreps noted many decades ago, "health communication is by definition an interdisciplinary area of inquiry, bridging social science, humanities, health professional, and health science knowledge" (1989, p. 12). The interdisciplinary nature of health communication is amply illustrated in this textbook's framework of WPHC. Recent work in health communication by researchers Hoffmann-Longtin and colleagues reiterates how the scholarship in the field of health communication reflects the field's interdisciplinary breadth, spanning contributions from the fields of communication, nursing, medicine, pharmacy, public health, and social work (2022). In her work centering the role of communication in health, Roxanne Parrott emphasizes the knowledge that arises from understanding the "informal and less intentional communication processes related to health" (2004, p. 751) emphasizing how communication behavior is central to achieving health outcomes.

### Domains of Health Communication

Health communication covers a range of topics such as disease control and prevention, emergency preparedness and response, injury and violence prevention, environmental health, and workplace safety and health (Parrott, 2011). At the national level, it emphasizes a developmental life-span perspective by focusing on domains such as adolescent health, elderly health, women's health, minority health, and reproductive health (Parrott, 2004). Such a diversity of perspectives and foci has often led to calls for systematization of the field and its different branches of study (Freimuth, 2012; Kreps et al., 2010; Ratzan et al., 1996). One of its primary foci is to understand how messages relating to health processes and healthcare delivery are created, sent, and received. These contexts situate the patient experience, patient-provider communication, healthcare teams, provider perspectives, caregiver and social support challenges, media effects, new technologies, campaigns, health and sociocultural factors in the examination of risky health behaviors, mental health and illness, ethical issues, and crisis communication. Contemporary health challenges have highlighted the multifaceted nature of the field of health communication (Hannawa et al., 2014). Health communication scholarship attends to issues of health equity, policy communication, public advocacy, cultural competence, and health literacy. In all these myriad and diverse aspects, health communication is challenged to account for the interdependence of the individual, social, and political factors related to health conditions in both advancing knowledge and designing implementations and interventions that make a measurable difference to health outcomes.

### Theories of Health Communication

#### Theories of Behavior Change

At the individual level, behavior prediction theories have been recognized in the development of behavior change interventions in providing a framework to help identify the individual determinants of behaviors and thereby develop successful interventions to change that behavior (Fishbein & Cappella, 2006). Theories of behavior prediction include the Theory of Planned Behavior (Ajzen, 1991; Ajzen & Madden, 1986), Theory of Subjective Culture and

Interpersonal Relations (Triandis, 1972), Transtheoretical Model of Behavioral Change (Prochaska & DiClemente, 1986), the Information/Motivation/Behavioral-Skills Model (Fisher & Fisher, 1992), Health Belief Model (Becker, 1974), Social Cognitive Theory (Bandura, 1986, 1997, 1994), Diffusion of Innovation (Rogers, 1983), and Theory of Reasoned Action (Ajzen & Fishbein, 1980).

Focusing on the determinants of intention, along with environmental factors, and skills and abilities, Fishbein (2000) proposed an integrative model of behavior. In this model, intention is predicted by determining the degree to which that intention (or behavior) is under attitudinal, normative, or self-efficacy control in the population. Overall, behavior change models emphasize the role of intention to perform the behavior, the skills and abilities required to perform the behavior, and the environmental context as it supports or prevents behavioral performance. Intention is determined by psychosocial variables like the attitude toward performing the behavior, the perceived social norms concerning performance of the behavior, and the self-efficacy with respect to performing the behavior. All these variables determining intention, in turn, depend upon the behavioral target and the population being considered (Fishbein & Cappella, 2006).

### Theories of Media Effects

Health communication professionals develop skills that facilitate at local, national, and global levels the goals of selling research, working with policymakers, persuading the public, and training healthcare providers and consumers (Hannawa et al., 2014). Health communication theories that guide approaches to prevention and care draw upon social psychological theories and models of behavior that are often individually focused (Airhihenbuwa & Obregon, 2000). They approach health prevention and promotion behaviors from an individual, linear, and rational perspective. Recent scholars have argued for centering culture in the planning, implementation, and evaluation of health communication and health promotion programs (Airhihenbuwa, 1995; Dutta-Bergman, 2005). Theories of media effects have been applied to communication campaigns for behavior change (Slater, 1999). These theories include agenda setting and multistep flow, theories of persuasion, such as the elaboration likelihood model (ELM) and protection motivation theory (PMT). These theories provide the health communication practitioner with a systematic way to segment audiences, select objectives, design campaign strategies, and design messages (Maibach & Cotton, 1995).

With social media, there is a proliferation of massive amounts of highly individualized information and the potential for health misinformation. Rains (2020) looks at big data and computational social science (CSS) techniques for examining public perceptions of health conditions or events, investigating network-related dimensions of health phenomena, and illness monitoring. Ruben (2016) examined the challenge of improving provider-patient communication specifically and health outcomes generally. Translation of theory into practice involves considering the complex and nuanced nature of the communication process that is not captured by the information-exchange perspectives. The translation challenge is made more challenging by the many channels of communication, changing healthcare and wellness landscape, and newer sources of health information services, sources, and settings.

Singelis et al. (2018) look at addressing the challenge of eliminating racial/ethnic health disparities by enhancing the cultural sensitivity (CS) of interventions to improve their effectiveness in diverse groups (IOM, 2003). The past two decades have seen an emphasis on the cultural component in communications, services, and interventions aimed at racial, ethnic, and cultural groups (e.g., Barrera et al., 2013; Healey et al., 2017; Nierkens et al., 2013). CS is defined as the

> extent to which ethnic/cultural characteristics, experiences, norms, values, behavioral patterns, and beliefs of the target population as well as relevant historical, environmental, and social forces are incorporated in the design, delivery, and evaluation of targeted health promotion materials and programs.

(Resnicow et al., 1999, p. 11)

Singelis et al. (2018) use the ELM (Petty & Cacioppo, 1986) to examine the surface structure and deep structure in the recall of oral health information from pamphlets varied in written messages and images. In their experimental study, they assigned Spanish-speaking, Mexican-heritage mothers of children under 6 to read pamphlets containing the same oral health information in Spanish. They define deep structure as found within the meaning of a message and the way it is presented and concerns the cultural, social, historical, environmental, and psychological factors related to a group's health behaviors. The deep structure of a CS message incorporates the values of a group targeted and offers explanations of events and consequences that are consistent with explanations commonly expressed and accepted in the targeted culture.

## Critical, Cultural, and Narrative Approaches to Health

### Critical Approaches

As health communication theory has matured in recent decades, it has aided in a deeper understanding of the complex ways in which communication shapes and is shaped by health contexts. Interpretive and critical perspectives have been employed in international, multi-methodological, cross-cultural research in communication contexts ranging from intra- and interpersonal, small group, organizational, and mass-mediated (Zoller & Kline, 2008). Such perspectives have broadened what health means and emphasized it from a contextual perspective.

*Review **Table 2.1**. Consider the information provided to illustrate how WPHC SJA principles could be applied to the contexts, careers, and resources that would be needed to address the contemporary challenges faced by health communication professionals.*

*Table 2.1* Settings of Health Communication Study and Practice

| Organization /Institution | Settings | Contexts | Careers |
| --- | --- | --- | --- |
| Academia | • Health communication programs housed in university-based departments of Communication | • Interpersonal communication<br>• Mass communication | • Researchers<br>• Academic professionals<br>• Educators<br>• Health counselors |

*(Continued)*

*Table 2.1* (Continued) Settings of Health Communication Study and Practice

| Organization /Institution | Settings | Contexts | Careers |
|---|---|---|---|
| Government | • CDC<br>• US Department of Department of Health and Human Services<br>• Federal government<br>• State/local government<br>• Agency of Healthcare Research and Quality | • Social marketing campaigns<br>• Audience segmentation<br>• Behavior change programs<br>• Policy development<br>• Crisis communication<br>• Risk communication | • Public health<br>• Ethics |
| Nonprofit organizations | • Social advocacy organizations<br>• Project Hope<br>• Joint Commission<br>• National Committee for Quality Assurance | • Message strategy<br>• Finance and business skills<br>• Accreditation and certification of healthcare organization and program quality and performance<br>• Client management | • Marketing<br>• Public relations<br>• E-health and new technologies |
| Private health organizations | • Center for Reproductive Rights<br>• National Association of Community Health Centers | • Web design<br>• Media relations<br>• Patient communication<br>• Presentation skills<br>• Writing skills<br>• Campaign planning<br>• Resource planning<br>• Tracking policy and clinical issues | • Marketing<br>• Public relations<br>• Advertising<br>• Campaign evaluation<br>• Health systems approaches<br>• Global health communication |
| International Organizations | • WHO<br>• WHO COVID-19 Pandemic Information Center<br>• Oxfam International | Medical care with goals ranging from:<br>• Promoting wellness<br>• Delivering medicines and supplies<br>• Health expertise and medical training during disasters<br>• Prevention of disease, saving lives around the globe<br>• Abolishment of poverty | • Social advocacy<br>• Research<br>• Global health communication |

## SJA Prompt

Table 2.1 provides the organizational and institutional settings and contexts of health communication education, careers, and practice. Consider what contexts, careers, and resources would be needed to address the contemporary challenges to the following:

1. Clinical determinants of health disparities (e.g., medical bias) through awareness of SDoH disparities
2. Creating a culture of equity across all domains of the healthcare system
3. Integrating health and health equity across community partners
4. Advancing social inclusion to reduce health disparities for diverse populations

Center recognition for systemic oppression at individual, group, cultural, and systems levels borne by specific populations as expressed in a disproportionate burden of disease, mortality, and morbidity.

*Principles of Critical Approaches*

Critical approaches are defined by opposition to established perspectives and especially social-scientific methodology, along with a refusal to legitimize the status quo. Critical theoretical approaches aim to

(a) change society according to ideas of enlightenment; (b) construct an opposition to the (mainly quantitative) research traditions influenced by "critical rationalism," (Popper, 1959); (c) [e]xpose the social status quo and thereby change society; and, (d) [further] an understanding of mass communication that distinguishes between harmful media that are instruments of suppression and beneficial media that promote ideas of enlightenment.

(Löblich & Scheu, 2011, p. 12)

For instance, Thompson and Duerringer (2020) employed a critical approach to study uncertainty for family members coping with contested illness in their relationships. They historicize cultural discourse implicated in individuals' contestations of family members' health complaints and find four central themes reflecting the Enlightenment Subject—you are not being rational; you are not trying; your symptoms do not make sense; you are not being yourself. Through this study, they hope to connect micro-processes to macrolevel discourses for people and their family members sharing similar experiences.

Critical theorists are interested in examining how the use of language and discourse sustains or perpetuates health inequities. Critical theorists focus on how language serves to promote interests while minimizing or excluding others. Critical health communication theory is concerned with challenging the factors that contribute to health disparities. As Lupton (1996) notes, critical theorists will ask, Whose values, beliefs, and concepts are being espoused, and whose are being neglected? Whose interest is the discourse serving at whose expense? What assumptions and pre-established knowledge or belief systems are being employed in meaning-making processes? How do forms of discourse create or perpetuate forms of social hierarchies?

Critical approaches contest the top-down approach toward knowledge dissemination from experts (e.g., those with medical or professional health knowledge) and their perceived role as disseminating the presumed knowledge to the masses, considered as ignorant and unreflective, for their good. Thus, its methods of persuasion, behavior change, and how to reach uniform, unmotivated populations represent a one-way model of communication. Critical scholars eschew the emphasis on campaign planning, cost-effectiveness, and evaluation of measurable effects to emphasize the ethical and political implications of such communication and its cultural implications (Lupton, 1996). Critical theorists also take a more nuanced view of culture as more than just lifestyle choices. Thus, critical approaches are inherently political in their inquiry and focus on the economic and historical factors shaping the language around health, disease, and treatment.

## Critical Cultural Approaches

*Emphases of Critical Cultural Approaches*

Critical cultural approaches in health emphasize the sociological, philosophical, historical, and feminist theories of the body, the practice of medicine, and the medical encounter.

Critical cultural approaches will emphasize how culture shapes understandings of health, illness, body, disease, and health communication contexts. It emphasizes experiences and context in meaning making and interpretation based on cultural and historical contexts (e.g., Ho & Bylund, 2008). For instance, Professor Mohan Dutta's CCA seeks structural transformations by positing alternative economic and political structures with the goal of achieving social change (Dutta, 2020). The CCA model imagines change through centering ownership in the empowered contributions of activists and communities at the margins of society.

### Discourse in Critical Cultural Health Communication

Discourse is described as "a pattern of words, figures of speech, concepts, values, and symbols that is organized around a particular object or issue and that can be located in wider historical, political, and social processes and practices" (Lupton, 1996, p. 61). Discourse is examined in macro-settings (e.g., bio-power) and interpersonal settings (e.g., agency). Feminist scholars will focus on the ways in which discourses enact control over the female body by opening and closing possibilities for agency. Dutta and de Souza (2008) challenge development initiatives that create essentialized categories homogenizing minority and marginalized cultures and pushing Western solutions in local cultures (Dutta-Bergman, 2004). The focus on agency and empowerment in critical cultural approaches is concerned with how the power balance and knowledge symmetry can be shifted to create an equitable relationship. Shamshad Khan's (2020) study on HIV interventions examines HIV/AIDS-related stigma and its power and structure implications.

As another example, Workman examines a fraternity's cultural practices of binge drinking as performance discourse in the form of drinking stories. Workman argues that the representations of drinking behaviors in their narratives "establish a set of meaningful practices for members of the culture" (2001, p. 429). He starts by laying out how drunken behaviors are learned socially and unconsciously (Bourdieu, 1990) and how gradually their meanings become concretized for a group as social practices. For example, he finds how adventure stories frame the behavior as risky to "make the situation more interesting, the danger more dramatic, or the behavior more outlandish" (p. 432). In an example of the pride in the telling of the stupid story that frames drunkenness as a form of recreational play, a member of the fraternity passed out and others drew a cat on his face, with whiskers

> and everything. And he woke up and he went back, started partying again, and he had no idea what happened to him…and everyone just laughed at him, because he thinks he's all cool, [and] the center of attention, but he's got that stuff drawn all over his face.
>
> (p. 434)

Workman's study emphasizes the need for "continued exploration of the culture using the language and construction of meaning by the culture itself" (p. 442).

### Social Constructionist Approach

The social constructionist approach to medicine has questioned assumptions guiding the biomedical push to improve doctors' and patients' communication competencies. Instead, the focus is on how the doctor employs symbolic and political power to wield control over knowledge and position the patient as seeking help and allowing access to their body. Professor Kenneth Gergen, an American social psychologist, has written and thought about the tenets of social constructionism in social, organizational, and personal contexts before turning his attention to its contributions to healthcare contexts.

*See Dr. Kenneth Gergen's interview in **Textbox 2.5** on the social constructionist approach. What avenues do you think this approach offers in making experiences and context more impactful and transformative?*

---

### TEXTBOX 2.5  Scholar Interview

### Dr. Kenneth Gergen
*Swarthmore College*

Q1. Your work foregrounds the relationship and the relational process as co-action. How does the relational perspective illuminate how we make meaning of health and disease?

A social constructionist approach calls attention to the ways in which health and illness are defined, who is making these definitions, how they are applied, and the cultural, political, and economic outcomes. The case of homosexuality is a classic example. In the United States, homosexual acts were long declared both illegal and symptoms of mental illness. Electroshock was one means of "curing the disease."

Q2. How would you describe the whole person approach to healthcare from the perspective of your work?

Constructionists pose critical questions of whose justice, whose diagnosis, and whose voices are excluded from this conversation? Constructionists also point to ways in which these meanings are generated within groups of people who may themselves feel justified. This is to recognize that there are multiple realities at play within a society and beyond. Inquiry is thus opened into optimal means of crossing boundaries of meaning and value, reforming realities, and opening new avenues toward reform.

Q3. Could you provide an example of how a social constructionist and humanistic approach can be designed and implemented to promote the goals of socially just, whole person healthcare?

While recognizing the significance of direct confrontation, constructionists work to develop less polarizing and more unifying forms of moving together. Constructionist efforts are especially prominent in the case of mental health and physical disablement. In the latter case, the concept of neurodiversity has been an especially powerful rhetorical tool.

Q4. Could you provide how the relational, whole person approach can help?

Constructionist inquiry also extends to the medical professions where concerns are directed, for example, toward biases in diagnosis and to ways in which patients' voices can be more fully honored in medical treatment.

## Narrative Theory

### Human Experiences and the Narrative Approach

Stories draw upon language and gestures and symbolism and storytelling to communicate human experiences and shape meaning making (Charon, 2006). Narrative theorists examine grand narratives of societies (e.g., what it means to have a "real job," Clair, 1996) and tease out relations of knowledge and power (Claire et al., 2014). Narrative scholars draw upon the idea of narration as the foundation of human communication understanding humans as a storytelling animal who uses symbols and narration as a metaphor for communicating human existence (Fisher, 1984). According to Fisher, the criteria of narrative coherence (how well the story "hangs together" by being free of contradictions) and narrative fidelity (how well the story "rings true" with listener experiences) offer the potential for understanding and assessing the rhetorical effectiveness of a story. Everyday stories exemplifying lived narratives and the intersectionality of marginalization (Allen, 1996) highlight the uniqueness of individual experiences. Allen, for instance, draws upon standpoint theory to describe her experience of being socialized into academia as a Black woman. Ellingson and Buzzanell (1999) listen to women's narratives of breast cancer treatment to cultivate a complex view of women's communication satisfaction with their physicians.

*Review* **Textbox 2.6**. *Apply the entertainment-education approach to the WPHC SJA prompts that follow.*

---

### Textbox 2.6   Entertainment-Education and Social Network Storytelling

#### WPHC Context

In entertainment-education (EE) approaches, characters in popular media moved from undesirable to desirable behaviors. Entertainment messages contain persuasive messaging that is effective through similarity with characters such as by creating involvement with a focus on the story, such as by identification or parasocial interaction, the phenomenon of becoming emotionally connected to characters. Amy Riley and colleagues applied an EE approach to present three cases of EE responses to the COVID-19 pandemic from leading global organizations, PCI Media, BBC Media Action, and Sesame Workshop. The EE theory utilized a planned behavior change approach and prosocial messaging to provide an evidence-based communication approach employing entertainment media for educational messaging. It is based on "the intentional placement of educational content in entertainment messages" (Singhal & Rogers, 2002, p. 117).

For instance, in transportation, audiences would become engrossed in the story world and temporarily detached from their present environment while experiencing the message. Narrative engagement, another EE construct, linked transportation with narrative comprehension theory, stating the media consumers are more involved when the story world has coherence. Sesame Workshop repurposed old content of handwashing to allow for low-cost distribution. Sésamo adapted its direct engagement by transitioning from in-person interventions to engaging with teachers and caregivers via WhatsApp.

For PCI Media, for example, tailoring messages meant working with partners to create content and call-in shows in local languages with local production teams. Others used a riddle approach to generate local solutions and allowed audiences to become active participants.

Some of the responses global EE campaigns advocated to address new challenges such as lockdowns and social distancing comprised three takeaways for EE as a health communication strategy:

**Takeaway #1**: Future EE programs for pandemic response may be well served by starting with existing infrastructure to quickly build capacity, support, and trust.

**Takeaway #2**: EE practitioners may wish to work with partners to tailor pandemic response programs to the local context.

**Takeaway #3**: EE should continue to focus on good storytelling while simultaneously considering evolving media formats and theoretical implications.

## SJA Discussion Prompt

EE leverages the appeal of popular media to educate and motivate viewers to improve their health, safety, or equality using popular media such as radio, television, and internet serials that allow viewers to engage with the content over a certain duration.

1. Can you think of ways an EE approach has been utilized over a social network such as Tik Tok, YouTube, or Instagram to build identification with health challenges that disproportionately affect minority audiences?
2. What are the strengths of such an approach in building identification? How can such identification be transformative and not perpetuate preexisting views and beliefs, such as by serving as an echo chamber?
3. How can EE approaches challenge established norms from the bottom-up?
4. How can digital storytelling tools co-opt traditional biases and create and circulate transformative narratives to bring about meaningful social and behavioral change?

## Resource

Singhal, A., & Rogers, E. M. (2002). A theoretical agenda for entertainment-education. *Communication Theory*, *12*(2), 117–135. https://doi.org/10.1111/j.1468-2885.2002.tb00262.x

Health communication researchers have employed narrative theory to understand topics such as physician-patient communication (Sharf, 1990). Sharf examines the rhetorical derivation of the word "compliant" to critique its assumption of clinician authority and suggest how physician-patient communication can be conceptualized as collaborative with active patient engagement. She employs Fisher's proposition of an overarching narrative philosophy to describe how patients most often recount their stories by providing a history of their experiences. Margaret Quinlan et al. (2020) conducted a study at the University of North Carolina (UNC) hospitals. They brought performing artists from a healing arts program called DooR-to-DooR (D2D) to hospital settings ranging from in-patient oncology wards, waiting rooms, and burn units. They employed a narrative theoretical approach to trace the historical development of contemporary hospital systems in the United States, the narrative and aesthetic potential of healthcare, and to situate art programming as disrupting the soundscape of UNC hospitals. They found the arts group's music performances helped distract patients from their troubling experiences and supported self-expression and storytelling among participants.

### Relational Health Communication Model

Many researchers have employed narrative approaches to understand health communication in different contexts. Query and Wright (2003) test Kreps's (1988) relational health communication model by examining the relationship between social support, communication competence, and perceived stress in a study of well-elders, elderly individuals with cancer, and lay caregivers by collecting participant narratives focusing on positive and negative expressions of social support. Kerr et al. (2020) explore identity negotiation and passing through the application of the skills of narrative medicine in the classroom. In doing so, they promote a narrative approach incorporating empathy in the medical curriculum to train future physicians in addressing social injustices and improving their patient relationships. Bute and Jensen (2011) interviewed 30 low-income women about their perception of formal sex-education experiences and how they related those experiences to their sexual health knowledge, beliefs, and behaviors. The researchers identify narratives of regret, narratives of satisfaction, and narratives of uncertainty and find that younger women were more likely to tell narratives of uncertainty than older women. Narrative inquiry has been used to examine photo-stories in doctor-patient communication with older adults who have limited health literacy by incorporating social learning theory and covering communication themes (Kroops van't Jagt et al., 2016). The researchers employed one-page photo-stories, narrated video clips using the original photo-story pictures, and interactive video clips covering participation and communication during PC consultations.

### Strengths of the Narrative Approach

Narrative approaches have in general been embraced as empowering and praised for their ability to incorporate nuance and person-centered perspectives in understanding complex contexts. For instance, in applying a narrative paradigm (Fisher, 1987) to Kreps's relational communication model, Query and Wright state that the complex and interwoven nature of relations among communication, social support, and health outcomes in a range of contexts warrants the employment of a narrative approach.

### Critique of the Narrative Approach

However, there are aspects that health communication practitioners need to be cautious about in employing narrative approaches. Narrative approaches have been applied to problematize therapeutic assumptions about narratives in post-conflict contexts (Cole, 2010). Cole argued the ways that narratives can also resist and undermine healing, reconciliation, and resilience. She suggests that the power of narratives to harm should also be acknowledged, particularly in post-conflict institutions such that those whose voices articulate subjugation, vulnerability, and judgment of public sharing of narratives are not silenced.

## Rhetorical and Humanistic Approaches to Health and Medicine

### Rhetoric of Health and Medicine (RHM)

The study of rhetoric in health is a new subfield in health communication. Researchers in this field focus on different health publics, their discursive practices, and the study of health, well-being, and medicine as a persuasive discourse (Scott et al., 2013; Segal, 2005). Scholars in RHM study health texts, artifacts, and practices to understand, as Jensen (2015) put it, "[T]he processes through which health-related ideas, assumptions, and arguments have been communicated by and in relationship with the technical sphere, public or mainstream audiences, counter-publics, and vernacular or lay constituencies" (p. 523). Practitioners in the field of RHM seek to improve the practice of medicine and positively impact health and well-being (Angeli, 2015; Arduser, 2017; Bernhardt, 2003; Hannah & Arduser, 2018). The goal of RHM researchers is to cultivate a deep understanding of what medicine is and to make it more humane. Efforts such as writing and medicine, neurorhetorics, and communication help us understand different facets of medical practice (Meloncon & Frost, 2015). Examples of the RHM approach include Katie Walkup and Peter Cannon's 2018 study of women's alcohol-and-other-drug treatment facilities findings that their health resembled a network of factors, including demographics, health experiences, and their own health literacy (Walkup & Cannon, 2018).

### Medical Humanities

Medical and health humanities are closely related to RHM. The goal of medical humanities is to inject humanism into the scientific practice and discourse of medicine in domains ranging from physician education, clinical encounters, treatment and diagnosis protocols, and medical discourse on patient compliance and adherence (Cole et al., 2014). According to the National Library of Medicine (2004), the medical humanities emphasize the "humane aspects of medicine and healthcare and [have] expanded to include research in social sciences disciplines that are informed by humanistic scholarship, such as cultural studies, anthropology, and medical sociology" [Institute of Medicine (US) Committee on Health Literacy; Nielsen-Bohlman et al., 2004]. The field of medical humanities draws upon institutional funding from schools of medicine and focuses on how medical training can improve health outcomes by integrating observation, empathy, and patient-provider communication. Medical humanists will draw upon literature, creative writing, history, and philosophy to challenge prevalent medical practices. For instance, disability studies scholars will draw upon the methods of advocacy and employ activism to change policies and environments, and argue for a shift in how medicine is practiced and conceptualized (Meloncon, 2013).

### Health Humanities

Distinct from, but related to, medical humanities, the field of health humanities (HH) has been defined as "the study of the intersection of health and humanistic disciplines (such as philosophy, religion, literature) fine arts, as well as social science research that gives insight into the human condition (such as history, anthropology, sociology, and cultural studies)"

(Health Humanities Consortium, 2021). To achieve its goals, HH scholars use methods such as "reflection, contextualization, deep textual reading, and slow critical thinking to examine the human condition, the patient's experience, the healer's experience, and to provide renewal for the healthcare professional" (Health Humanities Consortium, 2021).

HH includes health and wellness and is considered a more inclusive term. It was used by the Hiram Report (Berry et al., 2016) and scholars use the term to include the medical humanities, arts, and social sciences (Bleakley, 2015; Dolan, 2015). HH aims to help students develop a "critical understanding of social and cultural contexts, interpersonal skills, skillful communication, patient-centered attitudes, and enhanced ability to relate to others" (Gouge, 2018, p. 22; see also Mol, 2003). HH refers to both the medical humanities and the arts and social sciences to study their contributions to health and medicine (Dolan, 2015). As the Hiram Report states, students studying HH focus on health and healthcare delivery by paying attention to the social and cultural contexts of patient-centered care, ethics, and care of diverse populations by attending to relationships and reflective approaches. Improved communication is a fundamental skill that enhances integrated learning and the development of domain knowledge.

### RHM Orientation

Scholars in the field of RHM are application oriented, researching "current communication practices, and identifying best practices among healthcare providers" (Angeli & Johnson-Sheehan, 2018, p. 2). Both fields of RHM and HH, the authors note, share an interest in rhetoric and examine "narrative, metaphor, invention, identity, genre, collaboration, style, memory, rhetorical analysis, negotiation, and collaboration" (Angeli & Johnson-Sheehan, 2018, p. 2). Researchers Miriam and Andrew Mara (2018) sought to learn how Kenyan medical practitioners characterize their relationship between cancer and gender by probing how cancer is depicted artistically and perceived publicly in Kenya. In this way, they create a dialogue between Kenyan women and men who have cancer fictional narratives and the medical documents that document Kenyan cancer incidence (Mara & Mara, 2018). Their study explored medical practitioner attitudes toward patient experiences, cancer incidence, disease etiologies, and interventions.

Overall, by employing humanistic methods in the inquiry into health and the practice of medicine, the field of medical and HH aims to transform healthcare through deepening human connections, enhancing the capacity for empathy, and illuminating the cultural and social contexts in which health, illness, and care occur. As the alliances and intersections between these related fields develop, the burgeoning field of digital humanities offers promising new directions for including the role of social networks and technology in the understanding of health and well-being. **Chapter 9**, Technology and Health, provides a deeper look at the intersection of technology, the digital landscape, and health-related meaning making.

In conclusion, **Chapter 2, A Social Constructionist Approach to Health**, has explored the traditional and evolving theoretical frameworks defining the interdisciplinary and multifaceted field of health communication. It has provided an overview of the salient theoretical perspectives comprising the different historical traditions and traced their evolution to address present-day challenges and helping chart future directions.

*Textbox 2.7* provides a WPHC thought prompt on health competence and an SJA-applied exercise. Consider how you would apply this approach to applied community-based settings and to address health beliefs, stigma, health competency, and self-efficacy.

**Textbox 2.7   Present Challenges and Future Directions Exercise**

**Cultivating Health Competence**

*WPHC Context: Health Competencies Present Challenges and Call for Future Action*

Health communication scholars have argued for a collective responsibility view of health. For instance, Ratzan argues that we should all live in a health-competent society that values the individual so that the individual can make appropriate health decisions, that privileges communities so that we have policies that support health delivery and healthy behaviors, and that prioritizes a society that promotes innovation along with appropriate health resources, workforce, and infrastructure facilities that enable us to enact the fundamental values of supporting health. Ratzan reviews health competence as:

a. A framework for a balanced and comprehensive approach to health reform and development assistance
b. A change that implores people individually to change by behaviors, such as addressing obesity and preventive healthcare practices, as well as helps them make appropriate health decisions by building healthy, participatory communities and effective healthcare delivery systems, supported by good health policy

According to Ratzan, there are three principal domains of health competence: (a) the individual among communities, emphasizing connections between all sectors of the community; (b) the system of health, emphasizing connections between healthcare providers and patients, and systems and personnel; and (c) sociopolitical environment, emphasizing advocacy toward media or opinion leaders such as legislators to address public health challenges, advocate for quality, innovation, or to address complex and challenging issues.

*SJA Discussion Prompt*

1. What are some of the challenges that arise from health beliefs and attitudes, stigma, or self-efficacy in an area of chronic disease prevention, immunization, or prevention of infectious diseases?
2. Can you design a health program that focuses on health competence by strengthening partnerships among healthcare services and individual behaviors in the realm of maternal health in resource-poor communities?
   a. What components would such a program have?
   b. What kinds of effects do you envisage such a development of health competencies will lead to?

**Resource**

Ratzan, S. C. (2009). Health competent societies: Our challenge and future. *Journal of Health Communication, 14*(2), 99–101. https://doi.org/10.1080/10810730902791004

# References

Academic Consortium of Integrative Medicine and Health. (2021). *Introduction*. https://imconsortium. org/about/introduction/

Airhihenbuwa, C. (1995). *Health and culture: Beyond the Western paradigm*. SAGE Publications.

Airhihenbuwa, C., & Obregon, R. (2000). A critical assessment of theories/models used in health communication for HIV/AIDS. *Journal of Health Communication, 5*(Suppl), 5–15. https://doi.org/10.1080/10810730050019528

Ajzen, I. (1991). The theory of planned behavior. *Organizational Behavior & Human Decision Processes, 50*(2), 179–211.

Ajzen, I., & Fishbein, M. (1980). *Understanding attitudes and predicting social behavior*. Prentice-Hall.

Ajzen, I., & Madden, T. J. (1986). Prediction of goal-directed behavior: Attitudes, intentions, and perceived behavioral control. *Journal of Experimental Social Psychology, 22*, 453–474.

Allen, B. J. (1996). Feminist standpoint theory: A black woman's (re)view of organizational socialization. *Communication Studies, 47*(4), 257–271.

Angeli, E. L. (2015). Three types of memory in emergency medical services communication. *Written Communication, 32*(1), 3–38. https://doi.org/10.1177/0741088314556598

Angeli, E. L., & Johnson-Sheehan, R. (2018). Introduction to the special issue: Medical humanities and the rhetoric of health and medicine. *Technical Communication Quarterly, 27*(1), 1–6.

Arduser, L. (2017). *Living chronic: Agency and expertise in the rhetoric of diabetes*. Ohio State University Press.

Bandura, A. (1986). *Social foundations of thought and action: A social cognitive theory*. Prentice-Hall

Bandura, A. (1994). Social cognitive theory and exercise of control over HIV infection. In R. J. DiClemente & J. L. Peterson (Eds.), *Preventing AIDS: Theories and methods of behavioral interventions* (pp. 25–29). Plenum Press.

Bandura, A. (1997). *Self-efficacy: The exercise of control*. Freeman.

Barrera, M. Jr., Castro, F.G., Strycker, L.A., & Tolbert, D.J. (2013). Cultural adaptations of behavioral health interventions: A progress report. *Journal of Consulting and Clinical Psychology, 81*(2), 196–205. https://doi.org/10.1037/a0027085

Becker, M. H. (1974). The health belief model and personal health behavior. *Health Education Monographs, 2*, 324–508.

Bernhardt, S. A. (2003). Improving document review practices in pharmaceutical companies. *Journal of Business and Technical Communication, 17*(4), 439–473. https://doi.org/10.1177/1050651903255345

Berry, S., Lamb, E. G., & Jones, T. (2016). *Health humanities baccalaureate programs in the United States. Center for Literature and Medicine, Hiram College*. https://www.hiram.edu/

Bleakley, A. (2015). *Medical humanities and medical education*. Routledge.

Bourdieu, P. (1990). *The logic of practice*. Stanford, CA: Stanford University Press.

Bute, J. J., & Jensen, R. E. (2011). Narrative sensemaking and time lapse: Interviews with low income women about sex education. *Communication Monographs, 78*(2), 212–232. https://doi.org/10.1080/03637751.2011.564639

Center of Research Excellence in Ear and Hearing Health of Aboriginal and Torres Strait Islander Children. (2021). *What is otitis media?* https://www.earandhearinghealth.org.au/what_is_otitis_media

Charon, R. (2006). *Narrative medicine: Honoring the stories of illness*. Oxford University Press.

Clair, R. P. (1996). The political nature of the colloquialism, "A real job": Implications for organizational socialization. *Communication Studies, 47*(4), 257–271. https://doi.org/10.1080/036377596093763932

Claire, R. P., Carlo, S., Lam, C., Nussman, J., Phillips, C., Sánchez, V ... Yakova, L. (2014). Narrative theory and criticism: An overview toward clusters and empathy. *Review of Communication, 1*, 1–18. https://doi.org/10.1080/15358593.2014.925960

Cole, C. E. (2010). Problematizing therapeutic assumptions about narratives: A case study of storytelling events in a post-conflict context. *Health Communication, 25*(8), 650–660. https://doi.org/10.1080/10410236.2010.521905

Cole, T. R., Carson, R. A., & Carson, R. A. (2014). *Medical humanities*. Cambridge University Press.

de Souza, R. (2012). Theorizing the relationship between HIV/AIDS, biomedicine, and culture using an urban Indian setting as a case study. *Communication Theory, 22*(2), 163–183. https://doi.org/10.1111/j.1468-2885.2012.01403.x

DeLacy, J., Dune, T., & Macdonald, J. J. (2020). The social determinants of otitis media in Aboriginal children in Australia: Are we addressing the primary causes? A systematic content review. *BMC Public Health, 20*, Article 492. https://doi.org/10.1186/s12889-020-08570-3

Dolan, B. (Ed.). (2015). *Humanitas: Readings in the development of the medical humanities*. University of California Medical Humanities Press.

du Pre, A. (2002). Accomplishing the impossible: Talking about body and soul and mind during a medical visit. *Health Communication, 14*, 1–21. https://doi.org/10.1207/S15327027HC1401_1

Dutta, M. J. (2020). *Communication, culture, and social change: Meaning, co-option, and resistance*. Palgrave Macmillan.

Dutta, M. J., & de Souza, R. (2008). The past, present, and future of health development campaigns: Reflexivity and the critical-cultural approach. *Health Communication, 23*(4), 326–339. https://doi.org/10.1080/10410230802229704

Dutta-Bergman, M. J. (2004). The unheard voices of Santalis: Communicating about health from the margins of India. *Communication Theory, 14*, 237–263.

Dutta-Bergman, M.J. (2005). Theory and practice in health communication campaigns: A critical interrogation. *Health Communication, 18*(2), 103–122. https://doi.org/10.1207/s15327027hc1802_1

Ellingson, L. L., & Buzzanell, P. M. (1999). Listening to women's narratives of breast cancer treatment: A feminist approach to patient satisfaction with physician–patient communication. *Health Communication, 11*, 153–183. https://doi.org/10.1207/s15327027hc1102_3

Engel, G. L. (1977). The need for a new medical model: A challenge for biomedicine. *Science, 196*, 129–136.

Fishbein, M. (2000). The role of theory in HIV prevention. *AIDS Care, 12*, 273–278.

Fishbein, M. & Cappella, J. N. (2006). Role of theory in developing effective health communications. *Journal of Communication, 56*, S1–S17. https://doi.org/10.1111/j.1460 2466.2006.00280.x

Fisher, J. D., & Fisher, W. A. (1992). Changing AIDS-risk behavior. *Psychological Bulletin, 111*, 455–474.

Fisher, W. R. (1984). Narration as a human communication paradigm: The case of public mora argument. *Communication Monographs, 51*, 1–22.

Fisher, W. R. (1987). *Human communication as narration: Toward a philosophy of reason, value, and action*. University of South Carolina Press.

Freimuth, V.S. (2012). Reflecting on the accomplisments of health communication. *Journal of Health Communication, 17*(7), 745–746. https://doi.org/10.1080/10810730.2012.713841

Goffman, E. (1974). *Frame analysis: An essay on the organization of experience*. Harvard University Press.

Gouge, C. C. (2018). Health humanities baccalaureate programs and the rhetoric of health and medicine. *Technical Communication Quarterly, 27*(1), 21–32. https://doi/org/10.1080/10572252.2017.1402566

Guarneri, E.M. (2007). *The heart speaks: A cardiologist reveals the secret language of healing*. New York: Atria Books.

Hannah, M. A., & Arduser, L. (2018). Mapping the terrain: Examining the conditions for alignment between the rhetoric of health and medicine and the medical humanities. *Technical Communication Quarterly, 27*(1), 33–49. https://doi/org/10.1080/10572252.2017.1402561

Hannawa, A. F., Kreps, G. L., Paek, H-J., Schulz, P. J., Smith, S., & Street, R. L., Jr. (2014). Emerging issues and future directions of the field of health communication. *Health Communication, 29*(10), 955–961. https://doi.org/10.1080/10410236.2013.814959

Healey, P., Stager, M.L., Woodmass, K., Dettlaff, A.J., Vergara, A., Janke, R., & Wells, S.J. (2017). Cultural adaptations to augment health and mental health services: A systematic review. *BMC Health Services Research, 17*, article number 8. https://doi.org/10.1186/s12913-016-1953-x

Health Humanities Consortium. (2021). *About*. https://healthhumanitiesconsortium.com/about/

Ho, E. Y., & Bylund, C. L. (2008). Models of health and models of interaction in the practitioner client relationship in acupuncture. *Health Communication*, *23*, 506–515. https://doi.org/10.1080/10410230 802460234

Hoffman-Longtin, K., Kerr, A. M., Shaunfield, S., Koenig, C. J., Bylund, C. L., & Clayton, M. F. (2022). Fostering interdisciplinary boundary spanning in health communication: A call for a paradigm shift. *Health Communication*, *37*(5), 568–576. https://doi.org/10.1080/10410236.2020.1857517

Institute of Medicine (US) Committee on Health Literacy; Nielsen-Bohlman, L., Panzer, A. M., Kindig, D. A., editors. (2004). *Health Literacy: A Prescription to End Confusion*. Washington (DC): National Academies Press (US. 1, Introduction. Available from: https://www.ncbi.nlm.nih.gov/books/NBK2 16033/

IOM (US). (2005). Complementary and Alternative Medicine in the United States Washington (DC): National Academies Press (US); APPENDIX E, Model Guidelines for the Use of Complementary and Alternative Therapies in Medical Practice. Retrieved from: https://www.ncbi.nlm.nih.gov/books/ NBK83798/

IOM (US). (2009). *Integrative Medicine and the Health of the Public: A Summary of the February 2009 Summit*. National Academies Press (US); Models of Care. https://www.ncbi.nlm.nih.gov/books/ NBK219635/

Institute of Medicine (IOM). (2003). *Unequal treatment: Confronting racial and ethnic disparities in healthcare*. Washington, DC: National Academies Press.

Jensen, R. E. (2015). An ecological turn in rhetoric of health scholarship: Attending to the historical flow and percolation of ideas, assumptions, and arguments. *Communication Quarterly*, *63*(5), 522–526. https://doi.org/10.1080/01463373.2015.1103600

Kerr, A. M., Shaub, T., Casapulla, S., Smith, C., & Manzi, J. (2020). Addressing social justice and inclusion in the classroom: Using the principles of narrative medicine to discuss identity negotiation and passing. *Communication Teacher*, *34*(2), 97–102. https://doi.org/10.1080/17404622.2019.1625939

Khan, S. (2020). Examining HIV/AIDS-related stigma at play: Power, structure, and implications for HIV interventions. *Health Communication*, *35*(2), 1509–1519. https://doi/org/10.1080/10410236.2019. 1652386

Koenig, H. G., & Larson, D. B. (1998). Use of hospital services, religious attendance, and religious affiliation. *Southern Medical Journal*, *91*, 925–932. https://doi.org/10.1097/00007611199810000-00006

Kreps, G. L. (1988). Relational communication in healthcare. *Southern Speech Communication Journal*, *53*, 344–359.

Kreps, G. L. (1989). Setting the agenda for health communication research and development: Scholarship that can make a difference. *Health Communication*, *1*(1), 11–15.

Kreps, G. L. (2021). The role of strategic communication to respond effectively to pandemics. *Journal of Multicultural Discourses*, *16*(1), 12–19. https://doi.org/10.1080/17447143.2021.1885417

Kreps, G. L., Sparks, L., & Villagran, M. M. (2010). Editors' introduction, communication education, and health promotion. *Communication Education*, *59*, 215–219 https://doi.org/10.1080/036345210 03657734

Kroops van't Jagt, R., de Winter, A. F., Reijneveld, S. A., Hoeks, J. C. J., & Jansen, C. J. M. (2016). Development of a communication intervention for older adults with limited health literacy: Photo stories to support doctor-patient communication. *Journal of Health Communication*, *S2*(21), 69–82. https://doi.org/10.1080/10810730.2016.1193918

Last, J.M. (1995). Dictionary of epidemiology. IEA, 73. Retrieved from: chrome-extension://efaidnbmn nnibpcajpcglclefindmkaj/ https://pestcontrol.ru/assets/files/biblioteka/file/19-john_m_last-a_dictionary_ of_epidemiology_4th_edition-oxford_university_press_usa_2000.pdf

Leach, A. J., Morris, P. S., Coates, H. L. C., Nelson, S., O'Leary, S. J., Richmond, P. C. ... Torzilllo, P. J. (2021). Otitis media guidelines for Australian aboriginal and Torres Strait Islander children: Summary of recommendations. *Medical Journal of Australia*, *214*(5), 228–233. https://doi.org/10.5694/ mja2.50953

Löblich, M., & Scheu, A. M. (2011). Writing the history of communication studies: A sociology of science approach. *Communication Theory*, *21*, 1–22. https://doi.org/10.1111/j.14682885.2010.01373.x

Lupton, D. (1996). Toward the development of critical health communication praxis. *Health Communication*, *6*(1), 55–67.

Maibach, E.W., & Cotton, D. (1995). Moving people to behavior change: A staged social cognitive approach to message design. In E. Maibach & R.L. Parrott (Eds.), *Designing health messages: Approaches from communication theory and public health practice* (pp. 41–64). Sage Publications Inc. https://doi.org/10.4135/9781452233451.n3

Mara, M., & Mara, A. (2018). Blending humanistic and rhetorical analysis to locate gendered dimensions of Kenyan medical practitioner attitudes about cancer. *Technical Communication Quarterly*, *27*(1), 93–107. https://doi.org/10.1080/10572252.2018.1401344

Meloncon, L. (Ed.). (2013). *Rhetorical accessibility: At the intersection of technical communication and disability studies*. Routledge.

Meloncon, L., & Frost, E. A. (2015). Special issue introduction: Charting an emerging field: The rhetorics of health and medicine and its importance in communication design *Communication Design Quarterly Review*, *3*(4), 7–14. https://doi.org/10.1145/282697

Mol, A. (2003). *The body multiple: Ontology in medical practice*. Duke University Press.

Moncrieff, J. (2008). *The myth of the chemical cure: A critique of psychiatric drug treatment*. Palgrave Macmillan.

Nierkens, V., Hartman, M.A., Nicolau, M., Vissenberg, C., Beune, E.J.A.J., Hosper, K. … Stronks, K. (2013). Effectiveness of cultural adaptations of interventions aimed at smoking cessation, diet, and/or physical activity in ethnic minorities: A systematic review. *PLoS One*, *8*(10), e73373. https://doi.org/10.1371/journal.pone.0073373

Parrott, R. (2004). Emphasizing "communication" in health communication. *Journal of Communication*, *54*(4), 751–787. https://doi.org/10.1111/j.1460-2466.2004.tb02653.x

Parrott, R. (2011). Point of practice: Keeping 'health' in health communication research and practice. *Journal of Applied Communication Research*, *39*, 92–102 https://doi.org/10.1080/00909882.2010.536848

Petty, R.E., & Cacioppo, J.T. (1986). The elaboration likelihood model of persuasion. In *Communication and persuasion* (pp. 1–24). Springer Series in Social Psychology. New York. https://doi.org/10.1007/978-1-4612-4964-1_1

Pollett, S., & Rivers, C. (2020). Social media and the new world of scientific communication during the COVID-19 pandemic. *Clinical Infectious Diseases*, *71*(16), 2184–2186. https://doi.org/10.1093/cid/ciaa553

Popper, K. R. (1959). *The logic of scientific discovery*. New York: Basic Books.

Prochaska, J. O., & DiClemente, C. C. (1986). Toward a comprehensive model of change. In W. R. Miller & N. Neather (Eds.), *Treating addictive behaviors: Processes of change* (pp. 3–27). Plenum Press.

Query, J. L., & Wright, K. (2003). Assessing communication competence in an online study: Toward informing subsequent interventions among older adults with cancer, their lay caregivers, and peers. *Health Communication*, *15*(2), 203–218. https://doi.org/10.1207/S15327027HC1502_8

Quinlan, M. M., Harter, L. M., & Johnson, B. L. (2020). DooR to DooR's acoustics of care: Interrupting and transforming the biomedical landscapes of Western hospitals. *Health Communication*, *35*(9), 1113–1122. https://doi.org/10.1080/10410236.2019.161348

Rains, S. A. (2020). Big data, computational social science, and health communication: A review and agenda for advancing theory. *Health Communication*, *35*(1), 26–34. https://doi.org/10.1080/10410236.2018.1536955

Ratzan, S.C., Payne, J.G., & Bishop, C. (1996). The status and scope of health communication. *Journal of Health Communication*, *1*(1), 25–41. https://doi.org/10.1080/108107396128211

Resnicow, K., Baranowski, T., Ahluwalia, J.S., & Braithwaite, R.L. (1999). Cultural sensitivity in public health: Defined and demystified. *Ethnic Disparities*, *9*(1), 10–21.

Robinson, J. D., & Nussbaum, J. F. (2004). Grounding research and medical education about religion in actual physician–patient interaction: Church attendance, social support, and older adults. *Health Communication*, *16*(1), 63–85. https://doi.org/10.1207/S15327027HC1601_5

Rogers, E.M. (1983). *Diffusion of innovations*. New York: Free Press.

Ruben, B. D. (2016). Communication theory and health communication practice: The more things change, the more they stay the same. *Health Communication*, *31*(1), 1–11. https://doi.org/10/10410236.2014.923086

Scott, J. B., Segal, J. Z., & Keränen, L. (2013). The rhetorics of health and medicine: Inventional possibilities for scholarship and engaged practice. *Poroi*, *9*(1), 1–6. https://doi.org/10.13008/2151 2957.1157

Segal, J. Z. (2005). Interdisciplinarity and bibliography in rhetoric of health and medicine. *Technical Communication Quarterly*, *14*(3), 311–318. https://doi.org/10.1207/s15427625tcq1403_9

Sharf, B. F. (1990). Physician-patient communication as interpersonal rhetoric: A narrative approach. *Health Communication*, *2*(4), 217–231. https://doi.org/10.1207/s15327027hc0204_2

Singelis, T.M., Garcia, R.I., Barker, J.C., & Davis, R.E. (2018). An experimental test of the two-dimensional theory of cultural sensitivity in health communication. *Journal of Health Communication: International Perspectives*, *23*(4), 321–328. https://doi.org/10.1080/10810730.2018.1443526

Slater, M.D. (1999). Integrating application of media effects, persuasion, and behavior change theories to communication campaigns: A stages-of-change framework. *Health Communication*, *11*(4), 335–354. https://doi.org/10.1207/S15327027HC1104_2

Thompson, C. M., & Duerringer, C. M. (2020). Crying wolf: A thematic and critical analysis of why individuals contest family members' health complaints. *Communication Monographs*, *87*(3), 291–311. https://doi.org/10.1080/03637751.2019.1709127

Triandis, H. C. (1972). *The analysis of subjective culture*. Wiley.

US National Library of Medicine. (2004). Medical humanities. *U.S. National Library of Medicine collection development manual*. Retrieved from https://www.nlm.nih.gov/tsd/acquisitions/cdm/subjects57.html

Vanderpoll, T., & Howard, D. (2012). Massive prevalence of hearing loss among Aboriginal inmates in the Northern Territory. *Indigenous Law Bulletin*, *7*(28), 1–7. Retrieved from http://www.ilc.unsw.edu.au/sites/ilc.unsw.edu.au/files/articles/ILB%20728%20Hearing%20Loss%20-%20Vanderpoll_Howard.pdf

Vingilis, E., & Sarkella, J. (1997). Determinants and indicators of health and well-being: Tools for educating society. *Social Indicators Research*, 40, 159–178.

Walkup, K. L., & Cannon, P. (2018). Health ecologies in addiction treatment: Rhetoric of health and medicine and conceptualizing care. *Technical Communication Quarterly*, *27*(1), 108 120. https://doi.org/10.1080/10572252.2018.1401352

WHO. (2004). Chronic suppurative otitis media: Burden of illness and management options. Child and Adolescent Health and Development Prevention of Blindness and Deafness. https://www.who.int/pbd/publications/Chronicsuppurativeotitis_media.pdf

Workman, T. A. (2001). Finding the meanings of college drinking: An analysis of fraternity drinking stories. *Health Communication*, *13*(4), 427–447 https://doi.org/10.1207/s15327027hc1304_05

Zoller, H. M., & Kline, K. N. (2008). Theoretical contributions of interpretive and critical research in health communication. *Communication Yearbook*, *32*, 89–135.

## Additional Resources

Brooke-Weberling, M. (2014). The status of health communication: Education and employment outlook for a growing field. *Journal of Health Communication*, *19*(12), 1408–1423. https://doi.org/10.1080/10810730.2014.904024

Gergen, K. J. (2009). *An invitation to social constructionism* (2nd ed.), SAGE Publications.

Osher Collaborative for Integrative Health. https://www.oshercollaborative.org/

Riley, A. H., Sangalang, A., Critchlow, E., Brown, N., Mitra, R., & Nesme, B. C. (2021). Entertainment-education campaigns and COVID-19: How three global organizations adapted the health communication strategy for pandemic response and takeaways for the future. *Health Communication*, *36*(1), 42–49. https://doi.org/10.1080/10410236.2020.1847451

Wells, S. (2010). *Our bodies, ourselves, and the work of writing*. Stanford University Press.

# A Social Justice Activist Approach to Health

---

**Chapter Learning Outcomes**

Upon completing **Chapter 3**, "**A Social Justice Activist Approach to Health**," the student should be able to apply the WPHC SJA approach to:

1. Conceptualize engaged communication from an SJ sensibility to center advocacy and intervention.
2. Identify SJ values and principles, highlighting health inequities, disparities, and marginalized identities through an intersectional lens.
3. Design interventions for SJ in medicine to address health inequities in medical education, climate, policies, and guidelines.
4. Understand intersectionality in health equity and identify how cultural, institutional, and individual racism contributes to health inequities.
5. Explain the SJ approach to health through the lens of SDoH, distributive justice, and community empowerment.
6. Identify how health communication activism acts by dismantling racist ideologies, overturning oppressive structures, and transformational resistance.

**Consider the following context:**

> Titus Regional Medical Center (TRMC) was offering the COVID-19 vaccine, and I know a lot of the women, women that I work with that do not speak a lot of English, they were actually searching for a way to get the vaccine for themselves or their family members, but they were not able to find any resources in Spanish over how to get that vaccine.
>
> (Participant, Wagner et al., 2022)

> I have seen a lot and I have heard about many Hispanic people who don't have any way of going to the doctor and prefer to cure themselves with their own remedies, they prefer to go with their local remedies, they prefer to die. Some preferred to die of COVID before going there because they didn't have health insurance. Because we

DOI: 10.4324/9781003214472-4

are not aware of what the hospital offers, what the government through the hospital offers to help people with less opportunities. We need them to guide us more.

(Participant, Wagner et al., 2022)

Researchers Teresa Wagner and her colleagues completed a study during the pandemic in Mount Pleasant, Texas, which became a hotspot for COVID-19 cases in the Latinx community. The workers were employed by the local meat packing plant, agricultural, and manufacturing industries that required working in close quarters. Wagner's participants faced challenges with the use of masks, hand washing, and personal hygiene. Other researchers found that families of Latinx farmworkers in rural communities had incomplete knowledge of how transmission occurred and faced systemic barriers. These barriers added to the confusion when official guidelines contradicted or differed from the community's cultural practices, beliefs, and values. Reflecting the national trend in the rural communities' vaccination rate in the United States during the pandemic, the county's vaccination rate was a dismal 24.8% as compared to the state's 40.8%.

In another study, researchers Diana Burgess and colleagues found that healthcare providers' responses to patient narratives on racial disparities illuminated their struggle with accepting the "persistent racism" narratives. These narratives, which focused on patients' experiences with provider racism in direct ways, were found to be polarizing. They elicited resistance from those providers who scored low on the study item that assessed the degree to which they believed providers may contribute to healthcare inequality. Some of the patient comments from Burgess's study illuminate provider resistance to racism narratives:

He says many women decline treatment for potentially curable cancer that are African American. So that's a barrier he can't overcome? Like he can't get through to African American women? I would not say that at all. Yeah. I mean I would take each person separately.

(White female nurse practitioner (NP), Burgess et al., 2019)

It's possible based on the color of his skin, but on the flipside we're only getting one side of the story … it's entirely possible that this gentleman had experiences in his past that already kind of predisposed him to walking in with an assumption or a chip on his shoulder that he's going to get different treatment because of the color of his skin without taking each situation for itself. And he may also make that assumption when he doesn't get what he wants, oh, because of the color of my skin.

(White female NP, Burgess et al., 2019)

Burgess et al.'s study raised important questions about communication with healthcare providers. They found that engaging in a provider success narrative was appealing and built provider self-efficacy and motivation to engage in patient-centered communication. Alongside findings demonstrating how provider communication with non-White patients is of poorer quality (Gordon et al., 2006), the provider narratives reiterate that although it seems like a challenging task, tackling persistent racism narratives among providers is important, particularly when it is tailored to countering providers' preexisting beliefs.

## Chapter Organization

**Chapter 3**, "**A Social Justice Activist Approach to Health**" lays out the fundamental principles for engaging social justice (hereafter, SJ) in healthcare contexts. Chapter 3 is organized as follows: **First**, it will consider engaged communication scholarship from an SJ sensibility to highlight how SJ communication centers engagement and advocacy. It will provide a comprehensive look at SJ concepts and their definitions alongside SJA highlights and critiques. **Second**, it will outline SJ values and principles, framing SJ as an intersectional concept and encouraging students to construct a comprehensive framework of health inequities, SJA, and SDoH. **Third**, it will provide a comprehensive examination of SJ in medicine and SJA interventions to address health inequities in medical education, medical school climate, training, policies, and guidelines. **Fourth**, it will examine health equity and healthcare disparities from the perspective of collaboration and community empowerment. It will provide students with pathways for identifying structural practices to dismantle racial ideologies in public narratives and enact transformational resistance. It will provide an interventionist lens for conceptualizing change from oppressive structures to motivate collective action through collaboration and SJA. Along the way, students are provided multiple opportunities to engage with WPHC SJA contexts in discussion prompts, activities, and applied initiatives ranging from obesity to healthy school lunches, community-based self-governance, racial discrimination, intersectionality, social movements, and a critical examination of the work of federal agencies at the structural level. Health communication scholar interviews with Dr. Leandra H. Hernández, Dr. Brandi Lawless, and Dr. Kallia Wright highlight empowered community advocacy at the intersection of critical health communication in Chicana feminist approaches, health equity and disparities faced by the unhoused in San Francisco, and reproductive justice advocacy and Black women's agency in constructing reproductive justice to obtain optimal treatment and transform healthcare interactions. Discussion questions and thought prompts for reflection and present challenges and future directions exercises engage students in conceptualizing and enacting WPHC SJA through a reflective and critical lens.

## Engaged Communication Scholarship

### An SJ Sensibility

SJA scholars Kevin Carragee and Lawrence Frey call for an "engaged communication scholarship" where communication researchers, educators, practitioners, and students apply their knowledge, methods, and practices to work with and for the

> oppressed, marginalized, and under-resourced groups and communities, as well as with activist groups and organizations to intervene into unjust discourses and material conditions to make them more just, and documenting and reporting their practices, processes, and effects to multiple publics.
>
> (2012, p. 3976)

They define the SJ communication perspective as "the engagement with and advocacy for those in our society wo are economically, socially, politically, and/or culturally under-resourced" (Frey et al., 1996, p. 111). The steps that can help further engagement and advocacy should be grounded in an SJ sensibility, a term proposed by Frey et al. that "(1) foregrounds ethical concerns; (2) commits to structural analyses of ethical problems; (3) adopts an activist orientation; and (4) seeks identification with others" (1996, p. 111).

The confluence of recent social movements on racial justice, such as the Black Lives Matter (BLM) and the Blue Lives Matter movements with the global health crises illustrated how public health (PH), public safety, race relations, and community health are closely intertwined.

The BLM movement underscored the disproportionate burden of police violence as borne by communities of color (Black and Indigenous people are two or three times more likely to be killed in law enforcement encounters than White people). The racial disparities in the COVID-19 pandemic health outcomes illustrated how racism is a PH crisis requiring upstream solutions such as investment in health and economic security. The interplay of these diverse concerns highlights the interconnectedness of the relations between power, social context, and SJ. It shows how inequalities play out at the intersection of the multiple facets of an individual's identity such as race, class, gender, sexuality, and place of birth to position everyone differently in their ability to access opportunities necessary to cultivate good health and to thrive.

Review *Textbox 3.1*. Respond to the SJA discussion prompts that follow.

---

### Textbox 3.1   Obesity: Biological Factors, Food Deserts, and Food Swamps, and the Built Environment

#### WPHC Context

We take obesity for granted under the banner of many SJ contexts in the present moment. While the merits and necessity of such SJ contexts such as body positivity are unquestionable, there is no doubt that in those instances where poor diet and lifestyle choices lead to weight management challenges, PH outcomes and individual quality of life suffer. Consider the following context to obesity as a PH concern:

- In 1990 in the United States, the Behavioral Risk Factor Surveillance System (BRFSS) showed that every state had an obesity prevalence rate of less than 15%. In fact, ten states had obesity prevalence rates of less than 10%.
- In 2010, a mere two decades down the line, the BRFSS data showed that all 50 states had obesity prevalence rates greater than 20% (based on self-report). In fact, 12 states had prevalence rates greater than 30%.
- This data suggests that if the present trend continues, by 2030, half of all Americans will be obese. In other words, the body mass index, or BMI, a standard calculation of weight divided by height, of these Americans will be greater than or equal to 30 (for reference, the normal BMI is 18.5 to 24.9; overweight is 25 to 29.9).

Obesity is now considered a PH issue. Obesity leads to increased risk of many serious health conditions, such as coronary heart disease, stroke, and high blood pressure; type 2 diabetes; cancer; high HDL cholesterol; liver and gall bladder disease; sleep apnea and respiratory problems; osteoarthritis; and depression. Obesity also has economic impacts. The economic burden of obesity results from the preventive, diagnostic, and treatment services related to obesity and the indirect costs related to decreased productivity, disability, absenteeism, and loss of future income due to premature death. Biologically, obesity results from an energy imbalance (intake energy exceeds energy expenditure), genetic predisposition, and malfunctioning in biological systems designed to prevent weight fluctuation.

However, as the section on SJ values and principles shows, the role of social, environmental, and economical factors is an equally important consideration alongside the impact of biological factors on obesity. For instance, studies show that obesity can be facilitated or prevented by the "built environment," comprising easily accessible nutritious food and safe and accessible outdoor neighborhood spaces for physical activity. Likewise, an overabundance of fast-food restaurants and convenience stores (i.e., a "food swamp") is associated with increased community obesity rates. Not surprisingly, food swamps and food deserts are found in low-income, minority, and rural communities with limited access to affordable healthy foods and water and easy access to energy-dense, nutrient-poor foods, and sugary drinks. The data reflect this disparity. Over the past decade, it was found that adolescent non-Hispanic Black females and children are about twice as likely to be obese as their White counterparts (CDC, 2021).

### SJA Discussion Prompts

1. Under what conditions would obesity shift from being a biological health concern to one involving SJA and SJ principles?
2. How will a WPHC approach to obesity address some of its key SJ facets outlined earlier?
3. What communicative emphasis might a health communication message targeting adolescent non-Hispanic Black females employ to emphasize SJA in an initiative addressing obesity from a WPHC approach?

### Resource

CDC. (2021). *Health equity resource toolkit for state practitioners addressing obesity disparities.* https://www.cdc.gov/obesity/downloads/cdchealthequityobesitytoolkit508.pdf

### PH as Public Safety

In 2018, the American Public Health Association (APHA) passed a policy statement naming law enforcement violence as a PH issue. Conceptualizing PH and public safety as interrelated shows how safety is not limited to individual criminal activity or policing, persecution, and incarceration. Rather, it shifts focus to the ways in which people and communities are safer when affordable housing, healthcare, healthy food choices, green spaces, and quality education are available to help them flourish (APHA, 2022). Simonson (2021) points out how incarceration impacts the long-term intergenerational futures and communities.

*Table 3.1 categorizes the salient concepts in SJ in health and provides a definition of the terms along with how the terms have functioned to illuminate (or how they have been critiqued for their failings in being able to illuminate) the SJ gaps in healthcare. The left-hand column in Table 3.1 presents key SJ concepts and their definitions. The right-hand column explains how each concept emphasizes SJ concepts' impact on health outcomes in actionable and measurable ways. Respond to the SJA prompt provided.*

Table 3.1 SJ in Health: Concept Definitions, Illustrations, and SJA Critiques

| SJ in Health Concept/Definition | SJA Highlights/Critiques |
| --- | --- |
| **Health equity:**<br><br>*Definition 1:*<br>Health equity is defined as the absence of unfair and avoidable or remediable differences in health among population groups defined socially, economically, demographically, or geographically.<br><br>*Definition 2:*<br>The attainment of the highest level of health for all people. | Emphasizes:<br><br>• The unjust, unnecessary, and preventable nature of the differences in health.<br>• How social group differences in health, such as those based on race or religion, reflect an unfair distribution of health risks and resources.<br>• The SJ dimension of inequality. For instance, three times higher US infant mortality rates for non-Hispanic Blacks versus Whites are partially attributable to preventable differences in education and access to health and prenatal care (CDC, 2011). |
| **Health disparities:**<br>The preventable differences in the burden of disease, injury, violence, or opportunities to achieve optimal health that are experienced by socially disadvantaged populations (CDC, 2022). | • **Highlights inequities** while also relating inequities to the historical and present-day inequitable distribution of social, political, economic, and environmental resources.<br>• **Health disparities** have been critiqued for emphasizing health differences that adversely affect disadvantaged groups.<br>• **Health inequity** captures the moral dimension of health differences as they reflect injustice more than simply differences. |
| **Health inequality:**<br>References the differences in the health of individuals or groups such that any measurable aspect of health that varies across individuals or according to socially relevant groups can be called health inequality. | • Definitions of **health inequality** have been critiqued as posing the risk of neglecting issues of fairness and justice in the differences.<br>• For instance, the difference in **health outcomes** among those in their 20s as compared to those in their 60s (APA, 2022). |
| **Human rights:**<br>Defined as the rights inherent to all human beings, regardless of race, sex, nationality, ethnicity, language, religion, or any other status (UNHRC, 2022). | Illustrative examples include:<br><br>• The United Nations Human Rights Council (UNHRC) (USA) PH strategy aims to foster the conditions, partnerships, collaborations, and approaches that enable refugees to access healthcare and essential health services.<br>• The UNHRC also advocates for the inclusion of refugees into national health systems at affordable costs and provides guidance, infrastructure and capacity building, and other resources to increase access to healthcare (UN Refugee Agency, n.d.). |

**Participation:**
Understood as "involvement by those populations and individuals in decisions that affect the health of those populations and individuals. It implies the involvement and influence in the decisions affecting health status and healthcare services, implementation of decisions, evaluation, and monitoring, and … defining the problem" (WHO, 2022).

Social participation supports:

- Governance mechanism that provides opportunities for greater health equality.
- Raising awareness and recognition of the rights of groups with the highest level of health disadvantage.
- Transforming vulnerable groups into agents and protagonists of the policies and programs that affect them.
- Producing new collective knowledge that challenges dominant narratives.
- Promoting coherence, responsiveness, transparency, and rule of law.
- Facilitating the implementation and evaluation of strategies, programs, and activities.
- Promoting population consciousness of the private sector strategies used to promote products and choices that are detrimental to health (WHO, 2022, p. vii).

**Patient/community empowerment:**
**Empowerment:**
The process by which people gain control over the factors and decisions that shape their lives, by which they increase their assets and attributes and build capacities to gain access, partners, networks, and/or a voice, to gain control.

**Community empowerment:** References the process of enabling communities to increase control over their lives (WHO, 2022).

**Patient empowerment** is the process through which people gain greater control over decisions and actions affecting their health.

- **Patient empowerment** can be supported by dialogic relationships, co-production of knowledge, and collaborative care, where both providers and patients are equal and active partners in managing their healthcare.
- **Communities** are understood as groups of people who may or may not be spatially connected but who share common interests, concerns, or identities; could be local, national, or international; and with specific or broad interests.
- **Community empowerment** is more than the involvement, participation, or engagement of communities. It implies community ownership and action that explicitly aims at social and political change through a process of renegotiating power to gain more control.

**Shared decision-making:**
A model of patient-centered care that enables and encourages people to play a role in the medical decisions that affect their health (AHRQ, 2020)

Critiqued based on two assumptions:

- Individuals with good information can and will participate in the medical decision-making process by asking informed questions and expressing personal values and opinions about their conditions and treatment options.
- Clinicians will respect patients' goals and preferences and use them to guide recommendations and treatments.

**Access:**
Is concerned with helping people command appropriate healthcare resources as required to preserve or improve their health (Gulliford et al., 2002).

Critiqued based on the following assumptions:

- Services are available, and there is an equal opportunity to obtain healthcare.
- There is an absence of social, cultural, financial, and organizational barriers to the utilization of services.
- Utilization is not dependent upon affordability, physical accessibility, and not just adequacy of supply.

(Continued)

*Table 3.1* (Continued) SJ in Health: Concept Definitions, Illustrations, and SJA Critiques

| SJ in Health Concept/Definition | SJA Highlights/Critiques |
| --- | --- |
| **Inclusion:**<br>Refers to the intentional, ongoing effort to ensure that diverse people with different identities can fully participate in all aspects of the work of an organization, including leadership positions and decision-making processes (Tan, 2019). | • Assumes that inclusion is in and of itself grounded in SJ. For instance, inclusive health assessments by nurses must be intentional in upholding the principles of SJ and centering the humanity of all clients in their care, regardless of race, ethnicity, gender, sexuality, age, ability, and any other factor that makes them who they are.<br>• Invites healthcare professionals to consider their own personal biases, cultivate a safe environment of care, and go beyond standardized approaches to physical assessment based on the social construct of what it means to be "normal" (Braverman et al., 2011). |
| **Healthcare system:**<br>SJ in the healthcare system references equal healthcare services for all individuals and fair treatment, regardless of one's economic status, race, ethnicity, age, citizenship, disability, or sexual orientation (Habibzadeh et al., 2021). | Considers the following aspects for the delivery of safe, quality patient-centered care (Rosen & Mieres, 2020):<br>• Health literacy<br>• Language access<br>• Cultural competency |

**SJA Discussion Prompts**

SJ principles in WPHC contexts comprise numerous components as the left-hand side column of Table 3.1 illustrates. Discuss the SJ implications of the following situations for populations who are vulnerable and marginalized:

1. A situation where some of the SJ components are present but others are absent. For instance, what does SJ mean when collaborative participation is taken into consideration but not inclusion or shared decision-making?
2. A situation where SJ principles apply to some vulnerable populations but not others. For instance, what does SJ mean when members of low socioeconomic classification (SEC) populations are considered but individuals identifying as LGBTQIA+ are excluded?
3. A situation where the voice of vulnerable populations who are affected is not included or solicited in a collaborative and participatory manner.

Given the line of thinking of the previous SJA discussion prompts, consider the following:

1. What does WPHC mean in the context of SJ? Is one inextricably linked with the other? How so? Under what circumstances or conditions are they distinct and exclusionary concepts?

How does WPHC support the goals of SJ? What does SJ look like without WPHC? What would a health landscape where WPHC and SJ are missing look like for members of different populations?

## Resources

Agency for Healthcaree Research and Quality (AHRQ). (2020). *The SHARE approach.* https://www.ahrq.gov/health-literacy/professional-training/shared-decision/index.html

American Psychological Association (APA). (2022). *Older adults: Health and age-related changes.* https://www.apa.org/pi/aging/resources/guides/older

Braverman, P. A., Kumanyika, S., Fielding, J., LaVeist, T., Borrell, L. N., Manderscheid, R., & Troutman, A. (2011). Health disparities and health equity: The issue is justice. *American Journal of Public Health, 101*(Suppl 1), S149–S155. https://doi.org/10.2105/AJPH.2010.300062

CDC. (2022). *Adolescent and school health: Health disparities.* https://www.cdc.gov/healthyyouth/disparities/index.htm#:~:text=Health%20disparities

Gulliford, M., Figueroa-Munoz, J., Morgan, M., Hughes, D., Gibson, B., Beech, R., & Hudson, M. (2002). What does "access to healthcaree" mean? *Journal of Health Services Research and Policy, 7*(3), 186–188. https://doi.org/10.1258/135581902760082517

Habibzadeh, H., Jasemi, M., & Hosseinzadegan, F. (2021). Social justice in health system: A neglected component of academic nursing education: A qualitative study. *BMC Nursing, 20*, 16. https://doi.org/10.1186/s12912-021-00534-1

Rosen, S., & Mieres, J. (2020, August 3). Health care is long overdue for a social justice reckoning: Biases in the system put the lives and well-being of women and minorities at risk. *ScientificAmerican.* https://www.scientificamerican.com/article/healthcare-is-long-overdue-for-a-social-justice-reckoning/

Tan, T. Q. (2019). Principles of inclusion, diversity, access, and equity. *The Journal of Infectious Diseases, 220*(2, Suppl), S30–S32. https://doi.org/10.1093/infdis/jiz198

United Nations Human Rights Council. (2022). *Promotion and protection of human rights around the globe.* https://www.ohchr.org/en/hr-bodies/hrc/home

WHO. (2022). *Commission on social determinants of health, 2005–2008.* https://www.who.int/initiatives/action-on-the-social-determinants-of-health-for-advancing-equity/world-report-on-social-determinants-of-health-equity/commission-on-social-determinants-of-health

Research shows how negative health outcomes relate to health equity. For example, health inequities have been associated with shorter life expectancies, poorer physical and mental health, disproportionate mortality and morbidity burden, and systemic disadvantages that follow from poor education, higher crime environments, and an increased burden of chronic illness. The next section will discuss the concepts that comprise SJ with a focus on health outcomes.

### SJ Values and Principles

#### Understanding SJ as an Intersectional Concept

SJ refers to the "fair and proper administration of laws conforming to the natural law that all persons, irrespective of ethnic origin, gender, possessions, race, religion … are to be treated equally and without prejudice" (Universal Declaration of Human Rights, United Nations). The norms it draws upon are often derived from normative beliefs of what is right, good, and moral. It is based on the notion of fairness and the ethics that guide understandings of what it means to be fair. Such understandings are sometimes difficult to translate into practice as their meaning is often derived from the context in which they occur and are interpreted. SJ is composed of five principles: (a) diversity, (b) access, (c) equity, (d) human rights, and (e) participation (see Table 3.1 for their definitions and impacts).

*Review **Textbox 3.2** and try your hand at the SJA prompt that follows.*

---

**Textbox 3.2　Intersectionality and Health Inequities: SJ Implications**

**WPHC Context**

Understanding diversity enables an appreciation of the differences that exist among societal groups and how these differences can result in systemic disadvantages and inequities for those with marginalized identities. These disadvantages can, for instance, take the form of discrimination based on factors such as race, sexual orientation, age, gender, income, education, and other characteristics. In their discussion paper, López and Gadsden (2016) describe how an intersectional health equity lens helps to consider the interrelationships between these identities as a complex whole. It recognizes the ways in which race, gender, class, sexual orientation, disability, and other dimensions of inequality structure an individual's lived environment in particular ways to open and close opportunities to grow and access the institutional, social, and structural resources necessary to help them thrive.

Viewed from a critical lens, these differences constitute intersecting systems of oppression, producing specific lived experiences for categories of people.

---

**SJA Discussion Prompts**

Table 3.1 directs attention to the questions implicit in researchers López and Gadsden's essay. What are your thoughts on the following?

1. What kind of effort is needed to center the lives of groups that remain invisible at the intersections of the margins?
2. How will unpacking the multiple dimensions and systems of inequality promote the goals of health equity and SJ?
3. Can bringing together insights from health sciences, psychology, anthropology, art history, American studies, and law generate new forms of knowledge to develop a health policy based on equity?
4. Share your suggestions on the type of effort needed and its implications with a partner.
   a. What might you be missing? How does your perspective differ from your partner's? What SJ factors might be shaping the differences in your perspectives?
   b. Is intersectionality a factor in understanding the different types of effort that might be needed and its impacts?

**Resource**

National Academies of Medicine (NAM), López, N., & Gadsden, V. L. (2016, December 5). *Health inequities, social determinants, and intersectionality.* https://nam.edu/health-inequities-social-determinants-and-intersectionality/

To translate the principles of SJ in action, communication, and activism research (CAR) scholars Carragee and Frey advocate for an SJA approach that involves

action that attempts to make a positive difference in situations where people's lives are affected by oppression, domination, discrimination, racism, conflict, and other forms of cultural struggle due to differences in race, ethnicity, class, religion, sexual orientation, and other identity markers.

(Broome et al., p. 146)

The next half of this section will delve more closely into the SJ concepts as they apply to medicine as an institution and a practice.

*Review **Table 3.2**. Respond to the SJA prompts on the third right-hand column. How can the notion of intersectionality be incorporated in engaged ways through an SJA lens?*

Table 3.2 Health Inequities, SJA, and Social Determinants of Health: An SJ Audit

| WPHC Context: SDoH | SJ Context: Health Inequities | SJA Food for Thought: What Can I Do? |
|---|---|---|
| Racism | Racial and ethnic minorities experience higher rates of **morbidity and mortality** than any other US racial or ethnic group from a range of conditions including:<br>• Heart disease<br>• Cancer<br>• Cerebrovascular disease<br>• HIV/AIDS<br>• Diabetes. Hispanic Americans are almost twice as likely as non-Hispanic Whites to die from diabetes.<br><br>These differences have been found to be associated with:<br>• **Socioeconomic** differences<br>• Differences in **healthcare access** Environmental degradation<br>• Direct and indirect consequences of **discrimination** (IOM, 2003)<br><br>The Federal Office of Management and Budget has established five categories for **racial groups:**<br>• American Indian or Alaska Native<br>• Asian<br>• Black or African American<br>• Native Hawaiian or other Pacific Islander<br>• White<br>• Hispanic or Latino and not Hispanic or Latino. | **Community-specific, multisector interventions** in African American and Latino neighborhoods and Native American reservations address poverty, healthy environments, education, and housing.<br><br>**SJA Prompts:**<br><br>How would you:<br><br>• *Name and address racism?* How will your language reflect the fluid and dynamic nature of race as a social construct and its sociopolitical identity?'<br>• *Start an open and honest conversation about health equity within your organization, community, or agency?*<br>  • What strategies and approaches would you employ?<br>  • Who would you involve at your organization?<br>• What steps would you need to accomplish to facilitate an **institutional culture** of openness and accountability? |
| Education | **Health and longevity** have deteriorated among those with less education over the last few decades; less educated adults report worse general health, more chronic conditions, and more functional limitations and disability.<br><br>The **health effects** in the relationship with longevity are stronger for women than men and for non-Hispanic Whites than minority adults. The **pathways** through which education influences health lie in four categories:<br><br>1. Economic (better, stable jobs, higher income)<br>2. Health-behavioral (less high-risk behaviors such as smoking, unhealthy diet, poor exercise)<br>3. Social-psychological (social support), and access to healthcare (modest role) (Zajacova & Lawrence, 2019) | **SJA Prompts:**<br><br>• How can you bring about change in how we understand and communicate the long-term **educational processes** that precede the attainment of an educational degree and its effect on health?<br>• How can you **reconceptualize education** not simply as a vehicle for social success, valuable resources, and good health but also as an institution that reproduces *inequality across generations?*<br>• How can you situate historical, social, and policy contexts in understanding the relationship between **education and health?** |

| | | SJA Prompts: |
|---|---|---|
| Neighborhood environments | **Disadvantaged groups** (low-income and racially/ethnically minoritized people) experience greater harmful environmental exposures.<br><br>Evidence suggests that **low socioeconomic status (SES) groups** show greater health benefits if they live in a greener neighborhood (Rigolon et al., 2021) | Neighborhood environments shape and influence the daily conditions (under which people are born, grow, live, work, and age).<br>• How will you promote the **availability of** green spaces (trees and parks) in neighborhoods?<br>• How can **healthy behaviors** such as exercise be promoted in low-SES neighborhoods that lack safe and green open spaces for play? |
| Transportation | **Transportation barriers** lead to rescheduled or missed appointments, delayed care, and missed or delayed medication use.<br><br>**Consequences** may lead to poorer management of chronic illness and poorer health outcomes (Syed et al., 2014). | **SJA Prompts:**<br>• How can you identify **areas in your community** that face transportation barriers to **healthcare access?**<br>• Can you envisage a **collaboration** between your healthcare institutions, medical transportation services, and public transit authority to envisage public transit discounts or reimbursement and/or provision of cars to improve **healthcare access?** |
| Public Safety | The **intersectionality** of public safety and health highlights ways in which people can feel safer when they are provided with the healthcare, housing, infrastructure, and social services necessary to help them thrive while demonstrating the harm of focusing on safety as related to incarceration, crime, policing, and individual responsibility (Simonson, 2021). | **SJA Prompts:**<br>Identify the **structural factors** creating and perpetuating high crime conditions.<br>How can you:<br>• Join in **grassroots organizing** around the conditions of people's lives as a form of **collective care?**<br>• Link with similar efforts across the **country** and around the **world?**<br>• Help redefine the notion of a "**public**" whose health matters, including those who are incarcerated, their families, and their communities?<br>• Tackle the **inequitable distribution** of power, money, and resources (the structural drivers of the conditions of daily life).<br>• Measure the **problem** and assess the **impact** of action (develop a workforce trained in SDoH, raise public awareness of SDoH). |
| Housing | Racial and ethnic **housing segregation** is a by-product of both historic and contemporary racism and discrimination, as well as socioeconomic differences. | |

*(Continued)*

Table 3.2 (Continued) Health Inequities, SJA, and Social Determinants of Health: An SJ Audit

| WPHC Context: SDoH | SJ Context: Health Inequities | SJA Food for Thought: What Can I Do? |
|---|---|---|
| Food Choices | Evidence suggests that residences who have better **access to supermarkets** and limited access to convenience stores and limited access to fast-food restaurants and energy-dense foods tend to have healthier diets and lower levels of obesity. Residents of low-income, minority, and rural neighborhoods are most often affected by **poor access** to supermarkets and healthy food (Larson et al., 2009) | Low-income and **mixed-race neighborhoods** have a greater availability of fast-food restaurants. **SJA Prompts:** • How could you mitigate the negative health effects of the **distance** that residents typically have to travel beyond their neighborhood to purchase food? • What strategy can you device to **reduce disparities** by improving physical access to healthy, affordable food? • How will you garner neighborhood support for **healthy food** choices? |

## SJA Discussion Prompt

Conduct an SJ audit of your neighborhood based on the previous criteria.

1. How does your neighborhood fare on the SJA action steps as given in the third right-hand column in Table 3.2?
2. What steps will you need to take to improve its SJ score?
3. Is every neighborhood unique in its SJ score and challenges? How so? How are they similar? Why is the difference (if any) important?

## Resources

Larson, N. I., Story, M. T., & Nelson, M. C. (2009). Neighborhood environments: Disparities in access to healthy foods in the U.S. *American Journal of Preventive Medicine, 36*(1), 74–81.e10. https://doi.org/10.1016/j.amepre.2008.09.025

Rigolon, A., Browning, M. H. E. M., McAnirlin, O., & Yoon, H. V. (2021). Green space and health equity: A systematic review on the potential of green space to reduce health disparities. *International Journal of Environmental Research and Public Health, 18*(5), Article 2563. https://doi.org/10.3390/ijerph18052563

Simonson, J. (2021, August 5). *Blurring the line between public health and public safety.* Harvard Law Petrie Flom Center. Bill of Health—Examining the intersection of health law, biotechnology, and bioethics. https://blog.petrieflom.law.harvard.edu/2021/08/05/public-health-safety-blm-covid/

Syed, S. T., Gerber, B. S., & Sharp, L. K. (2014). Traveling toward disease: Transportation barriers to health care access. *Journal of Community Health, 38*(5), 976–993. https://doi.org/10.1007/s10900-013-9681-1

Zajacova, A., & Lawrence, E. M. (2019). The relationship between education and health: Reducing disparities through a contextual approach. *Annual Review of Public Health, 39*, 273–289. https://doi.org/10.1146/annurev-publhealth-031816-044628

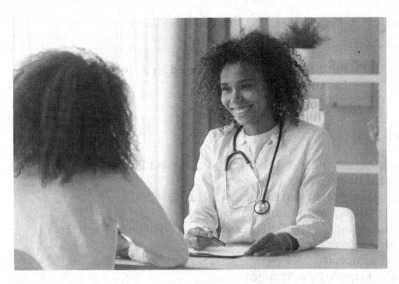

*Figure 3.1* A Push Toward SJ in Medicine Recognizes the Need for Racial Diversity and Equity in Medicine.

## SJ in Medicine

There is a growing recognition that SJ, which has often been considered the domain of liberal arts and social science courses, has been ignored or de-emphasized in medical education. Such studies reveal that the although the explicit curriculum (formal curriculum) may appear objective, the hidden curriculum (norms and informal practices) of medical schools often emphasizes and perpetuates discrimination, biases, and mistreatment that undervalues minority students through perpetuating racism, classism, sexism, and heteronormative values that reinforce health disparities.

Medical schools across the United States are taking steps to recognize this. In Hawaii, the John A. Burns School of Medicine has a Center for Native and Pacific Health Disparities Research (John A. Burns School of Medicine, 2022). The University of New Mexico's School of Medicine gives students hands-on experience with New Mexico's underserved populations and the historical-social context of SJs they face by providing opportunities for students to treat patient populations composed of homeless people and Spanish-speaking Mexican immigrant workers. The Association of American Medical Colleges' (AAMC) emphasis on integrating cultural competence education in medical education states how "cultural competence in healthcare combines the tenets of 'patient/family-centered care with an understanding of the social and cultural influences' that affect the quality of medical services and treatment" (2005).

*Review **Textbox 3.3**. Respond to the SJA prompt that follows.*

---

**Textbox 3.3    Federal Agencies Involved in Addressing SDoH Factors**

**WPHC Context**

- Federal Agency: Office of Disease Prevention and Health Promotion (ODPHP)
  Website: https://health.gov/
- Federal Agency: National Institutes of Health (NIH)
  Website: https://www.nih.gov/
- Federal Agency: Centers for Disease Control and Prevention (CDC)
  Website: https://www.cdc.gov/
- Federal Agency: Health Resources and Services Administration (HRSA)
  Website: https://www.hrsa.gov/
- Federal Agency: National Center for Health Statistics
  Website: https://www.cdc.gov/nchs/

**SJA Activity**

Browse through the websites of the federal agencies listed above:

1. What is the focus of each of them?
2. How do they work together to illuminate the barriers toward eliminating SDoH and to further the goals of achieving health equity through addressing the SDoH comprehensively?
3. Are there any other agencies you would involve?
4. If so, which ones would they be? Why?

---

One of the ways in which medical schools have responded to the national call for medical education reform and acknowledged the need for integrating SJ in medicine is by examining how the learning environment, curriculum, and faculty development can be transformed through collaboration and coordination with a range of stakeholders.

*Examine **Table 3.3**. The SJ intervention spaces are provided in the right-hand column. Please review and respond to the SJA prompts.*

*Table 3.3* SJ in Medicine and SJA Action Steps

| WPHC Context: Definition as Employed in Healthcare Settings | SJA Critique: SJ Intervention Spaces |
|---|---|
| **SJ in Medicine (Draper et al., 2020):** The idea that **healthcare workers are trained** in and promote fair treatment in healthcare so that health disparities are eliminated, discrimination is decreased, and bias, marginalization, and racism are addressed | **SJA Prompt:** <br> • What **responsibility do physicians and nurses** have toward understanding the struggles, such as poverty, sexism, and racism, faced by their patients? <br> • Should **promoting SJ** center the identity of what it means to be a physician? |
| **Anti-racism:** The **practices** of actively working to oppose individual and systemic racism | **SJA Prompt:** <br> White Coats for Black Lives (WC4BL) is a "medical trainee-run organization that aims to **dismantle racism** and accompanying **systems of oppression in medicine** and fight for the health of Black people and people of color" (https://whitecoats4blacklives.org/about/). <br> • How can medical professionals **disrupt systemic and interpersonal racism** in their practice and support the health of communities of color? |
| **Curriculum:** The **sum of learning activities** that are designed to achieve specific educational outcomes through a coherent structure and processes that link theory and practice in the professional education of a professional | Implementing **reforms** to medical school curricula is a multi-step complex process. Stanford Medical School approached this by working with course directors, faculty, students, and staff to revise existing course materials (https://med.stanford.edu/md/discovery-curriculum/social-justice-and-health-equity.html). <br> **SJA Prompt:** <br> • How can including **SJ and health equity** in medical school curricula meaningfully address the strengths and gaps in anti-racist education, health equity, and related SJ issues? |
| **Formal Curriculum:** The **learning experience** as constructed by the courses, lessons, and learning activities that the students participate in, as well as the knowledge and skills educators **intentionally** teach to students | **Formal curricula** emphasize class-based and clinical learning experiences that focus on the formal dimensions of learning in medical school. <br> **SJA Prompt:** <br> • To what extent can (or should) medical schools be responsible for **structuring learning environments** of students that go beyond their formal curriculum? |

*(Continued)*

Table 3.3 (Continued) SJ in Medicine and SJA Action Steps

| WPHC Context: Definition as Employed in Healthcare Settings | SJA Critique: SJ Intervention Spaces |
| --- | --- |
| **Hidden Curriculum:**<br>The informal and often **unintended lessons**, values, beliefs, and perspectives that students learn in school<br>Often comprises the **unspoken or implicit** academic, social, and cultural messages that are communicated to students while they are in school | **Hidden curriculum** messages oftentimes directly contradict those from the formal curriculum (e.g., surgery is too hard for women, it is okay to talk down to nonphysician staff, learning how to do a physical exam is more important than learning how to communicate with patients).<br>**Informal and hidden curriculum messages** are conveyed in the student lounge, in the elevator, in the cafeteria, and in a variety of ways.<br>Some schools have adopted **innovative approaches** such as coaching to help students **critically reflect** on and shine a light on the hidden curriculum (e.g., https://www.aamc.org/news-insights/navigating-hidden-curriculum-medical-school).<br><br>**SJA Prompt:**<br>• How can medical schools harness the **power of hidden curricula** in transformative ways? |
| **Implicit bias:**<br>The **attitudes** that affect our understanding, actions, and decisions in an unconscious manner. These assessments can be both favorable or unfavorable; they are activated involuntarily and without an individual's awareness or intentional control | **Implicit bias** in patient care can manifest itself in a range of situations, including racial bias, bias against LGBTQ+ individuals, obese patients, female patients, sexual minorities, and elderly patients.<br>Studies in a range of **healthcare contexts** have found that patient depression, life satisfaction, and outcomes are associated with the implicit biases of their physicians.<br><br>**SJA Prompt:**<br>• How can **advocacy**, meaningful interactions, and a climate of openness and fairness be created that allows for challenges, identification and reporting of biased attitudes and behavior to be facilitated in medical training and practice settings? |
| **Intersectionality:**<br>The complex, cumulative way in which the intersection of **different identities** overlap and intersect with systems in which they operate | **SJA Prompt:**<br>• How can the **health disparities** and **stigma** that transgender and gender-diverse people face be addressed in actionable ways?<br>• How can medical providers be **trained** to provide **affirming and comprehensive care** regarding body modification and clinical approaches to patients from the gender and sexual minority populations who face eating disorders and body dissatisfaction? |

**Marginalization:**
An abstract process through which people and groups have **limited access** to power, social and political resources, and are subjected to differential treatment because of their position in society

**Microaggressions:**
Defined as behaviors that **ambiguously disempower** racial minorities—that are brief and subtle verbal and/or nonverbal denigrating messages directed toward ethnic and/or racial minorities that carry the weight of the offending party's implicit bias, often below their own conscious awareness

**Healthcare microaggressions:**
Healthcare microaggressions refer to **implicit discrimination** within the healthcare setting, whereby treatment providers who are in positions of authority inadvertently marginalize members of minority groups through culturally insensitive interactions These may originate from **aversive racism** (denial of racist prejudices based on adherence to egalitarian ideals)

**SJA Prompt:**
Evidence suggests that the experience and **perception of marginalization** are linked to poor health through stress, anxiety, depression, occupational injuries, and limited access to healthcare.

- How can clinicians include **patient vulnerabilities** in the context of their personal needs and lived, everyday realities?
- How will **emphasizing vulnerabilities** allow clinicians to understand the proximal causes of their patients' disease process, promote respectful interactions that account for their everyday contexts, and allow for providers to experience the individual and health from the standpoint of the margins to develop appropriate, tailored interventions that highlight their resilience, personal agency, family support or other ways in which marginalized individuals thrive (Baah et al., 2019)?

**Experiential training** coupled with **consciousness raising** of providers has been recommended to work toward patient-centered and culturally informed practice. Such training calls for **reflective practice** that includes a **holistic appreciation** for the individual, the understanding of the oppressive nature of institutions against minorities and marginalized populations, and the acknowledgment of the power and privilege that may define the provider-patient relationship" (Cruz et al., 2019).

**SJA Prompt:**
- How can providers be **trained to recognize** the "moment-to-moment thoughts, feelings, and behaviors that may be inadvertently disempowering their patients."?
- How can providers be **trained to "empathize** with the lived experience of the patient's illness ... to try to understand the illness as the patient understands, feels, perceives, and responds to it"?

*(Continued)*

*Table 3.3* (Continued) SJ in Medicine and SJA Action Steps

| WPHC Context: Definition as Employed in Healthcare Settings | SJA Critique: SJ Intervention Spaces |
| --- | --- |
| **Discrimination:**<br>**Individual discrimination** is defined as:<br>**Differences in care** that result from biases, prejudices, stereotyping, and uncertainty in clinical communication and decision-making (IOM, 2003)<br>**Socially structured action** that is unfair or unjustified and harms individuals and groups.<br>**Structural discrimination** is defined as:<br>Macrolevel conditions (e.g., residential segregation) that limit opportunities, resources, and well-being of less privileged groups<br>Different **forms of discrimination** impact different population groups, including racial/ethnic minorities, women, LGBTQIA+ individuals, older adults, and people with disabilities (Healthy People 2030, 2022) | Experiences of **individual discrimination** have been documented to have numerous high physical and emotional health costs such as:<br>• Causing the body to be more **physically sensitive** in stressful social situations.<br>• Act as a **chronic stressor**, increase vulnerability to physical illness.<br>• Be related to **risky health behaviors** such as smoking and alcohol abuse while being related to **low participation in risk reduction behaviors** such as cancer screening, diabetes management, and condom use.<br><br>**SJA Prompts:**<br>• How might being a **part of several affected groups simultaneously** (e.g., intersectionality by race, gender, and place of birth) impact experiences of discrimination and lead to differential health outcomes?<br>• How can **residential segregation**, a form of **structural discrimination**, limit social and economic resources for individuals, families, and communities?<br>• In what way does **discrimination affect disparities** in access to quality education, with low-quality schools that have limited health resources, teacher support, and increased safety concerns, all factors that are **associated with** poor mental and physical health? |
| **Social accountability in medical schools:**<br>The **obligation** of medical schools to direct education, research, and service activities toward addressing the priority health concerns of the community, region, or nation that they are mandated to serve<br>These are **collectively identified** by governments, healthcare organizations, health professionals | **SJA Prompt:**<br>• What role might bear **witness to the injustices** and inequities that people face play in cultivating a socially conscious medical professional?<br>• Will **consciousness** of SJ-related issues encourage medical professionals to seek opportunities to serve those who they witness as being disenfranchised and underserved? |
| **SDoH:**<br>The conditions in the environment in which people are born, live, learn, work, play, worship, and age that affect a wide range of health, functioning, and quality-of-life outcomes and risks, such as availability of resources to meet daily needs; access to educational, economic, and job opportunities; and access to healthcare services | **SJA Prompt:**<br>• Should medical professionals **advocate** for better education and economic equality for their patients as research shows that these aspects are directly linked to better health outcomes?<br>• How does advocacy by medical professionals shape the ethics of the profession?<br>• Will it change your relationship with your provider in any way? |

**Structural Determinants of Health:**
The **policies, systems, and practices** that influence SDoH and health outcomes including racism and White supremacy, sexism and patriarchy, classism and capitalism, heterosexism, homophobia, transphobia, xenophobia, and imperialism

**Underrepresentation (UR):**
**UR** refers to population groups whose numbers in certain geographic areas or within a defined category or discipline) are disproportionately less than the general population (i.e., gender, race/ethnicity, sexual orientation, first generation, low income, veteran status, disabilities, people who identify with more than one race/ethnicity, and other identity groups

**SJA Prompt:**

- How can medical schools provide students with hands-on experience with **underserved populations** and the injustices they face through opportunities to work in local communities?
- How can engaging in **experiential work** that gives individuals a deeper insight into what it means to be a patient in underserved communities facilitate action and change?
- How can conceptualizing **SDoH** from the standpoint of margins illuminate the structural forces that shape marginalization?

**UR and Underserved Status:**

- Evidence suggests that "while diversity of the American population is one of the nation's greatest assets, one of its greatest challenges is reducing the profound disparity in health status of its racial and ethnic minority, rural, low-income, and under **underserved populations**" (NIMHD, 2021).
- For example, the American Indian and Alaska Native people experience lower health status (e.g., lower life expectancy and increased disease burden) compared with other Americans.
- **Underserved** status has been attributed to **structural factors** such as education and poverty, SDoH factors such as poor social and living conditions, as well as discrimination in the delivery of health services and cultural differences.

An **example of negative health outcomes** in a UR and underserved population:

- **American Indians** and **Alaska Natives** born today have a life expectancy that is 5.5 years less than the US all races population continue to die at higher rates than Americans in many other categories including chronic liver disease and cirrhosis, diabetes mellitus, assault/homicide, self-harm/suicide, and chronic lower respiratory diseases (IHS.gov, 2019).

**SJA Prompt:**

- Should medical curricula include knowledge of historical events, trauma, human rights violations that have historical and long-term consequences for underrepresented groups?

(Continued)

*Table 3.3* (Continued) SJ in Medicine and SJA Action Steps

| WPHC Context: Definition as Employed in Healthcare Settings | SJA Critique: SJ Intervention Spaces |
|---|---|
| **Underrepresented Minority (URM):** Defined as minorities employed in university or organizational contexts **includes race/ ethnic groups** who have been historically disadvantaged, in part, because of historical oppression: <br><br> • American Indian/Native American Asian/ Asian American Black/African American <br> • Hispanic/Latino/Latinx <br> • Native Hawaiian or Pacific Islander | **Mentoring:** <br><br> • **Mentoring** is the process through which a senior, experienced faculty member (mentor) provides guidance and support for a junior or less-experienced colleague (mentee). <br> • Mentoring is a critical element for **faculty career advancement** in academic medicine. <br> • Mentors in medical schools play a variety of **roles** in helping mentees delineate and accomplish career goals, enhance productivity, and provide education about the written and unwritten rules that govern the academic environment. <br><br> **Disparities in URM faculty mentoring:** <br> Many studies report that **URM faculty** receive less mentoring than their nonminority peers in medical schools. <br><br> **URM faculty challenges:** <br><br> • URM faculty are **challenged** to find mentors. <br> • URM faculty face marginalization. <br> • URM faculty face overt and covert racism. <br> • URM faculty report receiving **less mentoring** than their nonminority peers. <br> • URM faculty miss out on **activities** such as lunches, book discussions, seminars, and social hours—all activities that some medical school programs have implemented to support mentoring relationships (Kosoko-Lasaki et al., 2006). <br> • URM faculty are assigned a disproportionate share of **activities** that do not advance careers (e.g., serving on numerous committees). <br><br> **Disparities in professional advancement:** <br> A 2010 AAMC report suggests that non-White faculty are less likely to be **promoted;** another found that African American scientists are 10% less likely than their White peers to obtain **R01 grants** (Beech et al., 2013). <br><br> **SJA Prompt:** <br><br> • What are some aspects of the **mentor-mentee relationship** that should be addressed in mentoring programs to cultivate culturally appropriate mentoring relationships? |

## Underrepresented in Medicine (URiM):

The AAMC defines URiM as racial and ethnic populations that are **underrepresented** in the medical profession relative to their numbers in the general population

The **goal of URiM** is to foster student diversity in medical school admissions and the creation of a diverse healthcare workforce that is proportionate to and resembles the racial, ethnic, gender, and other identity-based profiles of the people they serve

## URiM populations include:

- American Indian/Native American, Black/ African American, Hispanic/ Latino/ Latinx, and Native Hawaiian or Pacific Islander
- Some medical schools will clarify Asian UR as defined as those who do NOT identify as Chinese, Japanese, Filipino, Korean, Asian Indian, or Thai

## SJA Discussion Prompt

- As you respond to the SJA discussion prompts on the right-hand side column of the Table 3.3, identify one example from media or personal narratives that illustrates the impact of those actions/inactions on the individual/marginalized identities referenced.

## Abstracted From

Draper, J., Malchuk, A. M., Vander Schaaf, E. B., Brown, S. H., Dent, G., Howard, N., Steiner, B., & Thomas, E. N., III. (2020, October). *UNC School of Medicine Task Force to Integrate Social Justice into the Curriculum: Final report*. https://colorusunited.org/wp-content/uploads/2023/01/Social-Justice-Task-Force-Report-and-Recommendations-Final-Final_12-9-20.pdf

URiM adoption by the AAMC on June 26, 2003, helped medical schools accomplish the following three important objectives:

a. Shift in focus from a **fixed aggregation** of four racial and ethnic groups to a **continually evolving underlying reality** ... by accommodating including and removing UR groups based on changing demographics of society and the profession.

b. Shift in focus from a **national perspective** to a **regional or local** perspective on UR.

c. Stimulate **data collection** and **reporting** on the broad range of racial and ethnic self-descriptions (AAMC, 2022).

AAMC's approach has been critiqued based on:

- Tension between **inclusive and exclusive** medical school admissions processes.
- Implications of tensions in admissions with respect to how the URiM definition increases **access to medical school**, in present-day and for historically underrepresented groups (Clay et al., 2021).

## SJA Prompt:

- Will broadening URM to URiM benefit all applicants? Who does it leave out?
- Does URiM promote justice and inclusion (Razak et al., 2015)?

What do you think?

The concepts in Table 3.3 reflect an awareness that clinical diagnoses and treatments are only as successful as their integration into the lived environment of the individual and the barriers posed by their social conditions. There is a growing recognition that medical professionals have a social and ethical responsibility to understand and respond to the lived conditions of their patients. Such care and knowledge should inform reflection on how medical care can help patients in sustainable and culturally sensitive ways. For instance, NYC Health + Hospitals, the largest PH-care system in the United States, partnered with the National LGBTQIA+ Health Education Center at The Fenway Institute to design and implement a novel sexual and gender minority (SGM) healthcare curriculum offered to employees between 2017 and 2020.

### Training and Medical School Climate

There is increased awareness of the need to address explicit and implicit bias in the medical school climate. Although less than 50% of heterosexual first-year medical students in a large United States study sample expressed some explicit bias against other students who identify as LGBTQIA+, greater than 80% held at least some degree of implicit bias against SGM. The evidence suggests that LGBTQIA+ patients too remain at risk of discrimination from even well-meaning providers. An underlying cause of such discrimination is providers' lack of training in interacting with diverse patient populations and in minority (e.g., LBGTQIA+-related) health issues. In the absence of training, providers may express stigma or unwittingly discriminate, may be unaware of SGM-health issues and terminology, and be lacking in SGM-appropriate communication skills. A lack of training in medical schools or poor-quality training also likely contributes to the presence of discomfort, poor-quality care, and lack of preparation. Provider implicit bias has been found with obese patients, female patients, and elderly patients.

### Significance of SJ Principles of Physician Training

The implications of examining SJ principles in medicine are significant. Physician bias against sexual and racial minorities, for instance, is linked to differential treatment of patients with potentially negative outcomes. For instance, in a study on patients outcomes with spinal cord injury, patient disability, depression, and life satisfaction were found to be associated with the implicit racial biases of their physicians. Although provider bias can have serious consequences, the relationship of provider bias with patient health outcomes in research findings is complex. For instance, there is little evidence correlating providers' implicit bias with bias in their treatment recommendations. Within medical schools, implicit and explicit bias can undermine the institutional climate for minorities, leading to the risk of a higher drop-out rate of minority members from medical school, with minorities reporting experiencing more burnout, or a reluctance to apply to medical schools altogether (Fallin-Bennett, 2015).

### Medical Education

In addition to individual medical schools, medical education has also seen changes at a structural level. The study of medicine has traditionally focused on biological determinants of health such as cellular metabolism, genetic markers, and vectors of infection. Acknowledging the need to bridge the "art and science of medicine for the betterment of public health," the American Medical Association (AMA), the nation's largest professional association of physicians, recently committed to a "dedicated, coordinated, and honest approach to target the systemic inequities in the healthcare system and social institutions." The AMA's 2021–2023 five-point plan for optimal health for everyone includes embedding racial and SJ in AMA's culture, systems, policies, and practices; building alliances and sharing power with marginalized and minority physicians and stakeholders; ensuring equitable structures and opportunities in innovation; addressing upstream determinants of health and root causes of inequities; and fostering pathways for truth, racial healing, reconciliation, and transformation.

Medical institutions are currently ranked by their social mission score. The AAMC has a "Tool for Assessing Cultural Competence Training" and a "Framework for Addressing and Eliminating Racism at the AAMC, in Academic Medicine, and Beyond" (2020). However, as UNC School of Medicine's task force report noted, challenges such as the optional nature of SDoH courses, short individual lecture-based trainings, often of poor quality, and ambiguity in key SJ principles in health and their teaching have prevented such efforts from being well-integrated and successful.

## Health Equity and Healthcare Disparities

### Impact of Health Inequities across the Life Course

Cultural, institutional, and individual racism is now recognized as a fundamental cause of adverse health outcomes for racial and ethnic minorities and racial and ethnic inequities in health; systematically advantaging Whites compared with other racial groups in the United States while creating conditions that are inimical to the health of all groups. Inequalities in health arise because of the differences in circumstances in which people grow, live, work, and age, and the systems put in place to deal with illness (WHO, 2022). Health inequities can have an impact across the individual's life course, intergenerationally, and societally (Arcaya, et al. 2015). For instance, social, political, and economic policies have a definitive impact on whether a child will grow up and live a flourishing life or whether their life will be full of struggles and systemic disadvantages (WHO, 2022). Health equity should be embedded in the decision-making processes of all facets of society. In Mount Pleasant in Texas, patient and community-centered care was made more effective through health communication that is culturally and linguistically sensitive to the language barriers that challenge members of diverse communities. They also integrated leadership training and training of healthcare providers in health literacy and cultural competencies (Wagner et al., 2022).

*As you read through **Textbox 3.4 Scholar Interview** with **Dr. Leandra H. Hernández**, consider how the Chicana feminist intersectional lens informs Dr. Hernandez's work. What does community advocacy mean for marginalized populations? How does this dynamic shift when we characterize those who are disadvantaged as vulnerable? Under what circumstances would it be appropriate to characterize marginalized populations as vulnerable? What does vulnerability imply in empowered community advocacy contexts?*

## TEXTBOX 3.4   Scholar Interview

### Dr. Leandra H. Hernández
*University of Utah*

1. Your scholarship has centered on communication and social change, emphasizing intersectionality, culture, and agency in addressing how community advocacy and activism can help conceptualize and articulate meaningful health outcomes. Can you share your thoughts on how power and health-based rights approaches can imagine collaborations that are owned and created by the marginalized?

   Historically, marginalized populations were positioned as those needing help, not necessarily those who have the expertise and agency to participate in creating their own community advocacy opportunities. In order to center the lived experience, agency, and expertise of community members to create better health outcomes, we need to directly engage with communities and relinquish researcher power and authority. For example, Dr. Sarah De Los Santos Upton and I published an article in *Frontiers in Communication* on critical health communication methods at the US-Mexico border. In this article, we advocated that scholars should (1) seek to historicize power relations contextualizing research engagement with minoritized communities; (2) refrain from characterizing research populations as vulnerable, which implies their inability to participate meaningfully in the research process; and (3) directly center community members as fellow experts and equal collaborators in the research and advocacy process.

2. How have theory and praxis centered and engaged SJA principles in action in your research?

   SJ is the heart of my research, teaching, and community service. It drives and fuels my community advocacy in multiple contexts as well. I have spent the past decade researching gender violence and reproductive justice at the intersection of critical health communication, media/journalism, and Latina/o/x communication studies. Most of my recent work has explored community resistance to *feminicidios* and violence against women in both the United States and throughout Latin America. I have also explored the ways in which resistance to reproductive feminicides are part of the larger enterprise of reproductive justice advocacy and community organizing efforts.

3. How do Chicana feminist approaches to Latina/o/x cultural health experiences address inequities and oppression and challenge the self-perpetuating disparities that have intergenerational health implications for marginalized and minority communities?

   Chicana feminist approaches to health communication interrogate the impacts of racism, colonialism, sexism, homophobia, and oppression on health outcomes and the ways in which Chicana, Mexican, and Latina/o/x communities have multiple, intersecting identities that shape their health beliefs and practices. Further, Chicana feminist approaches directly center the experiences of Latina/o/x/e communities and build upon concepts such as *nepantla, conocimiento,* borderlands, and *mestiza consciousness* in health spaces. By centralizing *Latinidad,* health communication researchers are able to grasp more nuanced findings about Latina/o/x/e health experiences in relation to power, agency, and oppression.

4. Can you give an example of how a project from your scholarship that means a lot to you personally illustrates the transformative potential between communication and health?

One project that is very meaningful to me explores the decision-making processes that Latinas experience when faced with the prenatal testing process. This project—my dissertation research—was my entry point into reproductive justice, and it utilized Chicana feminist and intersectional theoretical lenses. It was also informed by conversations I had with family members about their prenatal testing experiences; thus, I sought to disentangle the relationships among medical ethics, gender, power, culture, and disability. Multiple factors informed participants' shared decision-making processes about prenatal testing, genetic testing, and abortion: culture, relationships with family members, family histories and stories, lack of knowledge about prenatal testing, and a fundamental reconceptualization of what "healthy" means for a fetus or infant. Counter to preexisting research, participants were fully agentic patients who resisted power dynamics, unwanted health procedures, and incomplete health information. Participants ultimately developed a homegrown understanding of the prenatal testing process informed by their identities and cultural contexts.

## Understanding Health Equity

Health equity is when all people can achieve the highest attainable level of health. Addressing the SDoH, such as poverty, is essential to achieving sustainable improvements in health outcomes (WHO, 2022). Equally essential is addressing the social determinants of equity (as distinct from SDoH) to achieve SJ and to eliminate health disparities. Health communication professor Mohan Dutta (2008) emphasizes that although it is important to reduce individual risk by focusing on individual behavior change, a focus on the individual alone is not sufficient to mitigate the structural, interpersonal, social, and systemic disadvantages imposed on marginalized and minority communities.

### The Link between Health Equity and SDoHs

Health equity demands that greater attention and investment be made in marginalized and under-resourced communities, with input and equal representation of the community members in the decision-making processes. For example, transportation, education, availability of green space, healthy groceries and produce, and law enforcement are all essential for creating the conditions that enable all people and communities to attain and sustain good health. For instance, studies find that in rural Appalachia, people who knew someone who could provide rides to a member of their family reported a greater utilization of healthcare (Arcury et al., 2005). Conversely, Guidry et al. (1997) found that among cancer patients in Texas, 55% of African Americans and 60% of Hispanics identified poor access to a vehicle as a barrier that could result in missing a cancer treatment.

### Intersectionality and Health Equity

Health equity asks us to value all individuals and populations equally. It encourages intersectional efforts to address avoidable inequalities and to create conditions for optimal health for all, particularly for those who have experienced historical or contemporary injustices or socioeconomic disadvantages. Intersectionality attends to the ways institutional and social forces of racism, sexism, classism, ageism, and other-ism's intersect with individual identity dimensions such as those of race, gender, age, and class, to selectively afford privilege and to selectively disadvantage people at different social locations (Crenshaw, 1989). It also entails a responsibility to attend to the social systems and institutions that drive disparities. These include racially based clinical decision-making tools and health communication that spearheads programmatic efforts through campaigns, messages, and advocacy.

### Eliminating Healthcare Disparities

Efforts on addressing health equity challenges have focused on eliminating healthcare disparities through training programs that focus on teaching healthcare providers cultural competencies and enhancing their communication skills to bridge cultural differences, racial biases, and racism. For instance, Diana Burgess and colleagues conducted a study of healthcare providers at three Veterans Health Administration (VHA) Medical Centers in the Southern and Midwestern United States to develop and test communication strategies for motivating providers to engage in actions to reduce healthcare disparities in their own practice (2019).

Review *Textbox 3.5*. Attempt the SJA prompts that follow.

---

**Textbox 3.5　Discussion Questions/Thought Scenarios for Reflection**

**Healthy School Lunches, a Jab at Obesity, and Collective Participation**

**WPHC Context 1**

Healthy school lunch initiatives have been shown to have the benefits of increased healthy food consumption, healthy food purchases, and improved dietary choices in elementary and middle school children. These have resulted in improved nutrition, weight status, academic achievement, food security, and reduced emissions overall. Examples of these initiatives include the National School Lunch Program (NSLP), the Alliance for a Healthier Generation (national-level, nonprofit organization), Project Bread's Chefs in Schools (Massachusetts), and the Lunch Box's Rainbow Day Program (Colorado) that serve more whole grains, fruits and vegetables, low-fat milk and dairy products, and less sodium. Some of the communicative initiatives include attractive displays, verbal encouragement and prompts, and pre-slicing fruits. Such programs seek to implement a culturally sensitive approach to increase the effectiveness of obesity prevention efforts.

**SJA Prompt**

Imagine that you are a food service director for an elementary school in a minority neighborhood. Students in your community speak many different languages and come from families with nearly as many different food traditions. Your task is to ensure the diversity in the community is appropriately reflected in the diversity in the food served in the schools.

- What are some elements that your plan should include to recognize community needs and achieve them in an equitable manner? For example, your plan may include integrating more traditional dietary cultures, teaching children about native foods and their preparation, and building community engagement.

### WPHC Context 2

Health is determined by a complex array of social processes (WHO, 2019). A WPHC SJA perspective encourages participation in whole person health. WPHC prioritizes the SJ principles seeking to achieve the "promotion of social participation generally of governance in all policies. It signals a collective reflection by individuals or groups, deliberation and making decisions in collaboration with the institutions responsible, including involvement in planning and subsequent implementation of decisions" (WHO, vii). However, implementing participation in alignment with SJ principles is challenging.

### SJA Prompt

From the lens of social determinants of equity, considering the needs and challenges facing your community, discuss the following:

1. How will you evaluate that underrepresented groups, all affected stakeholders, invisible groups, and minorities are identified, contacted, and included?
2. How would you assess their participation opportunity and ability to articulate issues of concern to them?
3. How would you guide community discussions and decisions that relate to local action or policy to ensure their effectiveness?
4. What would such a participatory space look like? Think in terms of the ability of such a space to support reflexivity through "interaction, communication, information production, training, reflection, deliberation and appropriation, defining problems, and the agenda of priorities based on the needs of those who participate in the process, and not only on technocratic or administrative criteria" (p. 4).
5. How might such participation be transformative? In other words, how would such dialogue support a "change in the collective framing of the problem and priority setting to ... account for the most disadvantaged groups" (p. 4).

### Inspirational Example

Sparling, N. (2017, November 2). *For an inspirational community example, see: From Phô to fajitas, school lunches feed a diverse nation*. Civil Eats. https://civileats.com/2017/11/02/why-culturally-relevant-food-matters-in-school-lunch/

*The Burden of Health Disparities*

Health disparities place an overwhelming burden on the healthcare system. Most healthcare providers believe that healthcare disparities are primarily due to patient-level factors such as noncompliance with medical recommendations, lack of motivation, and having difficulty communicating. These have been attributed to the dominant framing of racial health inequality in the United States as a "White frame," which focuses on health problems experienced by people of color while ignoring the role of White perpetrators, racist practices, and institutional biases in creating these problems (Feagin & Bennefield, 2014). Hull, Stevens, and Cobb (2020) note that inequities in COVID-19-related morbidity and mortality are illustrated by the disproportionate morbidity and mortality burden borne by Latinx, Indigenous, and Black communities. For instance, Black Americans account for 13% of the US population but experienced 31% of COVID-19-related deaths. Similarly, Hispanic/Latinx people account for 13% but bore a mortality rate of 44% of COVID-19-related deaths. Indigenous communities account for less than 1% of the US population and experienced an overwhelming 22% of COVID-19-related deaths. They raise the questions of equity by asking how race, ethnicity, and insurance status might determine vaccination priority or whether Black, Indigenous, and Latinx people who experience long-term COVID-19 symptoms receive equitable diagnosis and care, given scholarly documentation of how racial stereotypes affect provider interpretation of patient symptoms (Yong, 2020).

## SJ Approach to Health

### Key Tenets of SJ

WHO's Commission on SDoH notes that SJ in health is often a matter of life and death. SDoH are defined as the factors that determine the conditions in which people are born, grow, work, live, and age and the wider set of forces and systems shaping the conditions of daily life. These forces include economic policies and systems, development agendas, cultural practices, social norms, and political systems. A key tenet of SJ is that everyone deserves equal rights and opportunities, including the right to good health. SDoH include income and social protection, education, unemployment, and job insecurity, working life conditions, food insecurity, housing, basic amenities, and the environment, early childhood development, social inclusion and nondiscrimination, structural conflict, and access to affordable health services of decent quality (WHO, 2022).

Healthy People 2030 categorizes the SDoH into five domains: (a) economic stability, (b) education access and quality, (c) healthcare access and quality, (d) neighborhood and built environment, and (e) social and community context. Studies show that SDoH account for between 30%–55% of health outcomes. Because an individual's environment shapes their ability to make healthy choices, Healthy People 2030's SDoH goal is to "create social, physical, and economic environments that promote attaining the full potential for health and well-being for all."

### SDoH and Health Inequities

SDoH have an important influence on health inequities. Health inequities are the unfair and avoidable differences in health status seen within and between countries. The APHA states that inequities are often the result of policies and practices that create an unequal distribution of power, money, and resources among communities based on race, class, gender, place, and sexuality, among other factors. SDoH must be addressed alongside structural forms of inequity, such as racism, for everyone in the community. Racism is defined as a system of structuring opportunity and assigning value to individuals and communities based on race that unfairly disadvantages some individuals and unfairly advantages others.

### Distributive Justice

To be healthy, the resources referenced by SDoH should be distributed in a fair manner that considers the need, capacity to benefit from, and the efficiency of access in lieu of the ability to pay or wield influence in society. This is the principle behind distributive justice, which focuses on a just distribution of resources needed for health, the human rights principles of nondiscrimination and equality, and the right to a standard of living adequate for health. From an SJ lens, health equity means striving to equalize opportunities to be healthy and working to close the gap between the disadvantaged and privileged groups by improving the health of the socially disadvantaged.

Review *Textbox 3.6* for a scholar interview with Dr. Brandi Lawless. How does her students' work with the health disparities faced by the unhoused in San Francisco incorporate SJA elements?

---

### TEXTBOX 3.6   Scholar Interview

**Dr. Brandi Lawless**
*University of San Francisco*

Increasing Water Access for Unhoused San Franciscans through Community-Engaged Learning

At the height of the pandemic, I taught Organizational Communication (designated as a Community-Engaged Learning class) remotely. I wanted the class to feel engaged, even though they would never set foot in my nonprofit partner's space. We conceptualized social justice as the equitable distribution of and access to resources. Through conversations with my community partner, it became apparent that water access was one of the biggest social justice issues in the community—one that led to health disparities among the unhoused.

My class worked with a local nonprofit to increase water access in the Tenderloin—the lowest-income neighborhood in San Francisco. Students learned about the United Nations Water Access, Sanitization, and Hygiene (WASH) standards and were asked to compare how the minimum guidelines for refugees as defined by the UNHCR could be applied to homeless residents in San Francisco. Using communication skill sets (e.g., social media strategies, persuasive writing, qualitative interviewing), students prepared an executive summary of their WASH assessment, drafted persuasive arguments to be used at public policy hearings, prepared slide decks for the nonprofit's use at city council meetings, and developed a social media campaign to raise public awareness around the issue. Students learned about organizational culture, power, privilege, and social justice in action through their relationship with a community partner.

Students were able to achieve the learning outcome of examining how organizational context(s) influence communication processes' by adjusting their work products for the unhoused community, nonprofit leadership, and public policymakers. They developed interpersonal relationships with members of the Tenderloin community that persisted beyond the course, challenged stereotypes they held about the neighborhood and its inhabitants, and developed a sense of action orientation around local policies. The students were empowered to learn more and *do* more with the knowledge they gained in class.

### An Intersectional View of SDoH

Healthy People 2030 addresses the SDoH from an intersectional and contextual perspective. This perspective considers the environment individuals live in to evaluate how it limits and supports their health outcomes. For instance, people who don't have access to grocery stores with healthy foods are less likely to have good nutrition. That in turn raises their risk of health conditions like heart disease, diabetes, and obesity, and lowers life expectancy relative to people who do have access to healthy foods. However, just promoting access to healthy food choices will not alone eliminate these and related disparities. Disparities are a function of the overall living conditions in an individual's environment. For instance, transportation barriers can hinder an individual's ability to travel to a grocery store. Alternatively, poor education quality may be associated with decreased awareness of the importance of making healthy food choices with good health. This illustrates the SDoH principle that improvement in related sectors like education, transportation, and housing are also required to achieve healthful outcomes.

### Addressing Health Inequities and Healthcare Disparities

The five categories of the SDoH act together. Research shows that any one SDoH is not by itself a unique predictor of health outcomes. Table 3.1 illustrates how each element of SDoH contributes to health inequities and disparities. It also shows how addressing any one element will not result in an improved health outcome. For instance, simply making affordable transportation available in low-income neighborhoods will not by itself decrease the rate of missed clinical appointments. Each of the elements needs to be understood from the perspective of the mutual interaction of the nonmedical factors that influence health outcomes.

### Fair Allocation of Resources

Fair allocation of community resources is at the center of creating health equity. These resources include affordable housing, good schools, healthy food choices, adequate public safety, low-cost and accessible transportation, safe and accessible parks and recreation spaces, and political voice. Related to these resources is the assumption of living conditions that are free from harmful pesticides, housing pollutants such as lead, and other vectors of infection. The emphasis on fairness in the allocation of resources highlights how health equity is at the center of good health outcomes.

Look at Table 3.2. Each of the elements of health equity identified in Table 3.2 is fundamentally connected with key issues of SJ. As opposed to SDoH, addressing social determinants *of equity* (SDoE) involves monitoring for inequities in all these categories as they impact discrimination, violence, education, access to nutritious foods, physical activity opportunities, language and literacy skills, and exposure to polluted air and water. For instance, structural racism would involve addressing the multilevel system of ideologies, institutions, and processes that have created and reified racial and ethnic inequities (Neely et al., 2020). Structural racism works across institutions to propagate racial injustice. The WHO emphasizes how achieving health equity involves the SDoE through an examination of the interrelated upstream factors, structures, policies, practices, norms, and values that underlie these disparities.

### Sustainable Development Goals

The United Nations' Sustainable Development Goals (SDGs) set the agenda for 2030 by labeling it a "decade of action," of connecting local action with global leadership, and of taking a whole person approach to health through tackling poverty, gender equality, clean water and sanitation, education, addressing climate emergencies, peace and justice, and good health and well-being along with investing in inclusive and sustainable economies (UN, 2021). The COVID-19 pandemic highlighted the vulnerabilities faced by disadvantaged communities globally. For instance, four out of every five deaths of children under age 5 occur in sub-Saharan Africa and Southern Asia, 94% of all maternal deaths occurred in low- and middle-income countries, and globally, adolescent girls and young women faced gender-based inequalities, exclusion, discrimination, and violence, putting them at an increased risk of acquiring HIV (UN, 2021). Engaging in the identification and examination of vulnerabilities to make a difference in health outcomes involves intervention in societal structures and attention to systems of power.

## Health Communication through an SJ Lens

### Collaboration and Community Empowerment

The preceding sections discuss how SJ and health are connected at the community and individual levels. They provide an insight into understanding disparities, such as those illuminating how African Americans and Hispanics are less likely to receive appropriate cardiac medication (e.g., thrombolytic therapy, aspirin, and beta blockers) or to undergo coronary artery bypass surgery, even when differences in factors such as insurance status, income, age, comorbid conditions, and symptom expression are considered. In a similar pattern, African American and Hispanic patients with bone fractures who are seen in emergency departments are less likely than Whites to receive analgesia, and African Americans with end-stage renal disease are less likely to receive hemodialysis and kidney transplantation (IOM, 2003). Addressing these disparities involves examining how the healthcare system comprising the continuum of services provided in traditional healthcare settings including public and private clinics, hospitals, community health centers, nursing homes, and other healthcare facilities, healthcare services, and healthcare professionals can collaborate to achieve quality of care that increases the likelihood of desired health outcomes and is consistent with current professional knowledge (IOM, 2003). It also includes community empowerment.

### Community Empowerment

Community empowerment is at the heart of achieving successful health promotion, disease prevention, and community health outcomes at an individual level (WHO, 2022). Communities are defined as groups of people who share common interests, values, goals, aspirations, and identities. Members of a community may or may not share the same geographical space but be spread across local, national, or international spaces. To empower community members is to enable communities to gain increased control over the factors, decisions, and circumstances that shape their lives. The process of enabling highlights how empowerment is a process of negotiation by which individuals increase their capacity to gain access to resources, build supportive networks and partnerships, gain a voice in political and civic affairs, and pursue other activities to gain control. It is a negotiation, as the process implies a realignment of existing power relations that were inequitable. To enable also highlights how one individual cannot empower another; individuals can only empower themselves by gaining power and control over their circumstances.

Examine **Textbox 3.7** for the WPHC context of racial discrimination and attempt the SJA prompt to discuss its SJ implications.

---

### Textbox 3.7    Racial Discrimination: SJ Implications

#### WPHC Context

Racial discrimination has been found to be significantly related to poorer health. Researchers Paradies et al. (2015) in their meta-analyses note that the experience of racial discrimination correlates with high blood pressure/hypertension, hypothalamic-pituitary-adrenal (HPA) axis dysregulation, which in turn damages bodily systems and leads to physical outcomes such as CVD and obesity. Likewise, their meta-analysis finds that the impacts of racism on the dysregulation of cognitive-affective regions such as the prefrontal cortex, anterior cingulate cortex, amygdala, and thalamus are like the pathways that lead to stress, anxiety, depression, and psychosis.

#### SJA Discussion Prompt

1. How might you imagine racial discrimination impacts poorer health outcomes in clinical settings?
2. How can communication interventions help address these factors?

#### Resource

Paradies, Y., Ben, J., Denson, N., Elias, A., Priest, N., Pieterse, A. ... Gee, G. (2015). Racism as a determinant of health: A systematic review and meta-analysis. *PLOS One*, *10*(9), e0138511 https://doi.org/10.1371/journal.pone.0138511

---

*Negotiation of Power Sharing*

Community empowerment, health promotion, and the SDoH are at the center of the negotiation of power sharing at the local and global levels to achieve equitable and socially just health outcomes for all (WHO, 2022). Communication is central to achieving the equitable and SJ objectives of such community empowerment and health promotion goals. For instance, health communication scholar Mohan Dutta and colleagues conduct ethnographic work in Aotearoa New Zealand to facilitate community participation spaces in constructing a response to the COVID-19 pandemic. By involving community advisory group members and grassroots dialogic work, the researchers suggest that the habit of "radical democracy in communities" is essential for preparing resilient communities that can anchor transformative futures through health crises (2020).

*In **Textbox 3.8**, **Scholar Interview**, **Dr. Kallia Wright** shares her thoughts about the impact of communication and culture on women's reproductive health. As she describes her research on Black women's reproductive health, consider how intersectionality and agency can contribute to suggesting transformative SJ contexts for underrepresented populations.*

---

### TEXTBOX 3.8   Scholar Interview

#### Dr. Kallia Wright
*University of Miami*

My qualitative research on communication about Black women's reproductive health has revealed that the cultural elements of gender and race intersect and influence experiences in the healthcare system. In my interviews, the Black women demonstrate awareness of the health disparities that plague their cultural group. They also know that encounters with medical practitioners can critically impact their health outcomes. Consequently, various women employ strategies to encourage optimal treatment. One such strategy illustrates that in conversations with doctors, Black women seek equitable interaction that also values their voices. My research has found that Black women use preemptive stereotype shields. These are verbal or nonverbal behaviors to reduce racism in interactions with medical practitioners, and the women consider these even before their appointments. These shields include code-switching, mentioning that they possess a degree of higher learning, using a loved one's credibility to verify their symptoms, and changing the physical environment of their hospital room, for instance, with scented oils so that medical personnel would treat them better. The use of these shields is demonstrative of agency, as described by the agency-identity model, and indicates that these women are aware of narratives of social injustice in the healthcare system. With Black women being three to four times more likely to experience maternal morbidity and mortality than other ethnicities, Black women's maternal health experiences are increasingly being publicized. I see participants in my studies as maternal health activists. They offer suggestions for medical practitioners, such as being more mindful of preemptive stereotype shields and determining why their patients use them. As a Black woman, I see this form of research as an opportunity to close the gap in women's maternal and reproductive health and potentially transform healthcare interactions with women in underrepresented groups.

### Communication in Achieving Equitable SJ Objectives

Communication can constitute both a supportive and disruptive factor in achieving health equity. Breakdown in "health communication processes and limited access to relevant health information" (Dutta & Kreps, 2013, p. 1) is a cause of health disparities. Breakdown in communication is associated with challenges (e.g., those stemming from racial bias) in the sociocultural translation of healthcare needs and values between communities and healthcare professionals. Vardeman-Winter's study of White women's communication to identify how systemic racism among primary healthcare grassroots communicators permeates their work with women experiencing health disparities cautions that health communication that reinforces the communicator-community member gaps (e.g., race, gender, class) perpetuates paternalism and racial disparities while undermining the goals of health equity (Vardeman-Winter, 2017). Her study participants, however, also enacted what she labeled "second generation health communication culture" by inculcating reflexivity, acknowledging privilege, defending local health beliefs, enacting listening-dominant dialogues, and making efforts to change the system.

### Communicating for SJ

WPHC that facilitates an individual and community's efforts to acquire power through increased ownership and action and through bringing about social and political change is in alignment with the goals of achieving health equity and SJ. Such WPHC centers dialogue, relationship building, participatory engagement, and critical examination between all stakeholders as central to community empowerment (see also, Broome et al. 2005). These approaches go beyond individual and member involvement to deliberation that raises awareness and consciousness of the inequitable and oppressive operation of power and seeks to shift these through increased knowledge, agency, and ownership of action for change.

## Health Communication SJA

### Targeting Structural Practices

Health communication SJA acts by dismantling the racial ideologies that are embedded in public narratives and enacted historically through structural policies and practices that perpetuate health inequities (Neely et al., 2020). Studies that examine structural racism, will for example, look for the historical and political contexts such as redlining and restrictive covenant policies rather than individual behavioral norms (e.g., drug use or alcohol consumption) that saw Black communities pushed into segregated and neglected contexts, alongside educational, economic, and social opportunities that resulted in a diminished culture of health to understand COVID-19 data revealing the disproportionately negative burden of COVID-19 on African Americans. International human rights agreements ask governments to respect, protect, fulfill, and promote all human rights of all persons, including the "right to the highest attainable standard of health" and the right to a standard of living adequate for health and well-being. The United States has signed but not ratified the International Covenant on Economic, Social, and Cultural Rights, which articulates the right to health or the "right of everyone to the enjoyment of the highest attainable standard of physical and mental health" (ICESCR, 1966). This right includes the right to equal access to all the SDoH. Braveman and colleagues emphasize that working to bridge the gap in health disparities through addressing

SDoH should be informed by knowledge and evidence to guide interventions. WPHC SJA can intervene effectively to reduce disparities by assessing feasibility, costs, and potentially harmful unintended consequences (2011) alongside governance and distribution of organizational resources.

### Transformational Resistance

Careful framing of the issue can cultivate transformational resistance. Transformational resistance critiques oppressive norms and practices and cultivates a desire for SJ. It is central to health communication activism. For instance, employing the conceptual lens of health disparities as a metric for guiding policy and practice and ensuring accountability will require a rigorous framing of the concept and the systematic associations with social disadvantage and negative health outcomes. Cultural racism, for instance, which refers to the installation of the ideology of inferiority in the values, language, imagery, symbols, and unstated assumptions of the larger society, creates an environment wherein racism can flourish and undergird both institutional- and individual-level racism, such as implicit bias (Williams et al., 2019). Such bias can often spread through commonplace and pervasive negative communication of racial and ethnic minorities through stereotypes, values, images, and ideologies that are consciously or subconsciously adopted and normalized (Jain, 2022). Critical communication shifts the focus from individual pathology and abilities to examining structural communication components that give rise to racial inequities is essential in countering and revealing the processes that perpetuate racist beliefs.

*Review **Textbox 3.9** to brainstorm how you might offer avenues for transformational resistance in a healthcare inequity context and target health disparities. What type of social movement organization might you create?*

---

**Textbox 3.9   Advocacy and Action for SJ and Health Equity**

**WPHC Context**

- **SJ Movement**: Freedom to Thrive
  **Website**: https://freedomtothrive.org/
- **SJ Movement**: White Coats for Black Lives
  **Website**: https://whitecoats4blacklives.org/
- **SJ Movement**: #FreeThemAll4PublicHealth
  **Website**: https://www.instagram.com/explore/tags/FreeThemAll4PublicHealth/?utm_source=ig_embed
- **SJ Movement**: National Council of Incarcerated and Formerly Incarcerated Women and Girls
  **Website**: https://givingcompass.org/fund/the-national-council-for-incarcerated-formerly-incarcerated-women-and-girls?gclid=Cj0KCQjw1tGUBhDXARIsAIJx01mc-CcXi230tBicPLgmm3P2Rn6N7aSpALJVwQaz-_4Yo-KtLWnbNw4aAkzcEALw_wcB
- **SJ Movement**: Unite Us
  **Website**: https://uniteus.com/

- **SJ Movement**: The Praxis Project
  **Website**: https://www.thepraxisproject.org/
- **SJ Movement**: Green Jobs Central
  **Website**: https://greenjobs.net/maryland/

### SJA Action Prompt

1. What are the health inequities that characterize a neighborhood where you live?
2. How can you apply your understanding of community empowerment to make a difference in these health outcomes?
3. What issue would a social media SJ movement you may design seek to impact? Create a hashtag for your SJ movement. What tactics would you employ to make a difference?

### *Conceptualizing Change from Oppressive Structures*

From an activist lens, as Neely and colleagues assert, transformational resistance involves considering the notion of how people of color could react to and demand change within oppressive structures in ways that do not conform to or perpetuate the social reproduction of oppression. The US Preventive Services Task Force (USPTF) recommends health communication that works to address disparities and to communicate gaps created by systemic racism in all dissemination efforts (2021). For health communication to address health inequities effectively, it must be coupled with activism that addresses not only the practices and conditions that characterize SDoH in the lived contexts where inequities and disparities are constructed and perpetuated but also in the structural and governance structures where they are articulated and organized. The goal of health communication SJA is to construct a health equity framework characterized by a culture of diversity and bridge the disproportionate burden of health risks and healthcare delivery gaps on poor health outcomes in Indigenous, Black, and Latinx communities and vulnerable populations. SJA illuminates the social causations of disease and addresses how the self-perpetuating cycle of social disadvantage, marginalization, and health disparities can be challenged and dismantled through action.

### *SJA and Collective Action*

SJA motivates collective action from all sectors of society including clinicians, health systems across the care continuum, guideline groups, professional and specialty societies, research funding agencies, PH agencies, policymakers, educators, community leaders, and community members. It supports collaboration that creates mechanisms for sharing best practices, using data to identify and address and monitor the metrics of success on anti-racism and health inequity. SJA, with an emphasis on transformative action, SJ, and communication frameworks focusing on message design, behavior change, and consciousness raising, is central to these efforts.

*As we conclude **Chapter 3, A Social Justice Activist Approach to Health**, consider **Textbox 3.10**. Attempt the SJA prompts that follow.*

**Textbox 3.10    Present Challenges and Future Directions: Principles of SJ**

### WPHC Context

Professional values guide action by members of the profession. They also provide a basis for evaluating the profession's standards and guidelines for appropriate action. The American Association of Colleges of Nursing (AACN, 2023) includes human dignity, integrity, autonomy, altruism, and SJ as its professional values. Education and training are recognized as key approaches in the development of professional values and helping nursing students understand the commitment for social factors affecting health such as lack of access to healthcare, inequitable distribution of healthcare resources, and societal violence. Current initiatives include cocurricular experiences, online learning, and digital storytelling to increase understanding of SJ issues. Some of the challenges in successfully embedding SJ concepts in nursing curricula include a lack of sufficient knowledge and experience in nursing educators to teach and institutionalize SJ. A second shortcoming in current curricular initiatives is the comparative ineffectiveness of traditional approaches such as lecturing in institutionalizing SJ in nursing graduates.

### SJA Discussion Prompt

1. There is increasing recognition of the need to transform medical curricula by integrating SJ training into the curriculum. Medical schools are prioritizing training in improving health equity and reducing health disparities. In addition, they are looking at how a just environment can support the goals of supporting a diverse learner group. Some schools have sought to include more effective and experiential approaches by educators trained in communicating SJ, ethics, and its components such as health literacy.
   a. Design one experiential approach for nursing students to understand what SJ means in a healthcare encounter.
   b. How does the initiative you designed disproportionately disadvantage those with marginalized identities (e.g., gender, LGBTQ+ status, race, income)?
   c. How will your experiential training bring the disadvantages faced by marginalized populations to light in a direct and experiential manner to nursing students?

2. The five principles of SJ include *equity*, *diversity*, *access*, *participation*, and *human rights*. What are some ways in which you can communicate to "amplify and integrate 'invisible-ized' narratives of historically marginalized" healthcare providers and patients" (American Medical Association, 2023) in a way that creates transformative beliefs, attitudes, and behaviors?

3. How would you answer scholars Carragee and Frey (2016) call that *"communication (professionals/researchers) have not intervened enough into social justice struggles,"* (p. 3989)?
   a. How can you imagine intervening in healthcare professional training to raise awareness of the SJ issues that arise in healthcare settings linked with class, gender, race, and sexual orientation, among others?

b. Do you agree with their thought that detachment from such engagement may mean being complicit in and supporting the continuation of oppressive processes and practices?

## Resources

The American Association of Colleges of Nursing. (AACN). Retrieved April 26, 2023, from https://www.aacnnursing.org/

American Medical Association. Retrieved April 26, 2023, from https://www.ama-assn.org/

Carragee, K. M., & Frey, L. R. (2016). Communication activism research: Engaged communication scholarship for social justice. *International Journal of Communication*, *10*, 3975–3999. https://ijoc.org/index.php/ijoc/issue/view/12

## References

AAMC. (2020). Tool for addressing cultural competence training. Retreived from https://www.aamc.org/what-we-do/equity-diversity-inclusion/tool-for-assessing-cultural-competence-training

American Public Health Association. (2022). *Social justice and health*. https://www.apha.org/what-is-public-health/generation-public-health/our-work/social-justice

Arcaya, M. C., Arcaya, A. L., & Subramanian, S. V. (2015). Inequalities in health: Definitions, concepts, and theories. *Global Health Action*, *8*. https://doi.org/10.3402/gha.v8.27106

Arcury, T. A., Preisser, J. S., Gesler, W. M., & Powers, J. M. (2005). Access to transportation and health care utilization in a rural region. *Journal of Rural Health*, *21*(1), 31–38.

Baah, F. O., Teitelman, A. M., & Riegel, B. (2019). Marginalization: Conceptualizing patient vulnerabilities in the framework of social determinants of health—An integrative view. *Nursing Inquiry*, *26*(1), e12268. https://doi.org/10.1111/nin.12268

Beech, B. M., Calles-Escandon, J., Hairston, K. G., Langdon, S. E., Lathan-Sadler, B. A., & Bell, R. A. (2013). Mentoring programs for underrepresented minority faculty in academic medical centers: A systematic review of the literature. *Academic Medicine*, *88*(4), 541–549. https://doi.org/10.1097/ACM.0b013e31828589e3

Broome, B. J., Carey, C., De La Garza, S. A., Martin, J., & Morris, R. (2005). In the thick of things: A dialogue about the activist turn in intercultural communication. In W. J. Starosta & G.-M. Chen (Eds.), *Taking stock in intercultural communication: Where to now?* (pp. 145–175). National Communication Association.

Burgess, D. J., Bokhour, B. G., Cunningham, B. A., Do, T., Gordon, H. S., Jones, D. M., Pope, C., Somnath, S., & Gollust, S.E. (2019). Healthcare providers' responses to narrative communication about racial healthcare disparities. *Health Communication*, *34*(2), 149–161. https://doi.org/10.1080.10410236.2017.1389049

Carragee, K. M., & Frey, L. R. (2012). Introduction: Communication activism for social justice scholarship. In L. R. Frey & K. M. Carragee (Eds.), *Communication activism: Vol. 3. Struggling for social justice amidst difference* (pp. 1–68). Hampton Press.

Clay, W. A., Jackson, D. H., & Harris, K. A. (2021). Does the AAMC's definition of "Underrepresented in Medicine" promote justice and equity? *AMA Journal of Ethics*, *23*(12), E960–E964. https://doi.org/10.1001/amajethics.2021.960

Crenshaw, K. (1989). Demarginalizing the intersection of race and sex: A Black feminist critique of antidiscrimination doctrine, feminist theory, and antiracist politics. *University of Chicago Legal Forum*, *1*, 139–167. https://chicagobound.uchicago.edu/uclf/vol1989/iss1/8

Cruz, D., Rodriguez, Y., & Mastropaolo, C. (2019). Perceived microaggressions in healthcare: A measurement study. *PloS One*, *14*(2), Article e0211620. https://doi.org/10.1371/journal.pone.0211620

Dutta, M. J. (2008). *Communicating health: A culture-centered approach*. Polity Press.

Dutta, M. J., & Kreps, G. L. (2013). Reducing health disparities: Communication interventions. In M. J. Dutta & G. L. Kreps (Eds.), *Reducing health disparities: Communication interventions* (pp. 1–4). Peter Lang.

Dutta, M. J., Moana-Johnson, G., & Elers, C. (2020). COVID-19 and the pedagogy of culture centered community radical democracy: A response from Aotearoa New Zealand. *Journal of Communication Pedagogy, 3*, 11–19. https://doi.org/10.31446/JCP.2020.03

Fallin-Bennett, K. (2015). Implicit bias against sexual minorities in medicine: Cycles of professional influence and the role of the hidden curriculum. *Academic Medicine, 90*(5), 549–552. https://doi.org/10.1097/ACM.000000000000066

Feagin, J., & Bennefield, Z. (2014). Systemic racism and U.S. health care. *Social Science & Medicine, 103*, 7–14. https://www.doi.org/10.1016/j.socscimed.2013.09.006

Frey, L. R., Pearce, W. B., Pollock, M. A., Artz, L., & Murphy, B. A. O. (1996). Looking for justice in all the wrong places: On a communication approach to social justice. *Communication Studies, 47*(1–2), 110–127. https://doi.org/10.1080/10510979609368467

Gordon, H. S., Street, R. L., Jr., Sharf, B. L., & Souchek, J. (2006). Racial differences in doctors' information-giving and patients' participation. *Cancer, 107*(6), 1313–1320. https://doi.org/10.1002/cncr.22122

Guidry, J. J., Aday, L. A., Zhang, D., & Winn, R. J. (1997). Transportation as a barrier to cancer treatment. *Cancer Practice, 5*(6), 361–366. https://doi.org/10.1016/j.clcc.2001.05.001

Hull, S., Stevens, R., & Cobb, J. (2020). Masks are the new condoms: Health communication, intersectionality, and racial equity in COVID-times. *Health Communication, 35*(14), 1740–1742. https://doi.org/10.1080/10410236.2020.1838095

International Covenant on Economic, Social, and Cultural Rights. (ICESCR). U.N. Human Rights. Office of the High Commissioner. (1966). Retreived from https://www.ohchr.org/en/instruments-mechanisms/instruments/international-covenant-economic-social-and-cultural-rights

John A. Burns School of Medicine. (2022). *Center for Native and Pacific Health Disparities Research.* https://native.jabsom.hawaii.edu/

Kosoko-Lasaki, O., Sonnino, R. E., & Voytko, M. L. (2006). Mentoring for women and underrepresented minority faculty and students: Experience at two institutions of higher education. *Journal of the National Medical Association, 98*(9), 1449–1459.

Neely, A. N., Ivey, A. S., Duarte, C., Poe, J., & Irsheid, S. (2020). Building the transdisciplinary resistance collective for research and policy: Implications for dismantling structural racism as a determinant of health inequity. *Ethnic Disparities, 30*(3), 381–388. https://doi.org/10.18865/ed.30.3.381

Razack, S., Hodges, B., Seinert, Y., & Maguire, M. (2015). Seeking inclusion in an exclusive process: Discourses of medical school student selection. *Medical Education, 49*(1), 36–47. https://doi.org/10.1111/medu.12547

United Nations. (2021). Sustainable Development Goals: Goal 3: *Ensure healthy lives and promote well-being for all at all ages.* https://www.un.org/sustainabledevelopment/health/

United Nations (n.d.). Universal declaration of human rights. Retreived from https://www.un.org/en/about-us/universal-declaration-of-human-rights

UN Refugee Agency. (n.d.). *Access to healthcaree.* https://www.unhcr.org/access-healthcaree

*U.S. Preventive Services Task Force.* (USPTF). (2021). Addressing racism in preventive services: A methods project for the U.S. Preventive Services Task Force. AHRQ Publication No. 21-05281-EF-2.

Vardeman-Winter, J. (2017). The framing of women and health disparities: A critical look at race, gender, and class from the perspectives of grassroots health communicators. *Health Communication, 32*(5), 629–638 https://doi.org/10.1080/10410236.2016.1160318

Wagner, T., Ramirez, C., Godoy, B. (2022). COVID-19 rural health inequities: Insights from a real-world scenario. *Journal of Communication in Healthcaree, 15*(1), 22–66. https://doi.org/10.1080/17538068.2021.1975472

Williams, D. R., Lawrence, J. A., & Davis, B. A. (2019). Racism and health: Evidence and needed research. *Annual Review of Public Health, 40*, 105–125. https://doi.org/10.1146/annurev-publhealth-040218-043759

WHO. (2022). *Social determinants of health*. https://www.who.int/health-topics/social-determinants-of-health#tab=tab_1

WHO (2022a). Health promotion. Track 1: Community empowerment. Retrieved from https://www.who.int/teams/health-promotion/enhanced-wellbeing/seventh-global-conference/community-empowerment

Yong, E. (2020, August 19). Long-haulers are redefining COVID-19: Without understanding the lingering illness that some patients experience, we can't understand the pandemic. *The Atlantic* https://www.theatlantic.com/health/archive/2020/08/long-haulers-covid-19-recognition-support-groups-symptoms/615382

## Additional Resources

Agency for Healthcare Research and Quality (AHRQ). (2020). *Strategy 6I. Shared decision making*. https://www.ahrq.gov/cahps/quality-improvement/improvement-guide/6-strategies-for-improving/communication/strategy6i-shared-decisionmaking.html

American Medical Association (AMA). (n.d.). Center for Health Equity. *AMA's Center for Health Equity mission and guiding principles*. https://www.ama-assn.org/about/ama-center-health-equity/ama-s-center-health-equity-mission-and-guiding-principles

AMA. (2021). *Organizational strategic plan to embed racial justice and advance health equity 2021–2023*. https://www.ama-assn.org/system/files/2021-05/ama-equity-strategicplan.pdf

Association of American Medical Colleges (AAMC). (2005). *Cultural competence education*. https://www.aamc.org/media/20856/download

AAMC. (2022). *Underrepresented in medicine definition*. https://www.aamc.org/what-we-do/equity-diversity-inclusion/underrepresented-in-medicine#:~:text=The%20AAMC%20definition%20of%20underrepresented,numbers%20in%20the%20general%20population.%22

CDC. (2011). CDC health disparities and inequalities report–United States, 2011. *Morbidity and Mortality Weekly Report, 60*, 49–51.

Healthy People 2030. (2022). *Discrimination*. https://health.gov/healthypeople/priority-areas/social-determinants-health/literature-summaries/discrimination

Indian Health Service (HIS). (2019). U.S. Department of Health and Human Services. *Disparities*. https://www.ihs.gov/newsroom/factsheets/disparities/

IOM. (2003). Committee on understanding and eliminating racial and ethnic disparities in health care. Introduction and literature review. In Smedley, B. D., Stith, A. Y., Nelson, A. R. (Eds.), *Unequal treatment: Confronting racial and ethnic disparities in health care*. National Academies Press. https://www.ncbi.nlm.nih.gov/books/NBK220344/

National Institute on Minority Health and Health Disparities (NIMHHD). (2021). *Overview*. https://www.nimhd.nih.gov/about/overview/

National LGBTQIA+ Health Education Center. (2022). *Health education*. The Fenway Institute. https://edhub.ama-assn.org/fenway-institute-eduLGBTQI+

WHO. (2019). *Participation as a driver of health equity*. https://apps.who.int/iris/bitstream/handle/10665/324909/9789289054126eng.pdf?sequence=1&isAllowed=y

# Section II

# Constructing Health

# Chapter 4

# Evolving Understandings of Health

**Chapter Learning Outcomes**

Upon completing **Chapter 4, Evolving Understandings of Health**, the student should be able to integrate the **WPHC SJA** perspective to:

1. Understand patient-centered care through the elements of integrative healthcare approaches and the therapeutic relationship.
2. Identify how diversity is central to the conceptualization, training, and delivery of healthcare.
3. Understand the elements of provider self-fulfillment, worker diversity, minority physician development, and uniform standards for graduate medical education.
4. Define the three different meanings of health in use and the distinctions between them.
5. Explain integrative medicine and complementary and alternative medicine as a part of the WPHC SJA framework.
6. Understand how interprofessional communication aids in the coordination of multiple systems of care.
7. Explain the collaborative approach principles guiding the ecological model of health and their contribution to the design of multilevel interventions in nature.
8. Situate how understanding the clinician-patient communication processes as socially constructed supports patient empowerment in ways that lead to concordance.
9. Explain how a value-based approach and integrated medical and social care offer a pathway for the future evolution of health from a well-being-centered WPHC SJA framework.

**Consider the following scenario:**

A medical resident pens an essay documenting his struggles dealing with the cancer diagnosis of his significant other.

(Posted by Jordan Michael Morrison-Nozik on the Health Humanities List Serv, January 19, 2023)

DOI: 10.4324/9781003214472-6

Time fractured when my first husband died.

There was a before, which no longer existed, and an after, which was unimaginable.

In between, the thinnest—unfathomably thin—line, was the today. The today meant putting one foot in front of the other. One today led to the next today. And finally the year was over.

(Time splintered by Scott-Conner, Carol, January 13, 2023, on PulseVoices.org)

In the poetic narrative, Carol Scott-Conner, a physician, shares her narrative of processing her spouse's death in a moving heart-felt essay. Narratives and storytelling such as Carol's acknowledge and recognize the healthcare provider as a human being and center their empathy, feelings, and vulnerability in the healthcare setting. Such recognition of both the healthcare provider and the patient's vulnerability is central to the WPHC-centered approach, an evolving understanding of how the practice of medicine should be embodied by patients, providers, caregivers, community members, and others collaborating in a shared effort to co-create a mutually constructed understanding of health.

## Chapter Overview

**Chapter 4, Evolving Understandings of Health**, will focus on an examination of how evolving understandings of health reflect diversity in understandings of health, healthcare approaches, and healthcare systems. It will explain how healthcare outcomes and delivery mechanisms are assessed to address disparities and advance health equity. **Chapter 4** is organized as follows: **First**, it will attend to how patient-care goals are achieved through WPHC in collaborative care and address provider stress and burnout and practitioner self-fulfillment. **Second**, it will focus on integrative medicine and complementary and alternative medicine as conceptualized through the lens of WPHC SJA approaches, highlighting interconnectedness, the therapeutic relationship, the multilayered nature of illness, interprofessional communication, and evidence-based inquiry. **Third**, it will focus on ecological models of health, emphasizing its components, the principles guiding the relationship between people and their context, emphasis on nature in designing complex interventions centering the individual in a situated context through mutual construction of collaboration and trust and concordance. **Fourth**, it will address evolving understandings of health through the lens of integrated medical and social care, vertical and horizontal integration, and the value-based WPHC IM care model centering well-being and inclusivity. Along the way, students will be engaged in discussion questions, case studies, present challenges and future directions exercises, and thought prompts for reflection. Students will be encouraged to apply the tenets of WPHC SJA in contexts ranging from patient care in graphic medicine to the employment of metaphors to address health equity as a structural problem, ecological approach to healthy campuses, and racial disparities in maternal mortality in the United States through the lens of the Quintuple Aim and health justice. A communication scholar interview with Dr. Maria Lapinski-LaFaive will highlight her perspective on interconnectedness in One Health with a social research and community participatory focus that brings people together globally.

## Diversity in Understandings of Health

As the chapters in Section I demonstrate, to deliver care that is equitable and addresses the contexts from which disparities arise, the healthcare provider cultivates an understanding of the patient as a whole person, with their attitudes and beliefs, values, cultural preferences, and family and community traditions. Delivering patient-centered care (PCC) in this manner wherein the patient is seen as a unique multidimensional human being, comprising the body, mind, and spirit, is the goal of WPHC.

### Whole Person Healthcare

#### WPHC and Emphasis on PCC

WPHC is PCC because it brings together a diverse range of healthcare resources to understand and meet the needs of each individual patient. In tailoring care to the individual patient, whole person care also considers the physical, behavioral, emotional, and social services that may be required to deliver the quality of care to achieve optimal well-being and health outcomes. WPHC seeks to respect each patient's individual values and beliefs and how they may impact their treatment choices.

#### WPHC and Emphasis on Diversity

A close understanding of diversity attends to the individual needs and backgrounds of each patient. Being aware of the distinct needs of diverse population groups plays a critical role in addressing the disparate risk factors (such as housing insecurity, lack of health insurance, low health literacy) facing disadvantaged, minority, and marginalized populations. Addressing these risk factors involves an intersection with the human services, housing, and social services functions of public health. Just as understanding diversity in patient populations is important to achieving successful health outcomes, it is important to build diversity in how healthcare and health are understood and conceptualized.

*Table 4.1 will give you a deeper look at the diversity of specialists, professionals, and approaches involved in WPHC.*

Table 4.1 Specialists included in WPHC Care Coordination

| Healthcare and Allied Healthcare Providers in WPHC | Elements of WPHC Approaches |
|---|---|
| Physicians and surgeons<br>Holistic nurses<br>Obstetrician gynecologists (OB-GYNs)<br>Social workers<br>Public health officials<br>Psychologists<br>Chaplains<br>Pharmacists<br>Massage therapists<br>Nutritionists and dietitians<br>Yoga and meditation therapists<br>Acupuncturists<br>Midwives<br>Dietitians<br>Audiologists<br>Nurse anesthetists<br>Speech, occupation, and physical therapists<br>Paramedics and emergency medical technicians (EMTs)EMTs include basic-level EMTs (EMT-As) and EMT-paramedics (EMT-Ps)<br>Counselors<br>Dental hygienists<br>Occupational therapists<br>Radiologic technologists and technicians (including nuclear medicine technologists, diagnostic medical sonographers, radiographers)<br>Physical therapists<br>Respiratory therapists<br>Medical record services<br>Wellness coaches | • A **WPHC** physician will treat the **whole person** across a **lifespan** instead of focusing on a specific disease. They seek to **restore** health, promote **resilience**, and **prevent disease** across a spectrum of **interconnected** biological, behavioral, social, and environmental areas (NCCIH, 2023).<br><br>• **WPHC coordination of care** involves healthcare, behavioral health, social services, public health, and complementary and integrative health professionals (AHCCS, 2023)<br><br>• **WPHC patient-centered approaches** emphasize health promotion, collaborative decision-making, patient resilience, and well-being.<br><br>• **WPHC coordination of care** is comprehensive across target populations, data sharing among systems, coordination of care in real time, evaluation of individual and population progress.<br><br>• **WPHC** focuses on **social risk factors** such as transitional housing, nonmedical transportation services for access to community-based services such as healthy food and employment.<br><br>• **WPHC service delivery** aims at reducing **social isolation** and partnering with health information exchange to have **a referral system** that enables healthcare providers to smoothly screen and refer members to **community-based** social service organizations. |

## Resources

Arizona Health Care Cost Containment System. (2023). *Whole person care initiative (WPCI).* Retrieved from https://www.azahcccs.gov/AHCCCS/Initiatives/AHCCCSWPCI/

National Center for Complementary and Integrative Health (NCCIH). (2023, February 4). *Whole person health: What you need to know.* Retrieved from https://www.nccih.nih.gov/health/whole-person-health-what-you-need-to-know

National Library of Medicine (NLM). (1989). *What does "allied health" mean? Allied Health Services: Avoiding crises.* Retrieved from https://www.ncbi.nlm.nih.gov/books/NBK218850/

*WPHC as Centering Humanistic Approaches in Provider Well-Being*

WPHC invites providers to acknowledge their own humanity in the healthcare relationship. Providers face stress and burnout because of emotional intensity, occupational hazards,

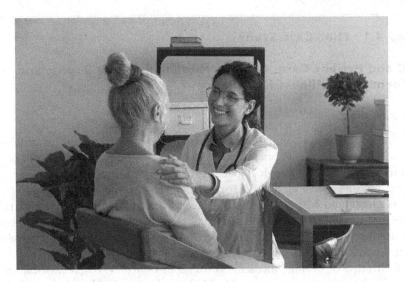

*Figure 4.1* Engaging the Self in Provider-Patient Interaction.

racism, discrimination, depersonalization, and lack of meaning in work (Agency for Healthcare Research and Quality,AHRQ, 2017; Brumback, 2022). Provider burnout can impact patient safety, quality of care, and continuity of care. Racism and discrimination faced by minority physicians and healthcare providers in the workplace aggravate stress, provider burnout, and lack of diversity in the medical profession (Serafina et al., 2020). The National Medical Association, which represents African American physicians and health professionals in the United States, lists among its priority issues on medical education to increase workforce diversity, minority physician recruitment and development, and development of uniform standards for graduate medical education for remediation, probation, and termination of resident physicians in training (2019–2020; National Medical Association, NMA, n.d.).

Acknowledging the humanity of the healthcare provider allows healthcare providers to cultivate a critical self-awareness of their beliefs, thoughts, and feelings, in the patient-provider interaction (Agarwal, 2019, 2018). For instance, Epstein suggests that doctors ask themselves: "What parts of your self are you engaging in the care of this patient, right now?," followed with, "Does it have to be that way?" Whole person medicine supports practitioner self-fulfillment by developing their analytical skills and ability to think in terms of an interconnected complex web of factors that make up an individual's health domain beyond the clinical isolation of causal factors (Thomas et al., 2018). The patient-centered medical home implementation seeks to enhance care coordination and improve physician satisfaction by placing patients at the center (AHRQ, 2022). This shift in considering a complex web of factors allows the physician to acknowledge the intersecting social, environmental, and behavioral factors that comprise the circumstances of each patient and include them in the clinical process, along with the biomedical factors (Welch-Cline, 2003).

*How does the mini-case study of graphic medicine presented in **Textbox 4.1** highlight innovative ways of imagining provider and patient self-fulfillment that transforms the patient illness experience and provider healthcare delivery and conceptualization experience?*

**Textbox 4.1    Mini-Case Study**

**WPHC and Patient Care: Graphic Medicine, Comic Books, and Transforming the Illness Experience**

*WPHC Patient Care*

Patient care is not always communicated in healthcare speak by medical professionals. Stories, anecdotes, narratives, poems, and even comics are entering the world of healthcare communication in the provider-patient realm. Graphic medicine is a new medium utilizing comics as a way of telling stories of illness through graphic pathologies. As Professors Green and Myers (2010) put it, graphic pathologies offer insights that may not come up in a clinical setting and thus may be instrumental in addressing communication misconceptions by shaping how we think about the experience of disease and treatment and ultimately, patient compliance and prognosis.

One illustration of graphic medicine is found in *Cancer Vixen*, a cartoon for *Glamour*, wherein the cartoonist, Marissa Marchetto, who was battling cancer while doing the cartoons, documents how her own cartoon alter ego helped her in her cancer journey from diagnosis to survivor. Visit the URL in the Resources section to see *Cancer Vixen's* description.

How does it embody the humanistic ethos in medicine and healthcare?

Other publications, such as *Pulse: Voices from the Heart of Medicine*, share personal experiences of healthcare providers and patients giving and receiving healthcare in intimate, authentic, and often candid narrative form. In her story, "Living and Letting Go in the ICU," author Margie Hodges Shaw, an associate professor of clinical bioethics in an Upstate New York academic medical center and medical school, writes about letting her mother go. During admitting her to the palliative care unit, when she asks the critical-care attending physician, "Does the hospital have a palliative-care unit?," and the attending says, "No ... we're prepared to navigate that process with you here in this room," she notes, "As kind as the response was, I wished for more–or less. Less monitoring, less intrusion, less intensive medicine. More peace and quiet. My mother craved peace and quiet."

Shaw's story embodies the form of self-reflection and other-directed perspectives WPHC-centered medical professionals seek in instances that involve suffering, differing values, and death.

*SJA Prompt*

• How can the stories WPHC providers tell make medicine more human and more patient-centered?

**Resources**

Green, M. J., & Myers, K. R. (2010). Graphic medicine: Use of comics in medical education and patient care. *BMJ, 340*. https://doi.org/10.1136/bmj.c863

Marchetto, M. (2007, March 5). *Cancer vixen*. Fourth Estate. Retrieved from https://bookshop.org/p/books/cancer-vixen-a-true-story-marisa-acocella-marchetto/6813383?ean=9780375714740

Pulse: Voices from the Heart of Medicine. (2023). *Stories*. Retrieved from https://pulsevoices.org/

Shae, M. H. (2023, February 3). *Living and letting go in the ICU*. Pulse. Retrieved from https://pulsevoices.org/index.php/stories/living-and-letting-go-inthe-icu

*Centering WPHC in the Meanings of Health*

As discussed in Chapter 1, the definition of health has expanded beyond the biophysiological to center psychosocial, communicative, historical, and environmental contexts. Early understandings define health as the absence of disease. A second definition emphasizes health as a state that allows the individual to cope with all the demands of daily life. The third definition of health, which reflects contemporary understandings, describes health as a state of balance or equilibrium that an individual has established within themselves and with their social and physical environment (Sartorius, 2006).

The emphasis in the third statement suggests that health includes living well with disease or impairment if there is the presence of balance or equilibrium that enables the individual to live a quality of life by their choice. For instance, the patient and the provider may work together to address the disease and restore balance with the internal and external environment. It also emphasizes the shift toward understanding how patients themselves feel about their disease and health as a condition of their clinical care. In this manner, the third statement takes an important step toward making the practice of medicine both clinical, patient-centered, and humanistic. Likewise, with health promotion efforts, the third statement emphasizes an empowered patient who is actively involved in undertaking decisions about improving their health. The third statement also emphasizes the environment such as the relationships (friends, family), the social context (media, politics, economics, community), legal (laws and policies), and so on in enacting health.

## Integrative Medicine

### Understanding Integrative Medicine (IM)

IM promotes health by nurturing the balance between mind, body, and spirit using evidence-based conventional and complementary treatments and services. As the landscape of medicine in the United States shifts toward a holistic and individualized approach to healing and health, the evolution of IM care captures the socio-cultural, regulatory, and structural changes in healthcare. The goals of IM go beyond treating a medical diagnosis in a human body to address the source of the imbalance or dysfunction before it presents as disease. Evidence-based complementary and integrative medicine (CIM) approaches are gradually shifting into mainstream medicine. IM incorporates both western and alternative forms of medicine.

### WPHC and IM

WPHC is foundational to IM approaches. Although IM is more expensive, the benefits it offers by offsetting future care and clinical treatments offer greater benefits to patient outcomes. For instance, patients with acute strokes who were managed by IM and those who were managed by biomedical approaches only had marked differences in outcomes at the 3- and 12-month mark after discharge (Park et al., 2018), In this case, those who were treated with IM had reduced all-risk mortality at the 3- and 12-month mark after discharge, which may have prevented future hospital admissions, and ultimately reduced patient costs.

*Using Complementary and Alternative Medicine (CAM)*

To treat the patient using WPHC, IM leverages a range of specialists, technologically sourced next-generation data sharing between the specialists, community partners, CAM professionals, and social services professionals. The interdisciplinary approach centers principles and treatments applied by CAM providers to clinical case management. IM protocols are implemented in a range of hospitals, healthcare systems, community health centers, and medical centers. Researchers Shin and Shim emphasize how health communication where expert accounts and lay accounts are both considered equally can help improve health outcomes from treatment using CAM recommended by both professionals and personal networks of family, friends, and coworkers (2019).

### Multidimensional, Integrated Approach

WPHC IM care is characterized by a multidimensional, integrated approach. IM care emphasizes biopsychosocial, holistic, and whole person approaches. The WPHC IM approach considers the individual in their context and goes beyond the biomedical to consider the mental, emotional, ecological, environmental, and spiritual aspects of the individual's life. It recognizes the interconnectedness of illness and disease with multiple facets of the individual life and allows for the integration of CAM approaches (e.g., acupuncture, mind-body therapies, and massage).

### Scientific Inquiry

Although it seeks to integrate a range of approaches, IM treatments are rooted in scientific, evidence-based inquiry. IM centers are available at multiple levels of care as consultation, PC, or comprehensive care. There are several criteria by which IM centers deliver improved care. First, patients from IM centers report overall improved healthfulness in symptom improvement during disease. This is illustrated in the case of breast cancer and other forms of cancer treatments. In these cases, patients were more likely to take ownership of their care and report an improvement in cognitive and emotional functioning along with overall global health. These improvements have been attributed to IM's focus on addressing the complexity of healing and palliative treatment necessary to address the emotional and spiritual components of the disease management process beyond the physical symptom and pain management.

*Review* **Textbox 4.2**, **Scholar Interview** *of* **Dr. Maria Knight Lapinski-LaFaive** *to understand how one communication researcher incorporates interconnectedness, context, and the environment in her scholarship.*

---

### TEXTBOX 4.2    Scholar Interview

**Dr. Maria Knight Lapinski-LaFaive**
*Michigan State University*

My interest in One Health scholarship started opportunistically to organize my thinking about how to approach communication research and to label the work I was doing in a way that others could more easily make sense of it. When I started my dissertation research in the late 1990s, I was working at the intersection of several major areas in the field: social influence, environmental, health, and intercultural communication. I needed a way to connect those different areas. I eventually saw One Health—or the ways in which the connections between human, animal, and ecological health are synergistic—as a way to frame my teaching and research in communication. Social research, and communication science research particularly, was not being talked about in the One Health/One Medicine sphere at that time and is still on the margins of that work, even though many scholars recognize its value. My own work in One Health involves a range of bringing people together to solve One Health challenges, working to help set a global agenda for One Health research and practice, and identifying solutions to the human behavior elements of One Health problems like watershed protection, zoonotic diseases, and domesticated animal health.

My own approach to research does not come from a social justice frame. I do not identify as a research activist, but I have, through my career, worked with activist communities to do research to inform problems. I have also centered culture in my research and as such have addressed health and environmental disparities. This includes work with communities on issues like HIV prevention, breast cancer risk reduction, access to maternal and mental healthcare, land and watershed conservation, and others. Fundamentally, I can best characterize my research approach as community participatory.

### Centering the Therapeutic Relationship

IM care centers the therapeutic relationship. The therapeutic relationship brings a collaborative approach to IM provider-patient relationship and emphasizes the relational domain of treatment and care (Agarwal, 2020). Emphasizing the therapeutic relationship also centers the provider's own attitudes, values, and beliefs (Agarwal, 2018). It also asks for the provider to be patient-centered by attending to the patient's values and beliefs, being compassionate, supportive, nonjudgmental, and listening to the patient's preferences. By recognizing the patient's personhood, the provider acknowledges what is unique in each patient. This implies being aware of the complex and multilayered nature of illness.

### Patient-Centered Care

The Institute of Medicine (IOM) defines PCC as being respectful of the patient and responsive to their preferences, needs, and values. In this manner, IM care includes storytelling, centering the patient's life journey, and shared decision-making as some of its key tenets. Communication researchers Fisher et al. (2019) examine how translational tools can be aided using metaphorical language by patients and providers in a family medicine setting to explain health experiences. They note that metaphors have been found to be counterproductive when discussing treatments that are unfamiliar, complex, or stigmatized as is often the case in IM settings where conventional medicine providers (e.g., family medicine physicians) offer patients CAM therapies like acupuncture (Bull, 2009). Communication studies such as those by Fisher and colleagues illustrate the power of metaphor in conventional medicine settings by allowing physicians and patients to collaboratively make sense of traditional Eastern medical practices by using familiar concepts.

*Review **Textbox 4.3** for an illustration of how a tree metaphor can illustrate health equity as a structural issue and attempt the SJA prompt.*

---

**Textbox 4.3    Discussion Questions/Thought Scenarios for Reflection**

**Critically Designing the Tree Metaphor to Address Health Equity as a Structural Problem versus an Individual Problem**

*WPHC Thought Scenario: Metaphors to Address Health Equity as a Structural Problem*

The Equity Lens in Public Health (ELPH) Research Project aims to address health equity by focusing on how we communicate about health equity. Inadequate and inaccurate representations of health equity can pose a barrier to constructing shared understandings. To do this, they focus on metaphors that "use images or phrases to communicate complex concepts..." and "to increase understanding and facilitate discussion of how to promote health equity and remove barriers that produce health inequities" (Shahram et al., 2017). Metaphors can help visually critique the health impact of injustice by showcasing politics, agency, power, and accountability (Krieger et al., 2012).

A metaphor is a communication device that encourages understanding of one thing or experience in terms of another (Lakoff & Johnson, 2008). Examples of a health metaphor might be the heart as a pump or the brain as a computer. Robert Entman incorporated metaphors in his definition of framing; thus, metaphors allow us to "select some aspects of a perceived reality and make them ore salient in a communicating text, in such a way as to promote a particular problem definition, causal interpretation, moral evaluation, and/or treatment recommendation for the item described" (Entman, 1993).

Shahram and colleagues recommend selecting metaphors critically, considering the audience, and the intended meaning of the message to promote active learning and reflection about health equity.

Shahram and colleagues recommend the following steps in their ELPH report:

1. **Frame the conversation**: Define health equity and its relationship with social justice values of challenging power and privilege, and socially constructed inequalities that stem from systematic oppression and disadvantage.
2. **Assess the intention**: Examine the metaphor for its communication about health equity focus on social conditions rather than individual characteristics.
3. **Deconstruct the metaphor**: For each piece of the visual, consider what each element might represent for your intended audience.
4. **Critically appraise the metaphor**: Examine the metaphor from the principles of social justice—what does access mean? How do SDoH position people for equitable access to resources for health?

5. **Reconstruct the metaphor**: Keep in mind the principles of social justice to reconstruct the metaphor. Identify what challenges present themselves.
6. **Envision effective action**: Create strategies to promote health equity that target structural factors that create inequities.

The Minnesota Department of Health provides the example of Dr. Camara Jones, MD, MPH, PhD, as she presents the cliff analogy to illustrate how people fall off the "cliff of good health." She uses a cliff to show the impact of social conditions, such as systems, structures, and policies; SDoH, such as race, poverty, gender, sexuality; and other inequities on health. She uses the cliff metaphor to call communities and professionals for action on the social conditions to eliminate health disparities to ask her audience: "what are the different parts of the cliff? What did you see?; What came to mind as you watched and listened?; What resonated with you? Where did you struggle?; Where do we spend most of our time and energy in public health?; What does the Cliff Analogy of Health ask us to do as public health professionals?"

## SJA Discussion Prompt

Craft the visual metaphor of a tree to communicate SDoH in action for a mental health theme: our environments cultivate our communities, and our communities nurture our health (source: Ramirez et al., 2008).

1. Use the following SDoH and outcomes to mark the roots, stem, and leaves of the tree:
   Poor quality schools, adverse living conditions, unemployment, tobacco and alcohol marketing, poverty, environmental toxins, discrimination, institutional racism, occupational hazards, segregation, disinvestment, disconnected members, restricted power, fragmented healthcare systems, heart disease, depression, obesity, stress, infant mortality, HIV/AIDS, substance abuse, smoking, and malnutrition.
2. Discuss the principles of SJ to see how you can use the health metaphor of the tree equitably, critically, and creatively:
   a. How can your visual communicate health equality?
   b. What can it say about health equity?
   c. What message does it communicate about the relationship between social and health equity? What should be said that is not said?

## Resources

Entman, R. M. (1993). Framing: Toward clarification of a fractured paradigm. *Journal of Communication, 43*(4), 51–58. https://doi.org/10.1111/j.1460-2466.1993.tb01304.x

Krieger, N., Dorling, D., & McCartney, G. (2012). Mapping injustice, visualizing equity: Why theory, metaphors, and images matter in tackling inequalities. *Public Health, 126*(3), 256–258. https://doi.org/10.1016/j.puhe.2012.01.028

Lakoff, G., & Johnson, M. (2008). *Metaphors we live by*. University of Chicago Press.

Minnesota Department of Health. (2022, October 3). *Cliff analogy of health*. https://www.health.state.mn.us/communities/practice/resources/equitylibrary/jonescliff.html

Ramirez, B. L. K., Baker, E. A., & Metzler, M. (2008). *Promoting health equity: A resource to help communities address social determinants of health*. Centers for Disease Control and Prevention. https://www.cdc.gov/nccdphp/dch/programs/healthycommunitiesprogram/tools/pdf/sdoh-workshop.pdf

PHABC Conference. (2016, December 12). *Workshop: Metaphor as a teaching tool for health equity*. https://phabc.org/wpcontent/uploads/2016/12/Metaphor-as-a-Teaching-Tool-for-Health-Equity.pdf

Shahram, S. Z., Dyck, L., van Roode, T., Strosher, H. W., Revai, T., Dang, P., MacDonald, M., & Pauly, B. (2017). *Health equity metaphors for effective communication*. The Equity Lens in Public Health (ELPH) Research Project. https://www.uvic.ca/research/projects/elph/assets/docs/KTE%20Resource%204%20%20HE%20Metaphors%20for%20Effective%20Communication.pdf

## WPHC and Interprofessional Communication

Achieving the goals of IM care implies the coordination of different systems of care. It involves effective interprofessional communication between multiple teams that may disagree on conflicting treatment approaches. Overall, IM approaches have been shown to increase patient satisfaction and provide patients with a greater sense of control over their treatment and health decision-making. For instance, most chronic care and cancer patients request CAM modalities in their care in addition to or alongside their biomedical treatment (Rajamma & Pelton, 2010).

### Barriers to Interprofessional Communication and IM

Several structural and social barriers exist at the interprofessional and literacy level in the achievement of the goals of IM. At the provider level, studies show that most doctors, nurses, and pharmacists in the oncology domain lack the appropriate knowledge to inform evidence-based CAM use (e.g., in a cancer care setting), suggesting a need to include research-based CAM education in medical education. The lack of provider knowledge often results in a dismissive attitude and discouragement of using CAM in their patient communication and practice (Keene et al., 2020). Researchers Broom and Adams (2009) identify the themes of risk, irrationality, seeking control, and desperation in oncology consultants as shaping CAM use, whereas nurses were perceived as CAM and patient advocates. Their study illuminates barriers in oncology care inherent in clinician-patient communication about CAM. Roberts et al. (2020) look at the communication model between acupuncturists and general practitioners to show that interprofessional communication can be facilitated through the systematic creation of a toolkit that contains elements of routine clinical practice for both clinical and CAM providers. Such research has the potential to integrate understandings across diverse workforce cultures in medicine.

*Examine **Table 4.2** to connect how clinician goals in a conventional medical system translate to the WHPC approach. How effectively does this translation counter systemic oppression and health inequities for disadvantaged and minority populations? Attempt the WPHC and SJA context of postpartum care for Black women that follows.*

Table 4.2 Collaborative WPHC Coordination in IM Settings

| Clinician Goals | WPHC Approach | SJA Critique and Health Equity Recommendations in Value-Based Payment and Delivery Reform* |
|---|---|---|
| Identify high-risk target populations | Integrate SDoH. Emphasizes housing instability, substance use disorders that integrate housing support, social services, and mental health services. | 1. Examine the **National Quality Forum's** road map for "disparities-sensitive" measures that ensure an accurate and complete collection of sociodemographic data.<br>2. Provide **patient engagement** incentives to improve documentation.<br>3. Improved data captures **intersectionalities** and improves quality through **stratified reports** and ensures action on disparities. |
| Embrace care coordination between multiple specialists and healthcare systems | Nurtures patient needs spanning social, emotional, and economic, and addresses the environmental conditions that affect their healthcare and quality of life. | 1. Enhance **healthcare organizations'** capacities and culture to collaborate with nonhealthcare and allied healthcare providers to bring in greater diversity that complements the cultural competency of clinicians and enhances governance structures.<br>2. Leverage community **health workers** to address social determinants of health and implement **virtual care options** to expand access. |
| Facilitate specialist referrals and referrals to community partners | Emphasizes a multidimensional, multisystemic, and collaborative care coordination approach. | 1. Integrate **structural reform** through screening patients for unmet social needs.<br>2. Partner with **community-based organizations** to organize structural modifications in housing and transportation.<br>3. Data sharing and cross-sector staff ensure effective **coordination of care** that is inclusive of health and social needs for disadvantaged and minority populations. |
| Evaluate clinician performance | Links performance measurement with careful consideration of which data elements to select for contextualizing data. For instance, labeling race, rather than racism, risks pathologizing race. | 1. Structurally, **payers** can consider increasing **upfront reimbursement** for organizations caring for **socially vulnerable populations** and higher-risk beneficiaries (e.g., Medicaid beneficiaries)<br>2. Include medical and behavioral diagnoses with social factors such as housing stability and neighborhood stress scores in evaluating clinician performance. |

*(Continued)*

*Table 4.2* (Continued) Collaborative WPHC Coordination in IM Settings

## WPHC Context: Postpartum Care for Black Women

**Postpartum care,** or care received by new mothers and their infants, is critical for ensuring maternal and newborn long-term health and well-being. Current recommendations state that all women should contact their OB-GYNs within the first three weeks of postpartum (The American College of Obstetricians and Gynecologists, ACOG, 2021). According to ACOG, rather than a single visit, postpartum care should be an ongoing process, concluding with a comprehensive postpartum visit not later than 12 weeks after birth. The comprehensive postpartum visit should include a full assessment of physical, social, and psychological well-being, including mood and emotional well-being, infant care and feeding; sexuality, contraception, and birth spacing; sleep and fatigue; physical recovery from birth; chronic disease management; and health maintenance. The change in scope of postpartum care as an ongoing process, not a single visit. Evidence suggests that enhanced ongoing postpartum care can make a significant difference for minority women: anticipatory guidance, or guidance given before hospital discharge, followed by a phone call at two weeks was found to reduce symptoms of depression and increased breastfeeding duration through six months postpartum among African American and Hispanic women (Howell et al., 2012).

## SJA Discussion Prompt

Research shows that Black birthing people are more likely to experience long-lasting mental health concerns after childbirth than their non-Black counterparts. Yet, Black mothers typically receive less mental health support for postpartum depression. The CDC's *Hear Her*™ campaign (2022) supports pregnant and postpartum women in their healthcare efforts. The campaign's website provides helpful content for postpartum women to identify warning signs, communicate effectively with their healthcare provider, and encourage women to receive postpartum care. Likewise, missed or delayed diagnoses of issues like hypertension and lack of action from providers of warning signs suggest that pregnancy-related deaths for Black and American Indian/Alaska Native women older than 30 were four to five times as high as they were for White women (CDC, 2019).

1. Research shows that expectant Black mothers were four times more likely to experience posttraumatic stress disorder (PTSD) than non-Black mothers. They were also less likely to seek or receive mental health treatment. Generational and systemic racism is a source of chronic stress (APA, 2022), a phenomenon researcher Neal-Barnett labels "weathering" (Neal-Barnett, 2010). Create a communication guide that can help healthcare providers to listen meaningfully to their Black women patients to identify environmental barriers in their lived contexts. These could range from housing instability to food insecurity and environmental toxins.
2. Create a vision board that can illustrate for a healthcare provider what it is like to be a pregnant Black woman in the twenty-first century.
3. What initiatives can healthcare providers take to build a more trusting relationship with Black women patients?
4. Black-centered group therapy and sister circles have reported positive health outcomes in expectant Black mothers. Design a community-centered approach that supports community ownership and empowerment in countering the chronic generational stress faced by Black women.
5. What initiatives can help healthcare providers engage in culturally sensitive postpartum care?
6. Make a list of SDoH and structural barriers that may impact postpartum care for Black mothers (e.g., flexible employment schedule, health insurance, safe neighborhoods).

## Resources

ACOG. (2021). Optimizing postpartum care. Retrieved April 26, 2023, from https://www.acog.org/clinical/clinical-guidance/committee-opinion/articles/2018/05/optimizing-postpartum-care#:~:text=The%20comprehensive%20postpartum%20visit%20should,recovery%20from%20birth%3B3B%20chronic%20disease

American Psychological Association. (2022). Focusing on maternity and postpartum care for Black mothers leads to better outcomes. Retrieved April 26, 2023, from https://www.apa.org/monitor/2022/10/better-care-black-mothers

CDC. (2019). Racial and ethnic disparities continue in pregnancy-related deaths. Retrieved April 26, 2023, from https://www.cdc.gov/media/releases/2019/p0905-racial-ethnic-disparities-pregnancy-deaths.html

CDC. (2022). Hear Her™ campaign: Pregnant and postpartum women. Retrieved April 26, 2023, https://www.cdc.gov/hearher/pregnant-postpartum-women/index.html

Howell, E. A., Balbierz, A., Wang, J., Parides, M., Zlotnick, C., & Levanthal, H. (2012). Reducing postpartum depressive symptoms among black and Latina mothers: A randomized controlled trial. Obstetrician Gynecology, 119, 942–949.

National Quality Forum (NQF). NQF issues quality roadmap for reducing healthcare disparities. Retrieved April 26, 2023, from https://www.quality forum.org/NQFs_Roadmap_to_Health_Equity.aspx

Neal-Barnett, A. (2010). Soothe your nerves: The Black woman's guide to understanding and overcoming anxiety, panic, and fear. Simon & Schuster.

Sandhu, S., Saunders, R. S., McClellan, M. B., & Wong, C. A. (2020, November 25). Health equity should be a key value in value-based payment and delivery reform. Health Affairs. https://doi.org/10.1377/forefront.20201119.836369

Welkin Health. (2021, April 06). Whole-person care comes full circle. https://welkinhealth.com/whole-person-care/

* Sandhu, S., Saunders, R. S., McClellan, M. B., & Wong, C. A. (2020, November 25). Health equity should be a key value in value-based payment and delivery reform. Health Affairs. https://doi.org/10.1377/forefront.20201119.836369

*Barriers to Implementation of IM in Institutional Settings*

Several barriers exist in the effective implementation of IM in institutional settings. The news media often frames CAM negatively as lucrative, unethical, and with a poor evidence base (Lewis, 2020). Because it is largely nonreimbursable, a system-level barrier in the integration of IM is the increased hospital costs of adding CAM programs and centers (Maruthappu et al., 2015). A third barrier to the successful adoption of IM programs is the lack of clinician training in the ideologies and practices of CAM integration. Fourth, the lack of provider knowledge of the IM modalities and implementation remains one of the central challenges. Fifth, health literacy also plays into the lack of acceptance of CAM modalities. Studies examining the relationship between health literacy and CAM use in low-income racially diverse patients show that those with higher health literacy were more likely to make use of CAM modalities such as relaxation techniques (Gardiner et al., 2013).

## Ecological Views of Health

### Ecological Model (EM)

EMs emphasize the interdependence of influences from one's environment and the contexts in which the behavior occurs. EMs attempt to address the limitations of health behavior change models, which place the onus of change on the individual, are based on purely objective, quantitatively assessed understandings of health and disease, and view health through the lens of deficits (Agarwal, 2020; Richard et al., 2011). EMs emphasize the complex factors comprising an individual's context as a key influence in shaping behavior. They foreground the interdependence between the individual and their environment as a dynamic process that shapes health. EMs are conceptualized through four components: (a) the relationship between people and their context, (b) the social construction of ecological knowledge, (c) the approach to collaboration, and (d) the social processes comprising the ecological settings.

### Relationship between Individuals and Context

From a WPHC perspective, ten main principles guide the understandings of the relationship between people and their context. These include (a) a shared and mutual understanding of how people appreciate their own context; (b) how people use their resources and negotiate constraints at the personal, organizational, and community levels; (c) how shared norms that guide the response to resources and constraints are understood; (d) how social settings define shared meaning and experiences of people; (e) how people enact behaviors based on how people employ and engage with available resources; (f) how people adapt their behavior based on situation and time; (g) how people enact relationships in a reciprocal manner taking into account the relationships between context and individuals; (h) how external settings shape the immediate context and the expression of norms and structures within it; (i) how interdependencies and relationships within one setting influence those in another setting; and (j) how social processes support or constrain interdependence of individuals and their social settings, roles, and norms (Kingry-Westergaard & Kelly, 1990). Select salient dimensions are discussed in detail in the following subsections.

*Look at the mini-case study presented in **Textbox 4.4** to consider an application of the ecological approach on college campuses. What does it tell you about your college campus?*

**Textbox 4.4   Mini-Case Study**

**A WPHC Approach: Healthy Campuses**

The American College Health Association (ACHA) provides an interesting application of the EM of **health on college campuses**. They ask, "What makes some students, faculty, and staff healthy and others unhealthy?"

At its heart, this question takes an ecological approach centered in WPHC because it considers how contexts shape health outcomes, takes an interest in the population but also in the individual, and looks for solutions that are community-based and not simply focused on the individual. Note also that it does not place the onus for being healthy or unhealthy on the students, faculty, and staff themselves. If it did, the question might ask, "What do some students, faculty, and staff do to be healthy and others do to be unhealthy?" In placing an emphasis on the context, the ACHA poses its second question: "How can we create a campus community in which everyone has a chance to be healthy and live long, healthy lives?" As they explain, their emphasis here is on understanding how the health outcomes of students, faculty, and staff are shaped by intersecting structural, interpersonal, and mediated frames. As such, it provides an opportunity to understand how WPHC, learning, productivity, and campus structures are interdependent with health outcomes.

*Look at the ACHA URL provided under the Resources section for specifics on this topic.*

**SJA Prompts**

1. How can you identify the following elements of the EM on your college campus?
2. What examples can you find of the following facets of the EM?
3. How does each of them interact to produce particular health outcomes?
4. Are these health outcomes different for specific groups of students, faculty, or staff? How so?
5. How can they be made more equitable?
6. Which other environmental, contextual, population-based, policy, and individual factors, among others, are missing?
   • **Public policy**: examples of local, state, national, and global laws and policies.
   • **Community**: relationships among organizations, institutions, and informational networks around the college campus such as local businesses, restaurants, cultural institutions, community leaders, parking, transportation, parks, and so on.
   • **Institutional factors**: rules and regulations as they operate on the campus such as financial policies, lighting, safety features, tobacco policies, campus climate, noise, lounge spaces, air pollution, and so on.
   • **Interpersonal factors**: formal and informal networks and social support systems including friend networks, family, and peer groups such as fraternities, clubs, and sororities. Roommates, supervisors, rituals, diversity, and Greek life are specific examples.

- **Intrapersonal factors**: includes factors such as religious identity, racial and ethnic identity, sexual orientation, age, genetics, time management skills, health literacy, and stigma. These are characteristics of the individual and include aspects such as knowledge, attitude, beliefs, and behavior.

### Resource

American College Health Association (ACHA). (2022). *Ecological model*. https://www.acha.org/ HealthyCampus/HealthyCampus/Ecological_Model.aspx

### The Environment in EMs of Health

First, EMs go to great lengths to take the environment into account in shaping WPHC-centered behaviors (e.g., Agarwal, 2020). Overall, they help researchers understand the inter-dependence between individuals and their context to develop approaches that are complex and multilevel in their methods (Sallis et al., 2008). They do not propose a cause-and-effect process between a factor and a health behavior or outcome; instead, grounding themselves in everyday relationships, organizational boundaries, social norms, and other community-level resources. They encourage us to examine everyone's context to design WPHC interventions and create environments and design policies that help individuals make healthful choices, rather than place the responsibility of making healthful choices on the individual. EMs do so by striving to create conditions that make it easy for people to enact healthful behaviors.

### Mutual Construction of Collaboration and Trust

Second, the individual is central in WPHC-centered EMs. EMs consider space, time, social context, and historical context in understanding the role of the individual and designing interventions (Kingry-Westergaard & Kelly, 1990). Likewise, how participants understand the resources and constraints available to them and the relationships that define the context are also important (Richard et al., 2011). Thus, for designing interventions that promote WPHC or help prevent disease, it is important to also understand how participants make sense of their own contexts and relationships. The emphasis on situated context and mutual construction of understandings in interaction illustrates the social construction of ecological knowledge. For instance, researchers Schofield et al. (2010) recommend the following steps to assist oncology health professionals to have respectful and informed discussions with their patients about CAM: eliciting patient understandings; respecting cultural and linguistic diversity and epistemological frameworks; asking questions about CAM use; exploring details and active listening; responding to the patient's emotional state; discussing concerns with respect for the patient's beliefs; communicating balanced and evidence-based advice; summarizing discussions; documenting discussions; and proper monitoring and follow-up.

*You may want to revisit* **Chapter 2** *on the social construction of health, which offers a deeper look at the social constructionist approach. How do you see the mutual construction of understandings in the ecological approach resonate with the need to address healthcare disparities and inequities?*

*Collaborative Approach in Ems*

Third, Ems state that the intervention should be designed through a collaborative approach with the individuals. The EM states that only by working together can researchers, community members, and individuals come to a shared understanding of context. Creating shared meanings is important for fully understanding the context in an unbiased manner that is fair to the members of the community. For instance, communication researchers Lobera and Rogero-Garcia (2021) examine how the public trust in CAM therapies such as homeopathy or acupuncture is shaped in different ways by the disinformation stemming from the scientific framing of alternative therapies (e.g., in prescription, communication, and marketing), which often leads to confusion about their scientific validation and distrust of the influence of big pharma on health policies, leading the general public to view CAM therapies as more effective. The authors also argue that media and pharmacies shape the scientific-like framing of CAM therapies, which contributes to the social construction of trust in their effectiveness.

## EMPOWERMENT, COLLABORATION, AND CONCORDANCE

Under collaboration, one innovative approach to addressing the barrier to the adoption of CAM is illustrated by Montana State University's (MSU) conceptual model of CAM health literacy (Schreffler-Grant et al., 2013). The model defines CAM health literacy as the information about CAM needed to make informed self-management decisions regarding health. The MSU conceptual model of CAM health literacy comprises the antecedents, such as the environment and demographics; the structural components, such as the health literacy components of information seeking, health and illness trajectory, and general health literacy; and the outcome, conceptualized as the informed self-management of WPHC. Communication researchers Bylund et al. (2010) focus on communication education as a means for improving the clinician-patient relationship and promoting health, with a focus on CAM users and the medically underserved. Taking a view of the clinician-patient communication process as socially constructed, the researchers emphasize patient empowerment as informed and collaborative partners in their communication in ways that will lead to concordance.

*Examine **Textbox 4.5** to consider how the concept of integrated healthcare can benefit from Quadruple Aim and vice versa in the conceptualization and delivery of equitable healthcare.*

---

### Textbox 4.5   A WPHC Perspective on Integrated Healthcare and Quadruple Aim

**Integrated healthcare** is also known as interprofessional healthcare (IPHC). It emphasizes a collaborative, team-based approach to patient care. Thus, communication among health professionals is important in the sharing of information, establishment of a comprehensive treatment plan, and coordination of the patient's biological, psychological, and social needs (APA, 2013). To achieve these collaborative interprofessional healthcare goals, an integrative healthcare team includes a diverse group of members ranging from physicians, nurses, psychologists, CAM professionals, and allied health professionals. The coordination of integrated WPHC delivery extends across the life span and to the different settings of healthcare delivery. These settings include PC, specialized medical settings (e.g., palliative care, rehabilitation units, cardiology, and surgical centers), long-term care settings, community-based health centers, and social service sites (APA, 2013).

Quadruple Aim (now Quintuple Aim) was adopted in 2014 from Triple Aim (Berwick et al., 2008) as a framework to optimize healthcare performance. The intent behind the Quadruple Aim is to guide the redesign of healthcare systems and the transition to population health by creating effective and efficient healthcare organizations. The Quadruple Aim of healthcare includes the goal of improving the experience of providing care through workforce engagement and includes reducing costs, improving population health, improving patient experience, and healthcare team well-being and productivity. The impetus behind Quadruple Aim is to reduce burnout in healthcare workers and counter the rising healthcare costs by improving efficiencies across the continuum of care (Arnetz et al., 2020). Thus, the Quadruple Aim focuses on the experience of joy, meaningfulness, and sense of importance in daily work perceived by healthcare workers.

## WPHC Application

Examine the Quadruple Aim (now Quintuple Aim) to healthcare delivery through a health equity and empowerment lens:

To address food insecurity, the Quadruple Aim does not simply stop at electronic medical records (EMRs) identifying those who are food insecure and improving access to food for individuals in a panel or clinical practice. It asks healthcare professionals to act on the purpose behind their actions by looking into how and why food insecurity is an issue and how health systems can intervene and advocate.

To design interventions, it asks healthcare providers to go beyond their position in the health system to gain input from the communities whom the intervention is to affect and to understand the benefits and burdens created by the intervention. It asks to go beyond analyzing data based on race, gender, and zip code to understanding how the community was affected and to design interventions to meet the needs of tailored populations.

It asks healthcare systems to understand how interventions are accessible given limitations of place, such as transportation.

And last, it asks how the process of intervention is empowering individuals and communities to understand who is being left behind or excluded and why. Thus, the health equity lens seeks to be inclusive in promoting population health, working with marginalized and disadvantaged populations in involving them in decisions affecting resource allocation, reconfiguring healthcare financing and provision to ensure coverage for all and equitable distribution of resources, and revitalizing primary healthcare to reinforce health equity promotion (Olayiwola & Rastetter, 2021).

## SJA Prompt

- How can the Quadruple Aim (with the inclusion of health equity) be applied to an economically disadvantaged and socially vulnerable population?

## Resources

American Psychological Association. (2013). *Integrated health care*. https://www.apa.org/health/integrated-healthcare

Arnetz, B. B., Goetz, C. M., Arnetz, J. E., Sudan, S., vanSchagen, J., Piersma, K., & Reyelts, F. (2020). Enhancing healthcare efficiency to achieve the quadruple aim: An exploratory study. *BMC Research Notes, 13*, Article 362. https://doi.org/10.1186/s13104-020-05199-8

Berwick, D. M., Nolan, T. W., & Whittington, J. (2008). The triple aim: Care, health, and cost. *Health Affairs, 27*(3), 759–769. https://doi.org/10.1377/hlthaff.27.3.759

Olayiwola, J. N., & Rastetter, M. (2021). Aiming for health equity: The bullseye of the quadruple aim. *Journal of Hospital Management and Health Policy, 5*. https://doi.org/10.21037/jhmhp-20-101

Sikka, R., Morath, J. M., & Leape, L. (2015). The quadruple aim: Care, health, cost, and meaning in work. *BMJ Quality & Safety, 24*(10), 608–610. https://doi.org/10.1136/bmjqs-2015-004160

### Social Processes in EM

Fourth, as Richard and colleagues note, the ecological approach pays attention to the social processes that contribute to shaping how we understand the meanings of WPHC. Collaboration and community intervention are also central facets of community-based participatory research (CBPR; see **Chapter 5, Healthcare Relationships**). Communication scholars have advocated for the use of precision in therapeutic terminology in the use of terms such as biomedical, holistic, integrative, and alternative to empower readers in making informed healthcare choices (Schreiber, 2005). Researchers Chan and colleagues examined how trained nutrition professionals such as registered dietitians (RDs) and non-RD professional bloggers communicated nutrition advice (2020). The researchers found that RD blogs emphasized healthy lifestyles, whereas non-RD blogs focused on emphasizing their credibility and legitimacy by challenging conventional medicine while promoting CAM.

## Evolving Understandings of Health

### Integrated Medical and Social Care

The previous conceptual threads illustrate a trend toward consolidation of different understandings, approaches, and philosophies of health in designing and delivering care central to WPHC. Integrated medical and social care is understood as the combination of vertical and horizontal integration. The coordination of care that is emphasized in an IM model is particularly well suited to meeting the goals of those needing chronic condition management or those with multiple comorbidities. Integrated medical care emphasizes clinical care in hospital-based settings, along with supporting social care and rehabilitation services. The WHO defines integrated medical and social care as "bringing together inputs, delivery, management, and organization of services related to diagnosis, treatment, care, rehabilitation, and health promotion" (WHO, n.d.). In this context, integration refers to the fragmentation in patient services and the lack of coordination and continuity in care. Its goal is to enable continuous and coordinated care with adequate financing, a shared vision, and a clear target audience. At a system level, it can be understood as vertical and horizontal integration. Integrated medical care offers a pathway for the future evolution of health as WPHC and medicine to address the challenges of population aging, growing medical complexity, increasing rates of chronic diseases and multimorbidity, rise in technology costs, and the attendant strain on healthcare systems (Maruthappu et al., 2015). The awareness of complex health and social needs is driving evolving understandings of health underlying the WPHC framework and WPHC-centered health systems.

*Advantages of IM and Social Care*

IM care bridges the gaps in the delivery of care with vertical and horizontal decentralization and specialization. Scholars Maruthappu et al. (2015) view vertical integration of care as the seamless structural integration of healthcare services within the health system ranging from process changes to physical colocation. Thus, vertical integration references integration between different levels of care ranging from single-site medical centers that have shared processes and EMRs for primary and secondary care provision. Horizontal integration covers the integration that happens between providers, organizations, networks, or groups in the healthcare system at the same level of care. Examples of horizontal integration might include collaboration between specialists in regional centers or the merger of PC centers to a spoke and hub model. IM care offers the advantages of reduced fragmentation of healthcare providers, lower barriers to access to care, increased efficiency, improved coordination and communication between care providers, and avoidance of duplication or contradictory decisions. By building in shared accountability, collaborative decision-making is improved (Kozlowska et al., 2018).

*Review **Textbox 4.6**. Attempt the SJA discussion prompt that follows.*

---

**Textbox 4.6   A WPHC Approach: Evolving Understandings in Care Coordination**

Table 4.1 provides an overview of the diversity of healthcare specialists who are involved in the conceptualization and delivery of WPHC in a range of healthcare settings. To achieve optimum health outcomes, it is essential to deliver care that is coordinated seamlessly across the care continuum. For instance, when all the specialists involved in WPHC share patient data through the care continuum, physical health services, behavioral healthcare services, and psychosocial healthcare services can be integrated to achieve optimal patient health and well-being outcomes. In evolving understandings of healthcare symbolized by WPHC, as PC approaches and wellness specialties overlap, care coordination is also becoming a collaborative, integrative practice.

Providers listed in Table 4.1 coordinate care through a WPHC model. In the WPHC model, the right care should be delivered, in the right place, at the right time. This emphasis on care coordination and data sharing that makes collaborative case management possible also makes it possible for patients to have easy access to healthcare systems, social services, and a range of specialized healthcare providers. The diversity in healthcare conceptualization, implementation, and delivery is especially critical for populations that are disadvantaged. For instance, for populations experiencing food insecurity, substance use challenges, or housing instability, the care team may prioritize behavioral health and housing support while engaging community partners to manage social determinants that affect a patient's well-being.

Integrative PC settings are, therefore, beneficial to disadvantaged, minority, and marginalized populations. They go beyond the PC practice to provide care where the patients can receive it in a manner that addresses their SDoH and by embodying the value systems that are reflected in their community and family settings.

## WPHC Discussion Prompt

Patients with complex chronic needs and multimorbid conditions must navigate between medical, behavioral health, and social service providers who are not adequately prepared to provide holistic WPHC in an integrative manner. To improve patient experience and reduce healthcare use and costs, coordination of medical, behavioral health, and social services for vulnerable populations is important.

Cross-sector care coordination requires all infrastructure elements to work together to achieve health equity and integrated healthcare delivery. These elements include care coordination staffing that meets patient needs, data sharing capabilities that support care coordination, standardized organizational protocols to support care coordination, and financial incentives to promote cross-sector care coordination (Chuang et al., 2019).

## SJA Prompt

Discuss how you would engage the individual patient in the structural implementation of the recommendations for cross-sector care coordination. For example, some healthcare pilots have developed innovative partnerships to improve the availability of services to vulnerable populations in the community. These include partnering with private homeowners to place people in new types of housing while priority placement for enrollees was being processed (Chuang et al., 2019).

1. How can person-centered practices effectively engage vulnerable patients in care?
2. What forms of patient-centered outreach would you design for vulnerable and disadvantaged populations?
3. How would you tailor communications in outreach and referral strategies to reach and effectively serve disadvantaged individuals (e.g., transitional housing and housing insecure members of society)?
4. What forms of partnerships can help address some of the challenges posed by SDoH such as housing insecurity?

## Resources

Chuang, E., O'Masta, B., Albertson, E. M., Haley, L. A., Lu, C., & Pourat, N. (2019). *Whole person care improves care coordination for many Californians*. UCLA Center for Health Policy Research. https://healthpolicy.ucla.edu/publications/Documents/PDF/2019/wholepersoncare policybrief-sep2019.pdf

*IM and Social Care as Patient-Centered WPHC*

The IM model has the potential of making healthcare more accessible in geographical locations or for patients with varying economic means and insurance coverage and offers promising pathways to address challenges in the delivery and conceptualization of patient-centered WPHC care. It is team-based, such as by involving providers within the same facility (the PC physician, specialist, physician assistant, or the nurse) or across facilities; integrates technology in diagnosis and treatment (e.g., virtual healthcare, by computer-assisted support, electronic health records (EHRs), apps to manage medication adherence, e-prescribing); and provides the option of online visits (e.g., patient visits via the internet, using a webcam and a telephone). Institutionally, from a WPHC perspective, the evolving healthcare landscape is shifting toward value-based care with a focus on patient experiences, population health, cost reduction, and lowering caregiver stress. The evolving WPHC-centered healthcare ecosystem also is shifting to an integrated healthcare delivery system by bridging analytics, data, and digital integration.

## Evolution of Health in the WPHC Framework

### A Brief Historical Overview of WPHC

A shift to value-based WPHC emphasizes outcomes and quality of care while reducing societal costs. The changing meanings of health are reflective of this changing structural and institutional healthcare landscape in line with the WPHC framework. In their review of the meanings of health, Badash and colleagues trace the evolution of health over time from its religious origins to holistic health to biomedical health and the more value-based understandings of the future. In ancient times, Badash and colleagues note, health was largely conceptualized in religious terms. People propitiated deities and offered sacrifices to ward off disease or cure illness. The rod of Asclepius, the international symbol of medicine, is a reminder of the religious origins of health as endowed by deities of medicine and healing. Hippocrates around the fifth century BCE shifted the emphasis to environmental/personal cleanliness and the origin of disease from imbalances in the four bodily fluids that could restore health through behavioral and medicinal actions. Galen, a physician in the Roman Empire, expanded upon the Hippocratic definition of health to include the whole patient like the holistic principles of health. Population health was also emphasized during the time of the Roman Empire. In the 20th century, WHO's definition of health and its modifications have dominated understandings of health. These have evolved from health as an absence of disease to mental, physical, and spiritual understandings of health, and inclusion of psychosocial concepts aligned with WPHC.

### Evolution of Meanings of Health in WPHC

Evolution in the understandings of health from a WPHC perspective emphasizes health as a dynamic state of well-being, emphasizing an individual's potential to meet the demands of life in a way that resonates with their age, culture, and personal responsibility (Bircher, 2005).

Value-based healthcare targets the structure of the healthcare system in the United States and conceptualizes health within a market-based delivery system. Evolving meanings of health seek to emphasize quality for the patient with respect to outcomes and value per dollar spent.

### Emergence of the Value-Based Approach

A value-based approach brings together the structural facets of reimbursement, cost of service, and the attainment of health outcomes that are valued by patients (Badash et al., 2017). The value-based system has six principles: (a) organizing into integrated practice units (IPUs) that provide the full cycle of care for the patient—addressing comorbidities, complexities, and other individual factors; (b) measuring costs and outcomes for each patient; (c) moving toward bundled payments that cover the full care cycle for acute medical conditions, the overall care for chronic conditions for a pre-determined period, or primary and preventive care for a specific patient population; (d) integrating healthcare delivery across separate facilities by assigning a single physician leader for each patient and adopting common protocols across sites; (e) geographically expanding healthcare providers' coverage through the use of satellite locations and affiliations with local community providers; and (f) supporting these changes with a healthcare information technology platform that is patient-centered, versatile, and makes it easy to negotiate medical data, while making the data accessible to all healthcare professionals (Badash et al., 2017).

### Addressing Inequities in Healthcare

Overall, evolving understandings of health under the WPHC paradigm include well-being, individual patient needs, and the organizational, value-based system that is required to meet those needs. Proponents of WPHC believe the value-based system is better equipped to address inequities in healthcare by providing a high quality of healthcare for the lowest cost. Its detractors argue that health outcomes envisaged in value-based healthcare are subjective and vary by individual patient needs and values. Thus, although some feel that the value-based system addresses WPHC more meaningfully by going beyond just stating positive outcomes to offer a more nuanced understanding of outcomes that is also patient-centered, others express a concern that the ability to meet the WPHC needs of all demographics in the population equitably might be challenged by economic disparities and inequitable access to technology. Because the value-based system relies on assessing the quality of care outcomes, their measurement and comparison become central. This raises the concern that based on a WPHC perspective, patient outcomes are subjective and may vary by each patient's unique condition and circumstances in tension with the criteria for well-being as defined as assessed by patients, payers, and society. A challenge for the evolving definition of health is to be inclusive in meeting the needs of disadvantaged groups (e.g., elderly, those with multiple comorbidities, the racially disadvantaged) while also being accessible in considering the meaning of what a good health outcome means from the perspective of each individual healthcare patient.

*As we conclude* **Chapter 4, Evolving Understandings of Health**, *consider Textbox 4.7 and respond to the discussion prompts.*

**Textbox 4.7   Present Challenges and Future Directions Exercise**

**Quintuple Aim and Health Justice in WPHC Delivery: Racial Disparities in Maternal Mortality in the United States**

### WPHC Challenges

CDC's data illuminate significantly higher pregnancy-related mortality ratios among Black and American Indian/Alaskan Native women (CDC, 2022). For instance:

- The data show that about 700 women die each year in the United States because of pregnancy or its complications.
- Statistics reveal that American Indian/Alaska Native and Black women are two to three times as likely to die from a pregnancy-related cause than White women.
- These disparities were constant across US states.
- The disparities increase with age, with disparities for Black and American Indian/Alaska Native women older than 30 years four to five times that of White women.
- The disparities increase with education; with the pregnancy-related mortality rate for Black women with at least a college degree five times more than that of White women with similar education.
- Black-serving hospitals have higher rates of maternal complications than other hospitals.
- Black women experience physical "weathering," i.e., their bodies age faster than White women's due to exposure to chronic stress linked to socioeconomic disadvantage and discrimination over the life course; making pregnancy riskier at an earlier age.

(Geronimus, 1992; National Partnership for Women & Families, 2018)

The Quintuple Aim focuses on enhancing patient experience, reducing cost, optimizing population health, addressing health equity, and including improvements to the work-life and experience of clinicians and care teams that provide care to patients. It is considered foundational to advance PC delivery in equitable and efficient ways. However, recent analyses, such as by Olayiwola and Rastetter (2020), have suggested that the Quintuple Aim is insufficient, in and of itself, to reducing health disparities, finding instead, that a stringent focus on the Quintuple Aim, in fact, has exacerbated health disparities rather than reducing them.

### SJA Discussion Prompt

Intersectionality advocates that we pay attention to the complex and nuanced ways in which social and political conditions of individuals are shaped by multiple intersecting factors, such as race, gender, class, and sexuality. It encourages us to examine how these intersections shape how systemic oppressions intersect and interact to produce major differences in embodied, lived race-gender experiences (López & Gadsden, 2016).

Based on the CDC data provided earlier (and accessible in the links that follow), consider the following questions:

1. How can you use the concept of intersectionality to enhance the Quadruple Aim in achieving equitable healthcare delivery?
2. What recommendations can you provide healthcare administrators to the inclusion of data based on your understanding of intersectionality that makes monitoring and reporting of healthcare disparities impactful in embodied ways?
3. What factors would you recommend healthcare providers attend to in assessing data on their patients from EMRs to deliver racially sensitive and culturally aware patient care?

### Resources

CDC. (2022, April 13). *Infographic: Racial/ethnic disparities in pregnancy-related deaths–United States, 2007–2016.* https://www.cdc.gov/reproductivehealth/maternalmortality/disparities-pregnancy-related-deaths/infographic.html

Geronimus, A. T. (1992). The weathering hypothesis and the health of African-American women and infants: Evidence and speculations. *Ethnicity & Disease, 2*(3), 207–221.

López, N., & Gadsden, V. L. (2016, December 5). *Health inequities, social determinants, and intersectionality.* National Academy of Medicine. https://doi.org/10.32478/201912a

National Partnership for Women & Families. (2018, April). *Black women's maternal health: A multifaceted approach to addressing persistent and dire health disparities.* https://www.national partnership.org/ourwork/health/reports/black-womens-maternal-health.html

Olayiwola, J. N., & Rastetter, M. (2020). Aiming for health equity: The bullseye of the quadruple aim. *Journal of Hospital Management and Health Policy, 5.* https://doi.org/10.21037/JHMHP-20-101

## References

Agarwal, V. (2018). The provider's body in the therapeutic relationship: How complementary and alternative medicine providers describe their work as healers. *Health Communication, 34*(11), 1350–1358. https://doi.org/10.1080/10410236.2018.1489201

Agarwal, V. (2019). The provider's body in the therapeutic relationship: How complementary and alternative medicine providers describe their work as healers. *Health Communication, 34*(11), 1350–1358. https://doi.org/10.1080/10410236.2018.1489201

Agarwal, V. (2020). *Medical humanism, chronic illness, and the body in pain: An ecology of wholeness.* Lanham, MD: Lexington Press.

Agency for Healthcare Research and Quality. (2017). *Physician burnout.* Retrieved from https://www.ahrq.gov/prevention/clinician/ahrq-works/burnout/index.html

AHRQ. (2022, August). *Patient-centered medical home (PCMH).* Retrieved from https://www.ahrq.gov/ncepcr/research/care-coordination/pcmh/index.html

Badash, I., Kleinman, N. P., Barr, S., Jang, J., Rahman, S., & Wu, B. W. (2017). Redefining health: The evolution of health ideas from antiquity to the era of value-based care. *Cureus, 9*(2), e1018. https://doi.org/10.7759/cureus.1018

Bircher, J. (2005). Towards a dynamic definition of health and disease. *Journal of Medical Healthcare Philosophy*, *1*, 335–341.

Broom, A., & Adams, J. (2009). Oncology clinicians' accounts of discussing complementary and alternative medicine with their patients. *Health: An Interdisciplinary Journal for the Social Study of Health, Illness, & Medicine*, *13*(3), 317–336. https://doi.org/10.1177/1363459308101806

Brumback, K. (2022, May 1). Black doctors say they face discrimination based on race. *AP News.* Retrieved from https://apnews.com/article/black-doctors-discrimination-f4c3e85f66880fe0e8869315610dc291

Bull, L. (2009). Survey of complementary and alternative therapies used by children with specific learning difficulties (dyslexia). *International Journal of Language & Communication Disorders*, *44*(2), 224–235 https://doi.org/10.1080/13682820802015643

Bylund, C., D'Agostino, T.A., Ho, E. Y., & Chewning, B. A. (2010). Improving clinical communication and promoting health through concordance-based patient education. *Communication Education*, *29*(3), 294–311 https://doi.org/10.1080/03634521003631952

Chan, T., Drake, T., & Vollmer, R. L. (2020). A qualitative research study comparing nutrition advice communicated by registered dietitian and non-registered dietician bloggers. *Journal of Communication in Healthcare*, *13*(1), 55–63 https://doi.org/10.1080/17538068.2020.1749351

Fisher, C. L., Ledford, C. J. W., & Crawford, P. (2019). Explaining acupuncture in family medicine: Patients' and physicians' use of metaphor. *Journal of Communication in Healthcare*, *12*(3/4), 180–188 https://doi.org/10.1080/17538068.2019.1683366

Gardiner, P., Mitchell, S., Filippelli, A. C., Sadikova, E., White, L. F., Paasche-Orlow, M. K., & Jack, B. W. (2013). Health literacy and complementary and alternative medicine use among underserved inpatients in a safety net hospital. *Journal of Health Communication*, *18*(S1), 290–297 https://doi.org/1080/10810730.2013.830663

Keene, M. R., Heslop, I. M., Sabesan, S. S., & Glass, B. D. (2020). Knowledge, attitudes, and practices of health professionals toward complementary and alternative medicine in cancer care: A systematic review. *Journal of Communication in Healthcare*, *13*(3), 205–218. https://doi.org/10.1080/17538068.2020.1755202

Kingry-Westergaard, C., & Kelly, J. G. (1990). A contextualist epistemology for ecological research. In Tolan, P., Keys, C., Chertok, F., & Jason, L. (Eds.), *Researching community psychology* (pp. 23–41). American Psychological Association.

Kozlowska, O., Lumb, A., Tan, G. D., & Rea, R. (2018). Barriers and facilitators to integrating primary and specialist healthcare in the United Kingdom: A narrative literature review. *Future Healthcare Journal*, *5*(1), 64–80. https://doi.org/10.7861/futurehosp.5-1-64

Lewis, M. (2020). Political citizens, consumers, or passive patients? Imagined audiences in the complementary medicine debate. *Communication Research & Practice*, *6*(3), 209–228. https://doi.org/10.1080/22041451.2020.1785192

Lobera, J., & Rogero-Garcia, J. (2021). Scientific appearance and homeopathy: Determinants of trust in complementary and alternative medicine. *Health Communication*, *36*(10), 1278–1285. https://doi.org/10.1080/10410236.2020.1750764

Maruthappu, M., Hasan, A., & Zeltner, T. (2015). Enablers and barriers in implementing integrated care. *Health Systems & Reform*, *1*(4), 250–256. https://doi.org/10.1080/23288604.2015.1077301

National Medical Association. (n.d.). *NMA Priority issues 2019–2020*. Retrieved from https://www.nmanet.org/page/NMA-Priority-Issues-2019-2020

Park, M., Hunter, J., & Kwon, S. (2018). Evaluating integrative medicine acute stroke inpatient care in South Korea. *Health Policy*, *122*(4), 373–379. https://www.doi.org/10.1016/j.healthpol.2018.02.004

Rajamma, R. K., & Pelton, L. E. (2010). Choosing non-conventional treatments: Consumers' attempts at controlling health care. *Journal of Consumer Marketing*, *27*(2), 127–138. https://doi.org/10.1108/07363761011027231

Richard, L., Gauvin, L., & Raine, K. (2011). Ecological models revisited: Their uses and evolution in health promotion over two decades. *Annual Review of Public Health, 32*, 307–326. https://doi.org/10.1146/annurev-publhealth-031210-101141

Roberts, K., Dowell, A., Nie, J.-B. (2020). From research to practice: Building bridges to enhance interprofessional communication between general practitioners and acupuncturists. *Journal of Communication in Healthcare, 13*(3), 234–244. https://doi.org/10.1080/17538068.2020.1769959

Sallis, J. F., Owen, N., & Fisher, E. B. (2008). Ecological models of health behavior. In Glanz, K., Rimer, B. K., & Viswanath, K. (Eds.), *Health behavior and health education: Theory, research, and practice* (pp. 465–485). Jossey-Bass.

Sartorius, N. (2006). The meanings of health and its promotion. *Croatian Medical Journal, 47*(4), 662–664.

Schofield, P., Diggens, J., Charleson, C., Marigliani, R., & Jefford, M. (2010). Effectively discussing complementary and alternative medicine in a conventional oncology setting: Communication recommendations for clinicians. *Patient Education & Counseling, 79*(2), 143–151. https://doi.org/10.1016/j.pec.2009.07.038

Schreffler-Grant, J., Nichols, E., Weinert, C., & Ide, B. (2013). The Montana State University conceptual model of complementary and alternative medicine health literacy. *Journal of Health Communication, 18*(10), 1193–1200. https://doi.org/10.1080/10810730.2013.778365

Schrieber, L. (2005). The importance of precision in language: Communication research and (so-called) alternative medicine. *Health Communication, 17*(2), 173–190. https://doi.org/10.1207/s15327027hc1702_4

Scott-Conner, C. (2023, January 13). Time splintered. *Pulse: Voices from the heart of medicine.* https://pulsevoices.org/index.php/stories/time-splintered

Serafina, K., Coyer, C., Speights, J. B. (2020). Racism as experienced by physicians of color in the health care setting. *Family Medicine, 52*(4), 282–287.

Shin, E., Shim, J.-M. (2019). Listen to doctors, friends, or both? Embedded they produce thick knowledge and promote health. *Journal of Health Communication, 24*(1), 9–20. https://doi.org/10.1080/10810730.2018.1554727

Spence, M., & Ribeaux, P. (2004). Complementary and alternative medicine: Consumers in search of wellness or an expression of need by the sick? *Psychology & Marketing, 21*(2), 113–139. https://doi.org/10.1002/mar.10118

Thomas, H., Mitchell, G., Rich, J., & Best, M. (2018). Definition of whole person care in general practice in the English language literature: A systematic review. *BMJ Open, 8*, e023758. https://doi.org/10.1136/bmjopen-2018-023758

Welch-Cline, R. J. (2003). At the intersection of micro and macro: Opportunities and challenges for physician-patient communication research. *Patient Education & Counseling, 50*(1), 13–17. https://doi.org/10.1016/S0738-3991(03)00073-9

WHO. (n.d.). Services organization and integration. Retrieved from https://www.who.int/teams/integrated-health-services/clinical-services-and-systems/service-organizations-and-integration

## Additional Resources

American Medical Association (AMA). (2021). *4 ways to include the whole health care team in telemedicine.* Retrieved February 6, 2023, from https://www.ama-assn.org/practicemanagement/digital/4-ways-include-whole-healthcare-team-telemedicine

Department of Veterans Affairs. (2022, December 30). *Whole health.* Retrieved February 6, 2023, from https://www.va.gov/wholehealth/

National Center for Complementary and Integrative Health (NCCIH). *NCCIH Strategic plan FY 2021–2025. Mapping a pathway to research on whole person health.* Retrieved February 6, 2023, from https://www.nccih.nih.gov/about/nccih-strategic-plan-2021-2025

Samueli Foundation. (2023). Retrieved from https://www.samueli.org/

The National Academies. (2023). *Transforming health care to create whole health: Strategies to assess, scale, and spread the whole person approach to health.* Retrieved February 6, 2023, from https://www.nationalacademies.org/our-work/transforming-healthcare-tocreate-whole-health-strategies-to-assess-scale-and-spread-the-whole-person-approach-tohealth

University of Minnesota. (2015, February 20). *Mental health and well-being ecological model.* Retrieved February 6, 2023, from https://mch.umn.edu/resources/mhecomodel/

Whole Health Institute. (2021). https://www.wholehealth.org/

# Healthcare Relationships

## Chapter Learning Outcomes

Upon completing **Chapter 5, Healthcare Relationships**, the student should be able to apply the WPHC SJA framework to:

1. Understand how provider-patient relationships can integrate patient-centered care and patient empowerment.
2. Apply the tenets of interprofessional team communication and culturally sensitive dialogue in healthcare relationships and digital health.
3. Critically evaluate the four models of the physician-patient relationship from an SJA perspective.
4. Understand the health implications of family relationships and family communication as exemplified in diverse racial contexts.
5. Understand how community engagement, communities of identity, and the active community engagement continuum contribute to equitable community health promotion approaches.
6. Identify how the elements of organizational wellness programs, medical professionalism, and workplace climate are affected by stigma.
7. Explain worker relationships, worker climate, and worker resilience as elements of WPHC.
8. Apply the different facets of healthcare relationships to a range of healthcare contexts from diabetes self-management to cancer care and social support in everyday health behaviors of minority and marginalized populations.
9. Apply community-engagement participatory approaches with an understanding of the difference between community-based and community-placed frameworks.

## Consider the following statistics:

The United States has the most expensive healthcare compared with other wealthy countries (Peterson Center on Healthcare and KFF). At the same time, the United

DOI: 10.4324/9781003214472-7

States ranks last overall in the 71 performance measures of healthcare including healthcare outcomes. The United States has the lowest life expectancy and highest suicide rates and chronic disease burden among 11 high-income Organization for Economic Cooperation and Development (OECD) countries. The United States has among the highest number of hospitalizations from preventable causes and the highest rate of avoidable deaths.

(Source: The Commonwealth Fund, 2021)

On the positive end, the United States outperforms its peers in terms of preventive measures with one of the highest rates of breast cancer screening among women ages 50 to 69. Americans also have the second-highest rate (after Britain) of flu vaccinations among people 65 and older. Finally, Americans use some of the most expensive and cutting-edge technologies, such as magnetic resonance imaging (MRIs), and specialized procedures, such as hip replacements, more often than their peers.

Such statistics on healthcare outcomes can be insightful and indicate the complexity of the healthcare landscape. They also indicate that more than the availability of technology and clinical procedures, at the heart of successful health outcomes are strong healthcare relationships. In fact, studies find that a strong patient-provider relationship predicts a significant portion of the success in the prevention, diagnosis, and treatment of disease, in supporting healthy lifestyle choices and medication adherence among marginalized and at-risk populations (such as among aging adults with a disproportionate burden of chronic diseases), and in adding value to the patient's experience of care (Olaisen et al., 2020).

Relationships are the bedrock on which healthcare delivery, implementation, and outcomes rest. Good communication skills are at the center of strong clinical interpersonal relationships, which have a direct and indirect impact on health outcomes (Epstein & Street, 2007). This chapter will examine healthcare relationships from the perspective of provider-patient relationships, family relationships, community engagement, and workplace relationships.

## Chapter Organization

**Chapter 5, Healthcare Relationships**, is organized as follows: **First**, it will cover provider-patient relationships with a focus on patient-centered care, patient empowerment, interprofessional communication, culturally sensitive dialogue, the four models of the physician-patient relationship, and digital health. **Second**, it will cover family relationships attending to family communication, supportive family ties, stressful family relationships, family health history, and long-distance communication. **Third**, it will cover community engagement with a focus on the community in health promotion efforts, community engagement approaches, culture and community relationships, the active community engagement continuum, and communities of identity. **Fourth**, the chapter covers workplace relationships with attention to the psychosocial factors comprising the work environment, organizational wellness programs, medical professionalism, workplace relationships and workplace climate, stigma, social support, and worker resilience. Along the way, students are provided valuable WPHC SJA context on the tenets of interprofessional communication (IPC), the SJA framework in healthcare relationship definitions and terms, patient-centered care and self-management support, critiques of the physician-patient relationship models, digital health and healthcare relationships, and family relationships in cancer management in action. In the scholar interview, communication scholar Dr. Eddah Mutua shares how her teaching incorporates African indigenous knowledge through the spirit of *sawubona communication* and a critical consciousness framework to racial justice. The discussion questions and thought scenario for the reflection exercise encourages students to think about enactments of social support in everyday health behaviors in the context of social support for marginalized and minority populations. The present challenges and future action exercise prompt students to apply the community-based participatory approach to understand the difference between community-placed and community-based initiatives. A practitioner interview with Dr. Kathryn Fiddler of TidalHealth Regional Hospital illustrates what social justice means to one hospital as it prioritized health equity and community engagement to build resilience and bring stakeholders together during the COVID-19 pandemic.

## Provider-Patient Relationships

### Patient-Centered Care (PCC)

PCC or person-centered care is a key healthcare approach that centers the patient in the healthcare interaction. PCC is central to WPHC. It emphasizes open and dialogic communication between patients and providers and shared decision-making. It envisions patients to be active partners who take ownership of their care in collaboration with their physicians. The Institute of Medicine (IOM) defines PCC as "providing care that is respectful of, and responsive to, individual patient preferences, needs, and values, and ensuring that patient values guide all clinical decisions" (2001). For PCC to be effective in WPHC, the patient should be empowered to take control of and act on their healthcare needs and priorities. Refer to Table 5.1 for a detailed look at how the PCC envisions empowered patients as those striving to create conditions for their own well-being and to engage in self-management support by taking shared responsibility for their healthcare outcomes (Pulvirenti et al., 2014).

### Eight Elements of PCC

PCC is composed of eight elements that support an empowered patient: respect for the patient's values, preferences, and needs; information and education; access to care; emotional support to relieve fear and anxiety; involvement of family and friends; continuity between healthcare settings; physical comfort; and coordination of care. Because the primary healthcare setting is central to addressing the health needs of patients at the community level, the primary care provider (PCP) relationship serves as a hub to center care, disease prevention, health promotion, and patient education communication. The PCP-patient relationship can significantly impact care access, preventive care, early detection, treatment, and chronic disease management.

*Browse **Text Box 5.1** to get an understanding of the key opportunities and challenges facing the primary care relationship in the context of the WPHC model. Respond to the SJA discussion prompt that follows. The mini-case study illustrates how interprofessional collaboration is an equally important aspect of successful PCC. It also touches upon how technology is impacting PCC, an aspect that is discussed in detail in **Chapter 9, Technology and Health**.*

---

### Textbox 5.1   WPHC in the Primary Care Relationship

The focus on WPHC reorients the primary care setting into realms such as whole person health and wellness, reflecting an awareness of the need for a comprehensive, integrated, holistic approach to supporting health and well-being. Such calls emphasize the long-term, sustained patient-provider relationship as the center of patient support for making healthy choices, both in the in-person and the virtual relationship domains.

Andrew Ellner, a cofounder of *Firefly Health*, a primary care service and technology company, notes the importance of providing primary care in the context of interprofessional collaboration. Interprofessional collaboration offers personalized PCC, which balances the inclusion of nonphysician health workers in a clinical team to serve primary care functions like diagnosis and management, along with care managers (e.g., nurses), community health workers, and patient navigators can help mitigate the use of emergency room (ER) visits and hospitalizations in a cost-effective manner. interprofessional collaboration is key to a patient-centered comprehensive care model. Interprofessional collaboration clinical teams are better positioned to ensure patient adherence to medical regimens and reduce disparities in care by helping patients with transportation barriers, literacy barriers, and access barriers. Integrated teams are also likely to be more successful in administering screening and brief interventions for conditions like alcohol use disorders, pharmacotherapy for opioid use disorders, and collaborative care models for treating depression and anxiety. However, as communication researchers Fox and colleagues observe in their study, communication challenges such as the power difference between physicians and nonphysician professionals and the increasingly broad scope of clinical activity in primary care practice can hinder collaborative activities.

### Challenges Facing Integrated Primary Care Settings

The emergence of technological advances in artificial intelligence (AI), poor patient-provider relationships from the perspective of consumer friendliness of providers, entry of telemedicine companies offering urgent transactional care over secure virtual platforms, and emergence of urgent care in retail pharmacies and stand-alone chains. The Centers for Medicare and Medicaid Services (CMS) are exploring innovative payment options (e.g., upfront per-member/per-month-PMPM) based on payment complexity to support care access, continuity, management, coordination, comprehensiveness, patient engagement, planned care, and population health. Such policies may allow evidence-based behavioral health interventions such as mindfulness and meditation, cognitive behavioral therapy (CBT) for insomnia, and diabetes prevention programs for weight management to be reimbursed and more widely available.

## SJA Discussion Prompt

1. To what extent can AI substitute for the interpersonal facets of your relationship with a PCP? What facets of your relationship with your family physician would not be replaceable by AI?
2. Would you recommend the primary care setting be integrated with wellness approaches such as meditation and lifestyle interventions for chronic conditions?
   a. How might such an integration be helpful to the patient's health and well-being?
   b. How would you ensure health equity for minorities and people who are socially disadvantaged in their ability to access and benefit from such an integration?

## Resources

CMS. (2022). *Innovation models*. Retrieved from https://innovation.cms.gov/innovation-models# views=models

Firefly Health. (n.d.). Retrieved from https://www.firefly.health/

Fox, S., Gaboury, I., Chiocchio, F., & Vachon, B. (2021). Communication and interpersonal collaboration in primary care: From ideal to reality in practice. *Health Communication, 36*(2), 125–135. https://doi.org/10.1080/10410236.2019.1666499

### Interprofessional Care Team Communication

Effective PCC relies upon a strong provider-patient relationship. Fox and colleagues underscore the need for attending to the interpretive actions that happen during informal interprofessional care (IPC) team communication and the organizational culture that supports open communication across different team roles and clinical settings. As the healthcare landscape becomes more specialized, effective PCC in WPHC implies navigating the interdisciplinary settings needed for effective engagement by the patient through the complex care continuum.

### Patient-Centered Communication

Delivering PCC across the care continuum means the WPHC provider attends to patient goals at each stage to ensure that the healthcare processes attend to the patient's preferences,

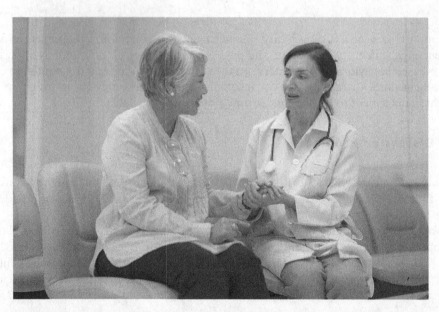

Figure 5.1 PCC strengthens the provider-patient relationship by emphasizing active listening and demonstrating empathy.

needs, and values. Demonstration of empathy, engagement, strong listening skills, and shared decision-making help strengthen the patient-provider relationship. Good PCC includes the patient and their family in care planning and increases patient satisfaction and quality of life (Finney-Rutten et al., 2016). PCC strengthens the provider-patient relationship by emphasizing active listening to patients' concerns, demonstrating empathy, explaining medical terms in simple and easy-to-understand language, and enabling patient self-management in decision-making (Anders et al., 2016).

Epstein and Street's (2007) cancer care model demonstrates the importance of an engaged patient. Their cancer care model centers communication in a multidimensional PCC framework around six key functions: foster healing relationships, exchange information, respond to emotions, manage uncertainty, make decisions, and enable patient self-management. This PCC framework promotes provider empathy, facilitates shared decision-making, and enables a shared understanding of the healthcare situation and goals of care.

*Examine **Table 5.1** for the definitions of key healthcare relationship terms and how they emphasize specific aspects of PCC, along with a critique of their application from a social justice framework.*

*Table 5.1* Definitions of Healthcare Relationship Terms and SJA Critique

| WPHC Context: Healthcare Contexts, Relationships, and Definitions of Key Terms | SJA Framework Emphasis/Critique in Healthcare Relationship Contexts |
| --- | --- |
| **Primary care:** <br> **Integrated, accessible** healthcare services by clinicians (**primary care providers**, PCPs) who are accountable for addressing a large majority of personal healthcare needs, developing a sustained **partnership** with patients, and practicing in the context of family and **community**. | **SJA Critique:** <br> • Emphasis on **clinician functions** of access, continuity, comprehensiveness, and coordination. <br> • The WHO's focus to achieve these SJ dimensions has been on **cost, quality, access,** and **equity** for patients to achieve a fair distribution of health outcomes among diverse populations. <br><br> **SJA Prompts:** <br> • *How would you describe your relationship with your PCP? Can you imagine circumstances whereby it could be (more/less) trusting, open, understanding?* <br> • *What might be the implications of expensive primary care services?* <br> • *How might poor primary care services impact disadvantaged areas?* |
| **Person-centered care/PCC:** <br> PCC is seen as an alternative to **paternalistic care models** in which medical experts analyze patients using tests and physical examination procedures to infer a diagnosis and establish a protocol of care based on a standard set of processes. | **SJA Critique:** <br> Critiqued for assuming that (a) patients have experiences and wants, that (b) it is possible for them to communicate these to others, that (c) (these) experiences and wants may be relevant for clinical decisions, and that (d) it is possible for patients and caregivers to interact in ways promoting the **inclusion of experiences** and wants of patients in **clinical decision-making.** <br><br> **SJA Prompt:** <br> *Do you agree with these critiques of PCC? How can these gaps be bridged to envision an empowered patient for effective PCC?* |

(Continued)

Table 5.1 (Continued) Definitions of Healthcare Relationship Terms and SJA Critique

| WPHC Context: Healthcare Contexts, Relationships, and Definitions of Key Terms | SJA Framework Emphasis/Critique in Healthcare Relationship Contexts |
| --- | --- |
| **Patient-centered communication:**<br><br>• **Communicative behaviors** that can enhance the quality of the relationship between the healthcare provider and patient or the patient's family in ways that balance the needs of healthcare professionals to diagnose and treat patients and the need to understand and involve patients.<br>• Includes **communication techniques** used by providers to care for patients based on concordant values, needs, and preferences while empowering patients to provide input and be active participants in their healthcare decisions (Epstein & Street, 2007).<br><br>**Shared decision-making:**<br>A model of PCC that enables and encourages people to play a role in the medical decisions that affect their health (AHRQ, 2022).<br>Its two central premises are<br>a. consumers with **good information** are more likely to participate in the medical **decision-making process** by asking informed questions and expressing personal values and opinions about treatments and options, and<br>b. clinicians **respect patients' goals** and preferences and use them to guide recommendations and treatments. | **SJA Critique:**<br>The IOM (2001) identifies patient-centered communication as one of six elements of **high-quality healthcare**.<br><br>• PCC is based on the goals of **patient empowerment** and **shared decision-making** set in a **collaborative, equitable setting**:<br>  a. Eliciting the patient's perspective on an illness<br>  b. Understanding the patient's psychosocial context<br>  c. Reaching shared treatment goals based on the patient's values<br>• Patient-centered communication builds on discussions that involve the following:<br>  a. shared deliberation,<br>  b. information sharing,<br>  c. empowering care,<br>  d. sensitivity to patient needs and values, and<br>  e. relationship-building.<br><br>**SJA Prompt:**<br>*How can PCC be supported by effective patient-centered communication to ensure equitable and inclusive quality of care?*<br><br>**SJA Critique:**<br>Envisions **mutual dialogue** in which both patient and physician are actively engaged in decision-making:<br>  a. The **physician** brings in medical training, knowledge, and expertise.<br>  b. The **patient** brings in experiential knowledge, subjective goals, and personal values through which to evaluate the risks and benefits of the different treatments for each patient.<br><br>**Patients** take responsibility for the following:<br>  a. **Identifying** and availing themselves of information<br>  b. **Speaking up** to share their concerns, goals, and questions with the healthcare team<br>  c. Enacting the role of a **proactive patient** effectively:<br>    a. reviewing information before/after a visit<br>    b. completing assessments of understanding and/or goals<br>    c. working with a coach or attending a support group or community-based educational program) |

**Healthcare providers** take responsibility to:

(a) **Communicate** risks and benefits clearly.
(b) **Elicit** patients' goals and treatment preferences.
(c) **Respect** patients' values, preferences, and needs when making recommendations for care.

**Organizations** take responsibility to:

(a) **Assess** meaningful patient involvement in decision-making.
(b) Patient **follow-up** on care and options.
(c) **Understanding** of risks and benefits.
(d) **Deliberation** of preferences for improvement.

**SJA Prompt:**

*How is the role and responsibility of the organization in shared healthcare decision-making significant?*

**SJA Critique:**

• Some researchers have critiqued patient empowerment for its inadequacy in supporting **vulnerable populations,** such as those in acute care or growing **older populations** with complex medical and social needs (e.g., Wakefield et al., 2018).

• **Empowerment** is central to the **patient–physician relationship** that encourages equitable partnerships with self-management and self-efficacy, and is best achieved with organizational commitment to measurement, assessment, and promotion of these qualities.

• **Patient empowerment** also implies **physician responsibility** to create the conditions for an empowered patient in both the informational and decision-making realms.

**SJA Prompt:**

*What might conditions facilitating patient empowerment for a patient from a marginalized and minority community involve?*

**Patient empowerment:**

• References the **engagement** and **involvement** of patients.

• Patient empowerment was previously defined as *"a process through which people gain greater control over decisions and actions affecting their health."* Its four components are:

(a) Understanding by the **patient** of his/her role.
(b) Acquisition by the **patient** of sufficient knowledge to be able to engage with the healthcare provider.
(c) **Patient skills.**
(d) Presence of a facilitating **environment.**

**Revised definition:**

*Patient empowerment is a process in which patients understand their role and are given the knowledge and skills by their healthcare provider to perform a task in an environment that recognizes community and cultural differences and encourages patient participation (WHO, 2009)*

(Continued)

*Table 5.1* (Continued) Definitions of Healthcare Relationship Terms and SJA Critique

## SJA Prompt

- How can the SJ critique in the right-hand column be translated to action for each of the dimensions of a healthcare relationship referenced by each definition?

## Resources

AHRQ. (2022). *Strategy 6I: Shared decision making*. Retrieved from https://www.ahrq.gov/cahps/quality-improvement/improvement-guide/6-strategies-for-improving/communication/strategy6i-shared-decisionmaking.html

IOM. (2001). *Crossing the quality chasm: A new health system for the 21st century*. National Academy Press.

Wakefield, D., Bayley, J., Selman, L. E., Firth, A. M., Higginson, I. J., & Murtagh, F. E. M. (2018). Patient empowerment, what does it mean for adults in the advanced stages of a life limiting illness: A systematic review using critical interpretive synthesis. *Palliative Medicine, 32*, 8. https://doi.org/10.1177/0269216318783919

WHO. (2009). *WHO guidelines on hand hygiene in health care: First global patient safety challenge clean care is safer care. 2, Patient empowerment and health care*. Geneva. Retrieved from https://www.ncbi.nlm.nih.gov/books/NBK144022/

### Patient-Centered Communication in the Physician-Patient Relationship

WPHC PCC emphasizes how providers and patients must both take responsibility for the healthcare relationship. PCC is associated with greater compliance with physician recommendations and medication, increased patient trust in providers, patient satisfaction, decreased uncertainty and anxiety, improved provider-patient relationship, and successful health outcomes (Dutta-Bergman, 2005a; Hong & Oh, 2020; Stewart, 2001; Trivedi et al., 2021; Wanzer et al., 2004).

For the patient, PCC implies taking ownership of their health. This involves engaging in health promotion behaviors such as healthy lifestyles, screening, medication adherence, and making long-term behavioral and lifestyle changes. For example, a patient with coronary heart disease might plan their lifestyle to incorporate a half-an-hour walk a day. Or a patient who has type 2 diabetes might download apps such as *Diabetes Journal* or *Accu-Chek* to help them consume balanced meals in appropriate portion sizes, test their blood sugar, and take their medications as prescribed.

### Patient-Provider Communication and Health Equity

#### PROVIDER PERSPECTIVE

Health disparities are not always an outcome of lack of access to treatments or availability of treatments. Oftentimes, these disparities manifest in conditions where treatments are available and accessible to patients. For instance, although pre-exposure prophylaxis (PrEP), a once-daily pill that protects patients from contracting HIV is available, only a few healthcare providers prescribe it to clinically eligible patient populations that are at risk for HIV such as people who inject drugs, men who have sex with men, transgender women, and people who exchange sex for resources. As Wilson and colleagues find, the reasons for its low prescription rates range from lack of provider engagement in PCC and poor patient-provider communication (Wilson et al., 2021). The lack of communication is exemplified by provider discomfort in discussing HIV-risk behaviors with patients. Similarly, Singh and colleagues find that race and ethnicity, age, and gender play a significant role in influencing PCC (Singh et al., 2018).

Furthermore, WPHC communication that acknowledges and acts upon each patient's SDoH can go a long way in building trust and overcoming barriers to a patient's ability to act on the information communicated in the patient-provider meeting. Effective communication can support an individual's self-efficacy or the individual's belief in their ability to engage in desired behaviors and take ownership of their health outcomes. Culturally sensitive structured dialogue employs narrative and motivational techniques to guide emotional feedback from patients.

#### PATIENT PERSPECTIVE

Central to WPHC is the belief that how patients perceive their physicians' PCC also shapes healthcare outcomes. Taking a sample of Caucasian and Arab participants, Jain investigates biases in the healthcare relationship from the perspective of both the provider and the patient (Jain, 2022). She examines the impact of a provider's biased perceptions on their patients and the impact of physician race and gender on patients' perceptions regarding the physician's communication, trust, competence, and intentions to visit. Her research finds that perceived physician competence and warmth mediate the effect of physician gender and race on

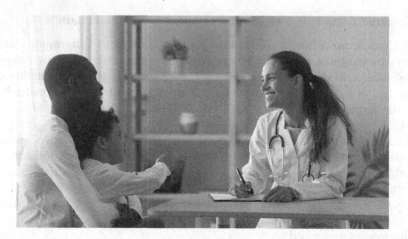

*Figure 5.2* A Good Provider-Patient Relationship Is Important for Positive Healthcare Outcomes.

perceptions of trust, physician's use of PCC, and intentions to visit. In other words, the effect of physician race on patient perception of trust, physician use of PCC, and their ultimate intentions to visit were mediated by physician warmth in their interactions. Jain's findings illustrate the importance of a good patient-provider relationship that is based on empathy and warmth in mitigating some of the negative causes of healthcare outcomes (Jain, 2022).

In another study, Anderson et al. (2021) find that Black women who were cancer survivors were less likely than White women to feel that their information needs were met. Black women who were cancer survivors were also more likely to report experiencing poorer communication with their providers. Being mindful of how income disparities, social exclusion, and racial discrimination in the daily experience of their patients' lives impact their material reality can help providers tailor their PCC in culturally sensitive ways.

*Textbox 5.2* *provides information on how diabetes patients can better manage their condition through education and support from providers and the healthcare team. Review the information provided and respond to the SJA discussion prompt provided.*

---

### Textbox 5.2   PCC and Self-Management Support

#### WPHC Context

Even with advances in the treatment of diabetes, achieving positive patient outcomes has remained challenging. In 2017, only 51.7% of adults aged 18 years and over with diagnosed diabetes had received formal diabetes self-management education and support. An increasing number of patients still experience devastating complications that result in a decreased length and quality of life. Increasing the number of persons with diagnosed diabetes who receive formal diabetes self-management education and support is an important focus area in improving health outcomes (Healthy People 2030, *Objectives and data. Increase the proportion of people with diabetes who get formal diabetes education*).

WPHC care centers self-management support. By receiving ongoing diabetes education and self-management support from their providers and healthcare team, people gain the knowledge, skills, and abilities they need to manage their condition. Patients gain clarity about their goals, values, and motivations. Patients who understand what their doctors tell them and participate in decisions about their care are better prepared to make daily decisions and take actions to make changes in their behaviors, solve problems, and make decisions by assuming responsibility for their care.

## SJA Discussion Prompt

PCC that enables patients to make good choices and sustain healthy behaviors is characterized by a collaborative relationship, participation between healthcare providers and teams, and patients and their families in a partnership that supports patients in building the skills and confidence they need to lead active and fulfilling lives (Institute for Healthcare Improvement, IHI, 2022).

1. What are some considerations healthcare providers should keep in mind to provide self-management support guidance and education to patients from diverse backgrounds? For instance, how will patient education, cultural beliefs, and economic status influence how effectively patients understand and utilize the information provided?
2. What WPHC-relationship factors might make the information shared in a healthcare setting with patients more effectively understood?

## Resources

AHRQ. (2022). *Self-management support*. Retrieved from https://www.ahrq.gov/ncepcr/tools/self-mgmt/self.html

Healthy People 2030. (n.d.-a). *Health literacy definition public comments, June 3, 2019–August 5, 2019*. Retrieved from https://health.gov/sites/default/files/2020-08/HP2030_Health-Literacy-Definition-Public-Comments_508.pdf

Healthy People 2030. (n.d.-b). *Objectives and data. Increase the proportion of people with diabetes who get formal diabetes education*. Retrieved from https://health.gov/healthypeople/objectives-and-data/browse-objectives/diabetes/increase-proportion-people-diabetes-who-get-formal-diabetes-education-d-06

IHI. (2022). *Partnering in self-management support: A toolkit for clinicians*. Retrieved from http://www.ihi.org/resources/Pages/Tools/SelfManagementToolkitforClinicians.aspx

*Four Models of Physician-Patient Relationship*

The healthcare relationship is a space for supporting patient autonomy and values and empowering the patient to take ownership of their health. In this manner, PCC is closely associated with patient self-management support. Moving through the paternalistic to the deliberative model outlines the arc toward WPHC characterized by greater patient autonomy, empowerment, and self-management. Through this process, the physician's role is as a dialogic partner who shares information in a collaborative manner to support shared decision-making in alignment with the patient's values, needs, and preferences.

## PATIENT SELF-MANAGEMENT SUPPORT

Self-management support in WPHC is a commitment to create the conditions that empower patients to take control of their own health and well-being (AHRQ, 2022). Healthcare professionals can facilitate self-management support by providing patients with clear, useful, and actionable information, helping them set goals and make plans to live a healthier life, putting a team of clinicians and administrative staff in place who clearly understand their roles and responsibilities, and using office systems that allow for timely follow-up and tracking of patients (AHRQ, 2022).

## PATIENT AUTONOMY

Table 5.2 provides a description and critique of the four models of the physician-patient relationship: the paternalistic model, the informative model, the interpretive model, and the deliberative model. Along with the definition and description of each model, Table 5.2 provides one approach to the physician role and responsibilities. It also provides the communication aspects associated with the physician role and responsibilities in each model in the center column. Finally, the right-hand side column provides the SJ framework implications that the physician role and responsibilities have in each model for patient autonomy, values, empowerment, and participation in care through shared decision-making and self-management support.

   *Review Table 5.2 with respect to the SJA critique provided in the right-hand column. Then respond to the SJA discussion prompt that follows.*

*Table 5.2* WPHC Context: Four Models of Physician-Patient Relationship

| Model | Central Premise | SJA Critique |
|---|---|---|
| Paternalistic model | • **Patients** receive interventions determined most appropriate by their providers for their health and well-being.<br>  • **Patient communication** may tend toward an authoritative view of providers and a passive view of patients.<br>• **Physicians** are considered experts who employ their knowledge to determine diagnosis and treatment plan.<br>  • **Provider communication** can be selective and geared toward patient consent to the interventions. | a. Seen as being a poor fit for patients who are **empowered**, educated, and independent decision-makers who value self-determination and liberty.<br>b. Poor fit for a medical system that values **patient autonomy** and participation in care.<br>c. Assumes that **patients and providers** share objective criteria for determining what is the most appropriate care.<br>d. Does not emphasize **patient autonomy** and choice. |

*(Continued)*

*Table 5.2* (Continued) WPHC Context: Four Models of Physician-Patient Relationship

| Model | Central Premise | SJA Critique |
|---|---|---|
| Informative model | • The **physician** provides the patient with all relevant **information** such that the patient can select the medical interventions per their choice, with the physician respecting the patient's choices in implementing their decision.<br><br>• The **physician** provides the diagnosis, nature of potential interventions, probability of risks and benefits, and uncertainties in knowledge.<br><br>• The **physician's responsibility** is to provide truthful, competent, and complete information. | a. Critiqued for assumption that **knowledge** is fully **objective** and that the **patient's values** are well-defined.<br><br>b. Critiqued for assuming **patient autonomy** is enacted through the **information giving** that will allow the patient to make the best possible decision aligning with their values.<br><br>c. Critiqued for not considering **physician's values or** understanding **patient values**.<br><br>d. Positions the **physician** as the one with the **technical expertise** who provides the patient with the means of control. |
| Interpretive model | • The **physician-patient interaction** serves to help elucidate the **patient's values** and desires and for the physician to help the patient to decide regarding the medical interventions that will support the patient's wants.<br><br>• The physician provides the patient with the information required to decide but also helps the patient articulate their values to help the **patient decide** in alignment with the values.<br><br>• The **patient's values** are not considered fixed or necessarily even known to the patient. | a. The **physician** is like a **counselor**, advising, providing information, and helping clarify the patient's values.<br><br>b. The **physician suggests** the medical interventions that support their values.<br><br>c. The physician is responsible for **engaging the patient** in a joint process of understanding.<br><br>d. **Patient autonomy** is conceptualized as self-understanding. |
| Deliberative model | • The **physician-patient relationship** is geared toward enabling the patient to choose the best health-related values for a given clinical situation.<br><br>• The **physician's role** is to provide clinical information and help elucidate the values embodied in the options.<br>  • The physician may suggest why certain health-related values should be pursued.<br>  • The **physician and patient** engage in deliberation to make a decision.<br><br>• The physician's input is limited to the health-related values as they bear upon the disease and its treatment and does not touch upon others that may be beyond the scope of the **physician-patient relationship**. | a. The **physician** acts as a teacher-friend and is positioned as **a dialogic partner** enabling **collaborative discussion** on the best course of action.<br><br>b. The **physician recommends** the best course of action, decision, and treatment.<br><br>c. **Patient autonomy** is exercised through moral self-development, empowerment to consider, through dialogue, a range of health-related values, and deliberate these in terms of their implications for treatment. |

*(Continued)*

*Table 5.2* (Continued) WPHC Context: Four Models of Physician-Patient Relationship

## SJA Discussion Prompt

1. Could you envisage a condition wherein the paternalistic model might be an effective model of patient-provider relationship? In what way might this model constrain patient ownership and control of their own health choices and behaviors?
2. How can the deliberative model effectively support patient autonomy in a patient-provider relationship where the patient and the provider share different cultural values?

## Resource

Emanuel, E. J., & Emanuel, L. L. (1992). Four models of the physician-patient relationship. *JAMA*, 267(16), 2221–2226. Retrieved from https://www.jama.jamanetwork.com/

### *Digital Health*

#### *Opportunities Offered by Digital Health*

Digital health supports WPHC by extending opportunities to attend to the patient-provider relationship in settings such as online portals. However, these need careful navigation. In cancer survivorship, for instance, where patients are faced with making sense of complex risk information, the use of online portals has been both supportive and challenging to the patient-provider relationship. Alpert et al. (2019) note that cancer patients report advantages in being able to control appointments, have a collaborative relationship with their oncologists, have a direct link to their care team, and have active communication that supports empowerment.

#### *Critiques of Digital Health*

At the same time, online portals are challenging for patients because they can be perceived as an inadequate substitute for in-person PCC. The empathic discussions between the provider and patient that promote patient understanding, satisfaction, and well-being that were essential components of PCC are seen as missing from the digital management of their healthcare process. With the increasing integration of patient portals in WPHC coordination of care, physicians need to understand the way individual patients want to be involved in their care, the shift in communication modes, and how patients make decisions about their treatment.

*Examine **Textbox 5.3** for a deeper look at the digitization of health and consider the discussion prompt in thinking about its impact on healthcare relationships.*

---

### Textbox 5.3    Digital Health and Healthcare Relationships

#### WPHC Context

The term "digital health" references the broad array of technologies and their use in health and healthcare. Digital health can encompass the use of data analytics, mobile health, wearables, and electronic health records.

Digital health is rapidly expanding how we access and consume healthcare. In doing so, it is also transforming how and when we communicate with our healthcare providers and the traditional healthcare relationship (Jongsma et al., 2021). Home telemonitoring, for example, is emerging as a promising alternative to in-person hospital visits. Digital technologies that can replace and support healthcare are becoming rapidly accessible in the consumer market. **Chapter 10** discusses technology and health in greater detail.

### SJA Discussion Prompt

There is a concern that the digitization of health will result in the overburdening of patients with greater responsibilities in managing their health by bearing responsibilities that are traditionally borne by physicians. Digital health may empower patients on the one hand by making digital data about their health visible and accessible directly to patients. On the other hand, how patients employ digital data is not certain. Digital data may be inconclusive or hard to interpret and may lead to confusion, anxiety, or complicated decision-making for both the healthcare provider and the patient.

1. Is there a caution with the digital health monitoring technologies that consumer wearables such as smartwatches promise to provide?
2. What should be the role and responsibility of a physician or healthcare provider in educating patients about how to interpret their digital health data?
3. What should patients keep in mind about communicating with their physicians or healthcare providers about their digital health data?

### Resource

Jongsma, K. R., Bekker, M. N., Haitjema, S., & Bredenoord, A. L. (2021). How digital health affects the patient-physician relationship: An empirical-ethics study into the perspectives and experiences in obstetric care. *Pregnancy Hypertension, 25,* 81–86. https://doi.org/10.1016/j.preghy.2021.05.017

## Family Relationships

Families are often the cornerstone of our lives from birth to old age. Scholarly definitions of family have focused on structure, such as biological or legal ties; function, such as caretaking or financial support; or transactions, such as creation of shared meaning through affective ties or symbolic communication such as stories and rituals. Family relationships are central to shaping an individual's health-related attitudes, beliefs, and behaviors. For WPHC, close and supportive family ties, such as those with partners, spouses, intergenerational family members, and siblings suggest association with strong caregiver coping skills, adaptability, and clear communication about illness and its management within families. They have been linked with positive health and well-being and stronger self-management skills. In addition, learning about the family can provide information about bolstering against the negative effects of stress. The experience of stress is associated with a higher incidence of CVD and unhealthy behaviors such as smoking, overeating, and depression. Family relationships also impact how individuals make decisions regarding prevention and screening, risk assessment, and clinical interventions (Baptiste-Roberts et al., 2007). Conversely, stressful family relationships, such as those characterized by conflict, blame, and lack of support have been associated with negative health outcomes.

WPHC is concerned with patients' lived contexts and values. One way of understanding the role of family relationships is through food-related beliefs and family rituals. Families are embedded in cultures, and family and cultural norms shape dietary choices. For example, family food rituals and beliefs mediated the association between the family conversation orientation and meat consumption and varied by race and ethnicity in Dorrance Hall et al.'s study. As the consumption of red meat is linked to a range of health concerns, family communication environments and their role in shaping beliefs about food consumption, such as of meat, become important (Dorrance Hall et al., 2021). The researchers found that in Hispanic and non-Hispanic White participants, an orientation toward conversation moderated the association between the orientation to conform and food beliefs.

### Family Communication

Family communication scholars have examined the diversity of family structures and social roles members adopt within families in the communication of health information. For instance, family communication studies suggest that African Americans are more likely than Whites to include extended family and fictive kinship in family. WPHC is interested in how family members engage in mutual influencing of healthy and unhealthy behaviors by observation and interaction and how different forms of social support can be utilized in reinforcing health outcomes in family relationships. Communicative tools such as sharing stories are one way of maintaining family closeness. Table 5.3 enumerates different forms of family relationships and their functioning. As shown in Table 5.3, the family systems theory views the family as an organized whole, where all members are interdependent, and where communication and behaviors are influenced and determined by the collective processes, structures, and values of its members (Minuchin, 1985).

### Family Health History (FHH)

Along with family ties, WPHC will also consider the FHH to get a complete understanding of an individual's health status. The FHH is a record of the conditions and diseases present within a family. It provides an understanding of the environmental, behavioral, and genetic factors shared across multiple generations of biological relatives. For instance, the family cancer history (FCH) is a starting point for decision-making during genetic counseling sessions and to guide recommendations for prevention (e.g., prophylactic mastectomy). The FHH is a known risk factor for many common chronic diseases and captures complex interactions between genes, the environment, and behaviors (Valdez et al., 2010). Although 96% of people consider FHH knowledge to be important to their health, fewer than 40% have actively collected their FHH (Yoon et al., 2003). Yoon and colleagues note racial disparities in health among African Americans and other minority populations are exacerbated by a lack of knowledge of their FHH (2002). Greater knowledge of FHH among minority and disadvantaged populations can guide message development strategies and interventions and improve health protective behaviors. African Americans, for instance, have lower disease risk perceptions than Whites and are less likely to believe FHH plays an important role in chronic disease development. Their beliefs make them particularly vulnerable to health risks as they are less likely to perform health protective behaviors or be aware of the FHH. Understanding how families communicate FHH and why they communicate and manage FH information is important in WPHC to support higher levels of health protective behaviors (Baptiste-Roberts et al., 2007).

### Family Cancer History (FCH)

As an example, lack of communication about FCH with relatives within African American communities may contribute negatively to prevention and early detection behaviors that can decrease cancer risk. Rositch and colleagues find that in their examination of the knowledge of FCH and factors that shape family communication of this history among African Americans in East Baltimore, Maryland, although most participants had at least one family member who had cancer, few families communicated openly about cancer history, and this information did not translate in the healthcare setting (2019). Others find that the interaction between awareness of FCH and cancer risk perceptions was significantly associated with mammography screening adherence (Hong et al., 2020).

### Personal Health Information (PHI)

Of relevance to WPHC is how family communication scholars have examined family communication of PHI. The notion of dialectical tensions or opposing ideas that coexist in the same frame (Baxter & Montgomery, 1998) is an important part of scholarship studying family communication and relationships. For instance, during illness management, family members report dialectical tensions as opposites such as autonomy versus connection (Baxter et al., 2002) or maintaining privacy versus the desire to share and express oneself. Dialectical tensions are at the core of the Communication Privacy Management (CPM) Theory. This theory says that managing privacy requires a complex array of rules and choices. Individuals are responsible not only for decisions regarding FHH but also to whom they give access to their own private information (Bylund et al., 2012; Petronio & Caughlin, 2006, p. 42). Look at Table 5.3 for additional information on the CPM and other family communication theories. For instance, using the CPM, focusing on the parent-child relationship in the family, Nielsen and colleagues find that parenting practices in households with young children are shaped by the ethnicity of the parents and reflected in how different sources of dietary advice were given salience to by the parents in making dietary decisions (2015). Others find that family communication acts require people to balance the dialectical tensions between disclosure and privacy (Baxter et al., 2002).

WPHC PCC is shaped by how individuals manage the disclosure of PHI. Studies find that individuals manage this dialectical tension through strategies such as denial, or discussing only one side of the issue, such as positive health information; segmentation, restricting discussion to one aspect or another, such as refusing to discuss sexual health but being open to discussing other topics; and integration, when people discuss both aspects of their health-related matters equally. Parent-child sexual health communication has been considered important in HIV and pregnancy prevention for young people. Addressing fear and discomfort among adolescents in African American families around discussing sexual information with religious parents could be offset by parents offering both religious and practical guidance to adolescents about sexual health (Williams et al., 2015). WPHC communication can be mindful of parent-child communication. As parents play an integral role in the sexual health development of their children, by communicating with children about sex, they have the opportunity to share information, as well as values, beliefs, and expectations, around sexual behaviors. Parent-child communication has protective effects for preventing risky behaviors and promoting healthy behaviors among adolescents (Lefkowitz & Stoppa, 2006). Marginalized family members can achieve resilience through five communicative processes, including (a) crafting normalcy, (b) affirming identity anchors, (c) utilizing communication networks, (d) reframing, and € downplaying negative feelings while focusing on positive emotions (Buzzanell, 2010).

*Table 5.3 provides the definitions, highlights, and critiques of some of the salient concepts and approaches and provides some applications from the perspective of cancer communication. Respond to the SJA prompts on the right-hand side.*

*Table 5.3* Family Relationships in Cancer Management

| Communication Concepts/Definitions | SJA Highlights/Critiques |
| --- | --- |
| **Family relationships:** Have been assessed with three domains—cohesion, expressiveness, and conflict (Moos & Moos, 1986). | **Family cohesion:** Refers to shared affection, commitment, helpfulness, emotional bonding, and caring among family members.<br>**Family expressiveness:** Refers to an open and direct style of verbal and nonverbal expression in family communications.<br>**Family conflict:** Refers to the open expression of anger, aggression, and interactions resulting from incompatible goals or violations of relationship expectations among family members.<br>**SJA Prompts:**<br>• *Identify one instance of positive influence of family relationships on health outcomes.*<br>• *Can you think of circumstances from recent health news whereby the health of members of minoritized identity LGBTQIA+ populations is supported or harmed by family relationships?* |
| **Family communication:** Understood as an interpersonal and intrapersonal process reflecting a family's interaction patterns, beliefs, and dynamics, which ultimately influence family cohesion and functioning (Braithwaite et al., 2015). | **Family communication contexts:**<br>• Cancer care research connects family communication with a positive association with patients' coping abilities and the quality of psychosocial support from their families.<br>• Family communication has been shown to increase family functioning and sustain the provision of support for the individual with cancer.<br>**Spousal communication research:**<br>• Includes examination of factors such as spouse reactions to negative disclosures, extent of communication about cancer-related issues, and protective buffering (hiding one's concerns from a spouse).<br>• Spousal research has focused mainly on married partners rather than on more diverse relationships, and most of the research has focused on breast cancer communication, with a growing body of literature on prostate cancer (e.g., Arrington, 2005).<br>**Parent-child communication:**<br>• Research has focused on challenges in the first year of a child's cancer diagnosis in both parents and siblings and continued challenges with a subgroup of family members.<br>• A gap in research on improving communication about cancer diagnosis among family members.<br>**Caregiver research:**<br>• Caregiving is understood as the provision of unpaid aid or assistance and care by one or more family members to another family member with cancer.<br>• Family member as a caregiver during active cancer treatment, survivorship, and end-of-life has been an important area of research (Harris et al., 2009).<br>**SJA Prompts:**<br>• *What may be one health risk in circumstances when a spouse is not supportive of a breast cancer survivor's journey?*<br>• *How might diverse relationships impact spousal communication of health issues?* |

**Coping:**

- Refers to a **transitional process of cognitive appraisal** and stress response within a person-in-environment perspective.
- Involves **culturally relevant** strategies for managing external and internal stressors related to an illness, such as cancer.

**Family communication in racial-ethnic minority groups:**

- Family communication and coping styles vary across minority groups, with open family communication contributing to effective individual and family coping in minority communities (Huang et al., 2022).
- Little research done in this area.

**Family communication:**

- Considered a central means of **adaptation** to managing cancer-related stress and coping.
- **Communication** experienced within families supports relationships, maintenance of social networks, and life satisfaction and is associated with a high quality of life across the life span.
- During **stressful life experiences** such as a cancer diagnosis, family members are often a critical source of social support and impact through, for example, helping manage stress, coping with traumatic challenges, and adapting to new circumstances in a healthy manner (Fisher & Nussbaum, 2015).

**SJA Prompts:**

- *Think of an example of a difficult diagnosis. What makes it difficult?*
- *What communicative strategies support its management?*

- Research indicates the importance of **open and constructive communication** among cancer patients and family members (Huang et al., 2022).
- Need to develop strategies to **minimize communication avoidance** and empower active conversations between patients and family members.
- **Minority family** communication:
  - **African American families'** concerns about privacy, along with pride or dignity, particularly between generations of family members noted as a barrier to communication.
  - Few families openly communicate their cancer history, and this information did not translate to the healthcare setting (Rositch et al., 2019).

**SJA Prompt:**

- *Family communication can be intimate and communal at the same time. Try to gain insight into a family communication strategy from a minority family.*
- *What resources did you draw upon?*

*(Continued)*

*Table 5.3* (Continued) Family Relationships in Cancer Management

| Communication Concepts/ Definitions | SJA Highlights/Critiques |
| --- | --- |
| **Family Communication Patterns (FCP) Theory:**<br><br>• Families create a shared reality for families to function and assign meaning to each other's behaviors.<br>• Conformity orientation and conversation orientation are measured to understand closed and open communication within the family and the family communication environment. | • **Conformity orientation**—refers to "the degree to which families create a climate that stresses homogeneity of attitudes, values, and beliefs" (Fitzpatrick, 2004, p. 173).<br>• **Conversation orientation**—refers to "the degree to which families create a climate where all family members are encouraged to participate freely in interaction about a wide array of topics" (Fitzpatrick, 2004, p. 173).<br>• Together, both conformity and conversation orientation help in assessing the degree to which **open or closed communication** is within the family.<br>• The **family communication environment** is believed to influence individual and family-level communicative and behavioral tendencies.<br><br>**SJA Prompt:**<br>*What are some health risks associated with both conformity and conversation orientation?* |
| **Family Systems Perspective (FSP):**<br>Families are understood as a unit, where communication serves as the medium through which shared beliefs, feelings, and emotions are transmitted, and family functioning is maintained (Bowen et al., 2004). | • FSP recognizes that family organization is important in **family functioning**.<br>• **Family organization** is understood as the way in which family members relate to one another. It consists of three domains:<br>  • **Cohesion**—the emotional bonds among family members.<br>  • **Flexibility**—the quality and expression of leadership and organization within the system.<br>  • **Communication**—the vector through which families attempt to balance cohesion and flexibility.<br>• During a **stressful situation**, such as a cancer diagnosis, the FSP maps onto the balanced or unbalanced dimensions of cohesion and flexibility. These in turn determine the implications for the family's well-being.<br>• **Communication** is understood as a **facilitating dimension** that helps families find balanced levels of cohesion and flexibility to achieve optimal functioning.<br>• Higher levels of family cohesion and flexibility have been associated with:<br>  • More open platforms for **sharing health information** and **greater support** for cancer discussion within families (Harris et al., 2009)<br>  • Individuals share family health information with those whom they felt close to, provide emotional support, and engage in contact more frequently (Rodriguez et al., 2016).<br><br>**SJA Prompt:**<br>*Consider a health condition that may be stigmatized for any reason. What communicative strategies might help in achieving a balance between cohesion and flexibility?* |

**Communication Privacy Management (CPM):**
Employs boundaries as a metaphor to understand how individuals manage the disclosure or concealment of private information (Petronio, 2002).

- Delineates processes to show how people **construct rules** for revealing or concealing information.
- **Family Privacy orientation** (Petronio, 2002):
  - Proposes that families adopt **privacy rules** to manage **privacy boundaries** that, if consistently used, can turn into orientations toward **disclosure** of private information for family members.
  - Further extended as general tendencies of family members toward **revealing and concealing private information** within and outside of the family.

**SJA Prompt:**

- *Under what circumstances can you imagine concealing private health information in family relationships may support positive health management?*
- *How can healthcare providers employ an understanding of CPM in managing patient relationships and disclosure?*

**Family history:**
Reflects shared genetic, behavioral, and environmental exposures.

Research has examined **family history communication** with the goal of understanding how individuals who have family members affected by certain conditions are at higher **risk** of developing those conditions.

**SJA Prompt:**

*Can you imagine an instance when family history communication has supported your health prevention or diagnosis behaviors?*

**Family:**
The organization and structure of a family as **a unit** can be understood as comprising closer or distant relations, and as existing at different levels (e.g., blood/nonblood, male/female, first-degree/second-degree).

- **Cancer risk communication** within a family can take place at different time points and in different forms.
- Research shows that **cognizance about cancer risk** facilitates information sharing among family members, often varying with time and with distance, with health-related cognitions, beliefs, and experience, and with older participants more likely to share genetic test results with family members (Chopra & Kelly, 2017).

**SJA Prompt:**

*How many diverse family organizations can you think of?*

(Continued)

Table 5.3 (Continued) Family Relationships in Cancer Management

## Resources

Arrington, M. I. (2005). "She's right behind me all the way": An analysis of prostate cancer narratives and changes in family relationships. *Journal of Family Communication, 5*(2), 141–162. https://doi.org/10.1207/s15327698jfc0502_5

Bowen, D. J., Bourcier, E., Press, N., Lewis, F. M., & Burke, W. (2004). Effects of individual and family functioning on interest in genetic testing. *Community Genetics, 7*(1), 25–32. https://doi.org/10.1159/000080301

Chopra, I., & Kelly, K. M. (2017). Cancer risk information sharing: The experience of individuals receiving genetic counseling for BRCA1/2 mutations. *Journal of Health Communication, 22*(2), 143–152. https://doi.org/10.1080/10810730.2016.1258743

Fisher, C. L., & Nussbaum, J. F. (2015). Maximizing wellness in successful aging and cancer coping: The importance of family communication from a socioemotional selectivity theoretical perspective. *Journal of Family Communication, 15*(1), 3–19. https://doi.org/10.1080/15267431.2014.946512

Fitzpatrick, M. A. (2004). Family communication patterns theory: Observations on its development and application. *Journal of Family Communication, 4*, 167–179. https://doi.org/10.1080/15267431.2004.9670129

Harris, J., Bowen, D. J., Badr, H., Hannon, P., Hay, J., & Regan Sterba, K. (2009). Family communication during the cancer experience. *Journal of Health Communication, 14*(S1), 76–84. https://doi.org/10.1080/10810730902806844

Harris, J. N., Hay, J., Kuniyuki, A., Asgari, M. M., Press, N., & Bowen, D. J. (2010). Using a family systems approach to investigate cancer risk communication within melanoma families. *Psycho-Oncology, 19*, 1102–1111. https://doi.org/10.1002/pon.1667

Huang, Y.-J., Acquati, C., & Monit, C. (2022). Family communication and coping among racial ethnic minority cancer patients: A systematic review. *Health & Social Care in the Community, 30*(3), e605–e620. https://doi.org/10.1111/hsc.13623

Moos, R., & Moos, B. (1986). *Family environment scale manual*. Consulting Psychologists Press.

Petronio, S. (2002). *Boundaries of privacy: Dialectics of disclosures*. SUNY Press.

Rodriguez, V. M., Corona, R., Bodurtha, J. N., & Quillin, J. M. (2016). Family ties: The role of family context in family health history communication about cancer. *Journal of Health Communication, 21*(3), 346–355. https://doi.org/10.1080/10810730.2015.1080328

Rositch, A. F., Atnafou, R., Krakow, M., & D'Souza, G. (2019). A community-based qualitative assessment of knowledge, barriers, and promoters of communicating about family cancer history among African Americans. *Health Communication, 34*(10), 1192–1201. https://doi.org/10.1080/10410236.2018.1471335

### Differences in Family Communication by Ethnic Group

Acknowledging and recognizing differences in patient lived contexts in WPHC involves respecting the diversity of family structures, definitions, and functions by ethnic group. Family communication research examines how these differences underpin health outcomes. African Americans are more likely to die from cancer than any other racial or ethnic group in the United States. Acknowledging the importance of family communication in health outcomes, the US Department of Health and Human Services (DHHS) recommends studying disparities in the use of FHH among different populations to achieve Healthy People 2030 goals. Despite disparities in health outcomes between African Americans and Whites in the United States, most research seeking to understand definitions of family, family structure, and family communication has centered on White families. Yet African American families face unique structural and psychosocial factors contributing to their use of prevention, screening, detection, and treatment services. Rositch and colleagues found that psychosocial factors such as fear/denial, pride/dignity, selflessness, and fatalistic attitudes about cancer were commonly reported barriers to sharing cancer histories with family members among minorities. Other findings suggest that low health literacy, shame, fatalism, worry, and cultural health beliefs may underpin disparities in FHC among minority communities (Ricks-Santi et al., 2016).

In African American families, women as mothers and grandmothers play an important role in promoting health. In WPHC contexts, findings that FHH communication is supported by awareness of a family history of disease, higher frequency of seeking health information, a belief that FHH is important, when someone in the family is diagnosed with a disease, or when disease-related risk and worry are higher (Hovick, 2014) gain relevance. Research shows that women in White families have served as gatherers and disseminators of information on family health histories, such as those at risk for hereditary breast and ovarian cancer. Not much is known about diverse families and the flow of health information or information about multiple diseases in diverse families. Such gaps have exacerbated health disparities. Thompson and colleagues study African American women's definitions of family and their family communication about health (Thompson et al., 2015). Their study finds that communication patterns differ in African American women depending on whether participants were collecting FHH information or discussing their own health more generally. In their study, women discussed their own health with a wide variety of people, and female relatives were important for both communication tasks, with a particular emphasis on older women. More research with disadvantaged populations can help refine WPHC.

### Long-Distance Caregiving

WPHC is concerned with understanding alternative relationships and their influence on health outcomes. Communication scholars Sparks and colleagues examine long-distance caregiving (LDC) in the context of families living at a distance. LDC family relationships are characterized by a lack of availability, a lack of intimate understanding of the caregiving needs at hand, and unknown financial burdens that are highlighted in evolving intimate family relationship needs across the life span. Sparks and colleagues' study highlights the role of the degree to which caregivers perceive the care recipients to be accommodating, respectful, polite, and trusting. PCC advocates care of the whole person in clinical settings and including family members in the decision-making process. (Epstein & Street, 2007). Family members provide decisional support to patients by assisting patients in seeking, organizing, and processing information for health decisions. In WPHC PCC, these decisions may involve finding a healthcare provider, receiving advice, or describing symptoms to providers.

In cancer communication, for instance, spouses are often the primary source of support (Miller & Caughlin, 2013). In African American communities, among men recently diagnosed with cancer, wives, daughters, or sisters were likely to relay health information and treatment options (Feltwell & Rees, 2004). Spousal support is associated with psychosocial outcomes, including distress and adjustment to diagnosis. Palmer-Wackerly and colleagues' study shows that partner support partly mediates the relationship between healthcare provider support and the patients' decision-making satisfaction within the cancer treatment context (Palmer-Wackerly et al, 2017). In WPHC PCC, the type of support given—emotional, informational, advice, or appraisal—influences patients' treatment decisions for both partner and healthcare provider support. For instance, partner support may not always be seen as positive. In some cases, patients do not seek or value support from their families. At other times, families do not always give the support that a patient desires from them (Krieger, 2014).

### Community Engagement

#### Community in Health Promotion Efforts

Along with the family, strong community relationships are a vital component of SDoH from a WPHC framework and are associated with improved health outcomes in a range of domains. Centering the community in health promotion efforts recognizes how culture and health are closely intertwined (Airhihenbuwa, 2007). This is particularly salient in minority and marginalized populations with a shared sense of socio-historic experiences and where community is a source of stability, mobilization, and resilience (see also Present Challenges/Future Directions Exercise). For instance, faith-based communities such as the African American church hold historic community significance since the times of slavery. The church serves as a sit of gathering for worship, community, and resource gathering (Lincoln & Mamiya, 1990). Many health promotion efforts targeting African Americans approach the church community to tap into existing social networks that facilitate recruitment and intervention.

Read **Textbox 5.4** to see what communication scholar and professor Dr. Eddah Mutua has to say about how she employs **sawubona communication** and critical consciousness in her teaching. What avenues does sawubona communication offer to think about WPHC?

---

### TEXTBOX 5.4    Scholar Interview

#### Eddah Mutua
*St. Cloud State Minnesota*

### Perspectives on Developing Healthy Relationships in Diverse Communities

My research and teaching interests are in the area of intercultural communication. Specifically, I am interested in exploring ways that create awareness of the environment in which communication occurs to promote healthy communication in a diverse world.

My teaching aims to center inclusive paths to acknowledge and actively support the struggles of marginalized groups, including Black, Indigenous, and people of color (BIPOC), people living with disabilities, LGBTQI, women, religious minorities, the poor, the elderly, non-White immigrants, and refugees, etc. These vast experiences call for new learnings about human communication in a diverse and dynamic world. In the last four years, I have been working on incorporating alternative perspectives and peda-gogical practices to promote a holistic approach to communication in diverse contexts.

My teaching incorporates African indigenous knowledge as a relevant framework to broaden theoretical perspectives that go beyond the Western-centric nature of current communication studies. I embrace the spirit of the African/isiZulu greeting "*sawubona*," which embodies the philosophy of African communication and demonstrates how it can be used to promote a holistic understanding of communication. Sawubona collo-quially translates as "We see you, respect you and value you." It is an ethical acknowl-edgment of one's existence, value, and life's worthiness. The exchange of this pleasant greeting is simple yet rich in spiritual and physical meaning. For example, the Greeter (Eddah) says, "*Sawubona Vinita*," and the response is "*Sawubona Eddah*." The greeting exemplifies the African practice of interconnectedness and community that brings vital-ity to human communication. Molefi Asante (2011) observed, "[O]ne cannot have a community without communication" (p. 145). When we commit to energetic engage-ment with our diversity then we can begin to see, respect, and value others, as well as tailor our communication to build community based on fairness, equity, empathy, responsibility, and freedom.

Closely related to the *sawubona communication* is the increasing critical consciousness about diversity, equity, and inclusivity/ inclusivity, diversity, equity, and accessibility (DEI/IDEA), and growing support for racial justice, social justice-oriented groups such as BLM. It calls for a nuanced understanding of what can be done for justice, equity, and inclusion when 'we see, value and respect' others. Undoubtedly, the murder of George Floyd has rekindled how we approach and practice good healthy communica-tion and social justice.

For me, a whole person health as conceptualized in this textbook, encompasses acknowledging the physical and spiritual aspects of our being as integral to communi-cation and the search and attainment of social justice. Frequently, I tell my students that communication does not occur in a vacuum. At all times, we must reflect on what is going on within and around us to develop healthier ways of perceiving self and others. For example, at any moment, one commits to showing a high regard for care and respect for self and others, their communication must be guided by the principles of respectabil-ity and responsibility for others. A respectful and responsible person endeavors to always do the best and recognize that their well-being and that of others is paramount. The quest for a whole person health requires us to ponder over questions such as, "What prompts what I say, how I say it, and why? Is the context for communication safe/healthy or hostile/unhealthy? Is this what is affecting my communication with others? How can I share my joy with others? How can I see others' pain? What can I do to find joy in me so that I can share it with others? What can I do to ease others' suffering? What can I learn from the courageous actions of other people?" These questions among others prepare us to work toward a holistic healthy being in a complex world.

You may be wondering how I engage my students with *sawubona communication* and critical consciousness about social issues. Our local community in central Minnesota has become more diverse following the influx of refugees, notably from East Africa, in the last 20 or so years. This context has become a site for developing innovative pedagogical practices that give students the permission to be inquisitive, investigative, and proactive about creating lifelong paths for empowering themselves to build healthy diverse communities. Service-learning pedagogy makes it possible to engage with students from diverse backgrounds. The goal of our collective participation is to acquire knowledge and skills to develop and sustain healthy relationships in a diverse community.

## Resource

Asante, M. K. (2011). Communication and the Pan-African dimension to community. *African Communication Research*, 4(1), 139–152.

*Community Engagement Approaches*

In centering the community, WPHC recognizes cultural competency or having knowledge of a group's cultural differences and behaviors or beliefs alone is not enough. Culture is dynamic and complex; to meaningfully incorporate it in WPHC contexts, a focus on the meanings that individuals share and on the explanatory models they use to discuss their health problems becomes salient to PCC. Doing so helps healthcare professionals gain a richer understanding of cultural meanings that are rooted in everyday lives (CDC, 2022). From this perspective, community-engaged approaches enable partnerships that can develop programs and research while staying consistent within the cultural framework of a people (Airhihenbuwa, 1995). This is vital for addressing health disparities, particularly among minority populations such as people from sexual and gender minorities (SGM). Researchers Flentje and colleagues' findings emphasize that safe community environments have a strong relationship with physical health among people from SGM (Flentje et al., 2021). Their study highlights how people from SGM experience physical health disparities attributed to greater exposure to minority stress, including experiences of discrimination of victimization, anticipation of discrimination or victimization, concealment of SGM status, internalization of stigma, and structural stigma. For minority populations, increasing WPHC PCC that provides a buffer against the effects of unsafe communities is important for positive health outcomes.

## THE SOCIAL-ECOLOGICAL MODEL

The social-ecological model for health promotion states that the health of individuals is affected by the interaction between the individual, the group/community, and the social, physical, and political environments (Israel et al., 2003; Wallerstein et al., 2003). This four-level model of health promotion has been widely used as a framework for designing WPHC-centered community interventions. It conceptualizes health broadly and focuses on integrating approaches to change the physical and social environments rather than modifying individual health behaviors. The first level of the model includes individual biology and personal characteristics such as age, education, income, and health history. The second level, relationship, includes an individual's closest social circle, such as friends, partners, and family members who influence a person's behavior and contribute to his or her experiences. The third level, community, explores the settings in which people have social relationships, such as schools, workplaces, and neighborhoods, and seeks to identify the characteristics of these settings that affect health. The fourth level looks at the broad societal factors that support or impair health such as cultural or social norms and the economic, educational, and social policies that create, maintain, or lessen socioeconomic inequalities between groups (CDC, 2022).

## ACTIVE COMMUNITY ENGAGEMENT CONTINUUM

Other approaches highlight the role of building community engagement as a dynamic and evolutionary process. The goal of community engagement approaches such as the active community engagement continuum is to encourage members to be change agents themselves (Russell et al., 2008). To do so, WPHC engagement moves from being consultative to cooperative to collaborative. Most WPHC PCC approaches seek to achieve community empowerment through collaboration with stakeholders such that all parties are mutually accountable for change.

### Diffusion of Innovation (DOI)

Another useful theoretical approach to WPHC that takes a community-centered approach is DOI. Diffusion has been defined as "the process by which an innovation is communicated through certain channels over time among the members of a social system" (Rogers, 1995). This theory employs communication about an idea or new health practice to drive community-engaged efforts. According to Rogers, there are different stages in the innovation process. Individuals progress through the stages of knowledge, persuasion, decision, implementation, and confirmation to decide whether to continue using the innovation. In knowledge, the community is exposed to an innovation but does not have enough knowledge about it. In the second stage, persuasion, the community is interested in the innovation and seeks out more information. In the third stage, decision, the community weighs the advantages and disadvantages of using the innovation and decides whether to adopt or reject it. If the community decides to adopt the practice, they apply it in the implementation stage to determine the usefulness of the innovation and if any additional information is needed. In the final stage, confirmation, the community decides whether to continue using the innovation and to what extent. According to this theory, the innovation process is also shaped by the individuals, who can be innovators, early adopters, the early majority, late majority, or laggards (who resist change and are often critical of others willing to accept the innovation). The characteristics of the innovation itself are also considered. These include (1) its perceived relative advantage over other approaches, (2) its compatibility with existing norms and beliefs, (3) the degree of complexity involved with adopting the innovation, (4) the trialability of the innovation or the extent to which it can be tested on a trial basis, and (5) the observability of the results.

*Review **Textbox 5.5**. Read through the SJA discussion prompt that follows and consider the role of social support and kinkeepers in your health and well-being.*

**Textbox 5.5   Discussion Questions/Thought Scenarios for Reflection**

**Social Support in Marginalized and Minority Populations**

*WPHC Thought Scenario 1*

**Social support**, such as in supportive interactions, is important during everyday relationships. Albrecht and Adelman define social support as verbal and nonverbal communication between recipients and providers that reduces uncertainty about the situation, the self, the other, or the relationship, and functions to enhance a perception of personal control in one's experience (1987). Supportive relationships can help mitigate stress. For instance, Leach and Braithwaite note families are important sources of social support. Their study finds that kinkeepers in families play an important role in keeping family members informed about one another. The kinkeepers do so by providing information, facilitating rituals, aiding, and maintaining family relationships.

On the other hand, a lack of close family relationships has been associated with negative health outcomes, such as an increased risk of depression in Hispanic individuals (Shim et al., 2014). Others have found that social support from family and friends positively influences self-management in chronic conditions, such as diabetes management. The development of social ties and utilization of social support within specific cultural communities, such as African Americans, impacts health in specific ways (Rees et al., 2010).

*SJA Discussion Questions*

1. In what ways has social support shaped your everyday health behaviors? For instance, does social network support (Textbox 5.7) or esteem support shape your dietary and physical exercise decisions?
2. How about decisions that concern disease prevention behaviors, such as obtaining a flu shot, consumption of alcohol in moderate amounts, or getting sufficient sleep every night?
3. What forms of social support did you receive?
4. Did your friends or family members offer encouragement, make you accountable to your goals, or serve as a role model for you?

**Resources**

Albrecht, T. L., & Adelman, M. B. (1987). *Communicating social support*. SAGE Publications.

Barnes, M. K., & Duck, S. (1994). Everyday communicative contexts for social support. In B. R. Burleson, T. L. Albrecht, & I. G. Sarason (Eds.), *Communication of social support* (pp. 175–194). SAGE Publications.

Leach, M. S., & Braithwaite, D. O. (1996). A binding tie: Supportive communication of family kinkeepers. *Journal of Applied Communication Research*, *24*, 200–216. https://doi.org/10.1080/00909889609365451

Rees, C. A., Karter, A. J., & Young, B. A. (2010). Race/ethnicity, social support, and associations with diabetes self-care and clinical outcomes in NCANES. *Diabetes Education*, *36*(3), 435–445. https://doi.org/10.1177/0145721710364419

Shim. R. S., Ye, J., Baltrus, P., Fry-Johnson, Y., Daniels, E., & Rust, G. (2014). Racial/ethnic disparities, social support, and depression: Examining a social determinant of mental health. *Ethnic Disparities*, *22*(1), 15–20.

*Community-Based Participatory Research (CBPR)*

CBPR is widely used for community engagement. In CBPR, all the collaborators respect the strengths that each brings to the partnership, and everyone in the community participates fully in all aspects of the research process. Its aim is to achieve social change to improve health outcomes and eliminate health disparities, and thus, provides a useful framework for WPHC contexts. CBPR literature makes a distinction between community-based and community-placed (Peterson, 2010). Communities of identity, for instance, refer to groups of individuals who share language, worldviews, values and norms, geography, and/or simply a commitment to common interests and needs. The tenets of CBPR are understood as parallel with culturally sensitive, culturally appropriate, or culturally tailored research.

Of relevance to WPHC contexts is the understanding of culturally tailored research that seeks to understand the cultural dimensions that can be integrated into health messages with an aim to bring about individual behavioral change in a targeted population. For instance, researchers Julie Maertens et al. (2017) in their study culturally tailor their web-based intervention for Latinos about the human papillomavirus (HPV) vaccine to incorporate suggestions from community members in the messaging. Doing so enabled them to modify the health information presented by reducing the amount of text, using brighter and more appealing colors, creating an eye-catching logo, and depicting how the HPV vaccine works with the immune system using graphics.

The CBPR approach illustrates how WPHC practitioners can construct relationships that demonstrate an understanding of and incorporate the community meaningfully in care contexts. Cultural sensitivity includes the dimensions of surface and deep structure. Surface structure refers to attempts to imbue health interventions with superficial characteristics of a target population such as language, food, and music. Deep structure seeks to imbue messages with core cultural values and environmental, social, and historical factors that shape health behaviors. Dutta-Bergman (2005b) focused on subaltern and indigenous communities to propose a culture-centered approach (CCA). The CCA seeks to center community by asking, "What does it mean to be healthy in your community?" "What is stopping you from realizing that vision?" and employing these facets to center the active role of the community in developing health applications (Dutta, 2007).

*Translational Research*

A final approach of relevance to the WPHC framework that includes community participation is translational research. **Chapter 6, Healthcare Systems**, will go into the clinical research aspects of translational research and challenges posed to optimal care delivery by lack of minority participation in greater detail. As proposed by the National Institutes of Health (NIH), translational research is focused on participatory research that can go from "the bench to the bedside and into the community." One framework utilized in translational research comprises its segmentation into four phases labeled T1–T4. T1 alludes to the translation of basic science into clinical research and includes phase 1 and 2 clinical trials, T2 represents the further research that translates its relevance in patient care and includes the phase 3 trials, and T4 is the movement of "scientific knowledge into the public sector … thereby changing people's everyday lives" through public and policy changes. The participation of the community members and stakeholders as equal partners is essential to the success of the premise of translational research.

### Workplace Relationships

*Organizational Wellness Programs*

In understanding context in the WPHC framework, work contexts, stress, and health are seen as intimately related, especially for disadvantaged and minority populations. An estimated 78% of US employees say that work is their biggest source of stress. These place a disproportionate burden on healthcare costs due to lost productivity. The workplace environment consists of the location of work, psychosocial factors that relate to the workers' roles and relationships at work, factors related to the job, and organizational policy. Racial and ethnic minorities disproportionately work in low-paying jobs and face increased risks of work-related injury or disability. Policies and benefits such as paid sick leave and unemployment compensation are associated with improved health outcomes. Psychosocial factors of the work environment include characteristics of the job (e.g., workload, job control, repetition, or monotonous tasks, mental and cognitive demands, clear job definitions), organizational structure (e.g., communication issues), interpersonal relationships (e.g., relationship with employer, supervisor, coworkers), temporal aspects of work (e.g., shift work, cycle time of tasks), financial and economic aspects (e.g., salary, benefits), and community aspects of the occupation (e.g., prestige, status). Organizational wellness programs focus on physical and mental health with little attention paid to social health comprising the quality of their network of professional and personal relationships. Poor physical and social working conditions are associated with chronic illnesses such as hypertension and work-related accidents. Organizational communication researchers Farrell and Geist-Martin (2005) find that social health focus in workplace wellness programs was constituted by building camaraderie with peers, communing with superiors, and reconnecting with family.

*Check out the **practitioner interview** with **Dr. Kathryn Fiddler**, vice president of population health at TidalHealth to see how one hospital system navigated its role in the community. How did TidalHealth's collaboration with community stakeholders and community empowerment improve healthcare outcomes at the height of the COVID-19 pandemic crisis?*

---

### TEXTBOX 5.6    Practitioner Interview

#### Dr. Kathryn Fiddler, DNP, MBA, RN
*Vice President of Population Health, TidalHealth*

1. When the COVID-19 pandemic hit, what brought about the realization that there were gaps in the populations whose healthcare needs were not being met? How were these needs and gaps identified? Were there gaps in the healthcare needs of these populations prior to the pandemic as well? How did TidalHealth work to integrate health equity as part of the practice, process, action, innovation, and organizational performance and outcomes?

    When the pandemic hit—TidalHealth was experiencing exceptionally high volumes of non-English speaking individuals with COVID. We had large populations of Haitian individuals living in the area and many were arriving to our ED very sick. These individuals had limited access to healthcare resources, often worked in agriculture, or were related to individuals in agricultural roles. We recognized the gaps in education related to COVID and significant financial challenges. We worked on supporting improved access in three ways.

Individually—took a small team to the community, with masks, sanitizer, education in local language, to support those community members most affected by COVID.

Community—Engaged with local poultry plants, local health department, and community organizations to share information, understand challenges, and develop mechanisms to provide access for those most challenged. We educated poultry plants on the need to approve time off (paid) for sick employees to prevent spread, conducted pop-up and drive-up testing at prioritized locations to support those communities most impacted.

System-wide—we developed a COVID-19 dashboard, which included demographics of race, gender, ethnicity, language, and tracked COVID testing, hospitalization, deaths, vaccination (when available) and reported this weekly to local health department, providers, and community organizations to raise awareness of the impact of COVID.

Mid-2020, we also engaged with Institute for Healthcare Improvement, a national healthcare quality improvement organization in their "Pathway to Health Equity" program with 20 other healthcare institutions across the country. We had a stakeholder group educated on racism, health equity, diversity, inclusion. We wrote a TidalHealth history of racism and shared; we began to build dashboards to understand our TidalHealth team, our patients, and our community as it relates to REAL-G data.

2. How did TidalHealth proceed with this knowledge? How did the key stakeholder network community, Tri-County Mediation, emerge as a center of coordination for these efforts? What communities are involved? How is coordination among the key stakeholders in these communities maintained? These might include all the components that make a thriving community—transportation, housing, public safety, education—and other elements.

TidalHealth has had a team focused on population health for several years. There was little community awareness of the work of the team. COVID brought to light some of the work we were doing, and in concert with the Tri Community Mediation—Vulnerable Population Group—teams from across the region came together to learn, grow, share alongside each other. Oftentimes, assumptions [were] made by groups about others' role in the system. TidalHealth grew in the role of "convener" as the size of the system allowed it to be able to bring stakeholders together. Tidal-Health also became aware of some of the connectedness of all the social determinants of health. The teams were better able to speak to the importance of education, childcare, safe housing, and others through these engagements with the community. As COVID evolved and grants became available, we were able to write for collaborative grants to support housing, workforce development, and other aspects of health equity.

3. Within TidalHealth, what efforts were made to identify and train medical and healthcare personnel with the consciousness, tools, and resources to confront inequities as well as to embed and advance equity within and across all aspects of the health system?

We used the IHI tools to train our board, executives, and stakeholder teams. We also had all employees educated on DEI, implicit bias, and health equity as part of annual training.

4. Can you speak a little more about TidalHealth's initiatives in the community during the pandemic and after in the post-acute COVID-19 crisis phase with addressing health disparities among key populations in the Eastern Shore? How were key priorities determined? How did these priorities shift during the course of the pandemic? What role did communication play in the initiatives designed to challenge disparities?

TidalHealth supported communication through a joint COVID-19 hotline with the County Health departments, we did two town halls with the community and also had healthcare leader quarterly meetings to educate and update the community. Our lead physician had weekly meetings with all local healthcare providers and sent a weekly email as well.

We did mass drive-through testing events, pop-up testing, community education and outreach as well as operating a vaccine clinic. We engaged with local churches and church leaders, met with the local Haitian community leaders, and went on many radio and TV stations.

5. Social justice in healthcare involves equity, access, participation, diversity, and human rights. How was your work emblematic of these principles in action during the pandemic and beyond? What were some of the biggest challenges in this journey? What were some of the most noteworthy outcomes that were achieved?

For us, social justice in healthcare starts with access. Early in the pandemic, we worked to provide those most challenged by COVID to have access to testing, education, and then vaccines. We broadened definitions of frontline workers to those who supported the community, allowing our rates of vaccination for our BIPOC population to be higher than many other communities. We now are engaged as board members for our local Haitian Development Center, we have Memorandums of Understanding with several community agencies to provide community health workers and social workers to support improvement in chronic disease and recently were awarded a $1.2 million grant through the Maryland Health Care Commission to reduce healthcare disparities for hypertension and diabetes in five local zip codes.

6. The work of the collaborative, Tri-County Mediation, continues. Where do you see it headed? How will TidalHealth's operations continue to work to challenge existing systems of privilege and oppression to improve health outcomes in marginalized communities on the Eastern Shore?

Our population health team has continued to grow. We have begun building bridges of trust through shared commitment to our community. Through our work with our health equity dashboards, explicitly calling out evidence of systemic racism and disparities, and sharing this data thoughtfully with our healthcare team and community—we will continue to move this work forward. There is much to do, and with these teams continuing to learn, grow share, be vulnerable, and work toward collaborative answers focused on "*getting it right*" versus being right, we can continue to improve outcomes.

## ORGANIZATION AS FAMILY

Organizational communication scholar Erika Kirby argues that organizations are increasingly appropriating family-like roles in their employees' lives through initiatives such as work-life or work-family programs, flexible work options, and dependent-care benefits (Kirby, 2006). Such concern is exemplified in organizational physical and mental health programs. Physical health programs such as health screening and education, nutrition, fitness programs, and meditation classes are instances where organizational resources extend into domains such as cardiovascular health, nutrition, weight loss, stress management, and fitness levels. Mental health programs offered by organizations include counseling for personal, emotional, and psychological concerns, lifestyle counseling, stress management training, and relaxation practices. Organizations are also increasingly appropriating a spiritual role (Buzzanell & Harter, 2006) through strategies like integrating philosophical spaces for meditation, reflection, and prayer in the workplace; doing work that honors one's personal values and corporate values; standing up for what is right; living by the Golden Rule; and honoring one's employer by doing an honest day's work. Although these are helpful initiatives, Kirby cautions of a need to remain aware of how employees may be co-opted in unhealthy work schedules under the guide of cultivating balance in their lives, whereby the responsibility of the health outcomes remains on the individual employee while the organization sidesteps the issue of workplace stresses and harmful workplace exposures (e.g., chemical exposure or repetitive motion problems).

## MINORITY STRESSORS

Employees who belong to minority groups are more likely to face infringements on their professional boundaries and to face increased scrutiny over their professional actions within the workplace. Studies show that women, staff, racial/ethnic, and sexual and gender minority groups working in a professional capacity in academic institutions are significantly more likely to consider changing jobs due to unprofessional behavior that manifests as bias and discrimination (Alexis et al., 2020). To address this concern, it is important to apply professional standards equitably and avoid stigmatizing minority and marginalized populations. An inequitable environment is more likely to increase minority perceptions of isolation and to contribute to a lack of engagement. Organizational tensions between inclusion and assimilation place an unfair burden on minority groups to confirm, even though they may be challenged to feel a sense of belonging. Inclusivity supports diversity and is the opposite of conforming or assimilation. For instance, professional standards are not inclusive when underrepresented members of an organization must conform or assimilate to adhere to them.

## MEDICAL PROFESSIONALISM AND STIGMA

Understanding the perception of difference and identity in terms of social acceptance was addressed by Erving Goffman in his work on stigma (Goffman, 1963). Stigmatized individuals are in some way excluded from complete social acceptance, often stemming from characteristics that stem from prejudice or bias. For instance, homosexuality, one of the categories of stigma that is covered by Goffman, was once defined as a medical condition and criminalized. In 1974, it was removed from the list of psychiatric disorders recognized in the United States, even as the gay movement shifted homosexuality from a stigma to a politicized identity. The concept of "covering" was coined by Erving Goffman and alludes to how individuals with known stigmatized identities perceive greater pressure and put more effort into down-playing those identities to assimilate better into majority groups. Identifying and addressing covering by minority groups can help break down barriers and lead to a culture of inclusion and authenticity. The converse is also true. For instance, medical professionalism and its standards are vulnerable to being mobilized with a degree of strictness among marginalized groups (e.g., racial, or religious minorities in the medical field), thus displaying what is known as weaponization in their unequal application. This weaponization can damage individuality and identity and cause conformity, shrink efforts to increase the diversity of the workforce, create harmful environments, and force marginalized populations to assimilate to be included.

### WORKPLACE CLIMATE

From a WPHC perspective, healthy workplace relationships support healthy behaviors in many ways. For instance, exclusive breastfeeding for the first six months and continuation with supplementary feeding for up to two years and beyond is recommended by the WHO. However, this is a challenge for new mothers seeking to return to work earlier than the Family and Medical Leave Act of 1993 provision of 12 weeks. Returning to work after maternity leave poses significant challenges for breastfeeding, suggesting that working women face significant obstacles when combining work and motherhood in the postpartum period. The perception of coworker support greatly influenced women's beliefs about overall organizational support. According to the US Department of Labor, women's participation in the US labor force has increased from 32.7% in 1948 to 56.8% in 2016. Given that over 70% of mothers with children under the age of 18 are employed, the workplace climate can make a significant difference in parenting patterns. In their survey-based study with 500 working mothers, Zhuang and colleagues found that mothers' perception of supportive coworker communication has an impact on sustained breastfeeding. A supportive environment can help women maintain work-family balance. Workplace climate and a perception of social support or stigma can shape mothers' decisions to breastfeed.

### Role of Social Support

Social support is defined as the assistance and protection given to individuals as the functional content of relationships (Cohen & McKay, 1984). Social support can shape health promotion and disease prevention behaviors while mitigating the effects of stress. Zhuang et al. (2019) use the social support stress-buffering model, which posits that social support received by individuals protects them from the detrimental effects of stress. This protective effect may happen at the time of stress appraisal such that an individual may not perceive a potentially stressful event as stressful because social support buffers the process or inhibits maladaptive responses and facilitates adjustive counter responses (Cohen & Wills, 1985). Textbox 5.5 provides an insight into the role of social support in minority and marginalized families.

Social support has protective health functions (Cassel, 1976). Research shows positive links between support and mental and physical health (House et al., 1988). Social support comprises listening support (listening without giving advice or being judgmental; emotional comfort or comforting workers and indicating that others care about their well-being, and emotional challenge or challenging workers to evaluate their own attitudes, values, and feelings. Verbal and nonverbal messages sent by managers and coworkers can communicate support or disapproval of minority identities and behaviors.

STIGMA AND MARGINALIZED POPULATIONS

In the example of the workplace climate for lactating mothers returning to work, the lack of coworker support was a major barrier to continuing to pump breastmilk. Social support in the workplace can help in countering stigma or for marginalized populations to internalize stigma. WPHC settings are mindful of context, including workplace support or stress. Internalized stigma is defined as the "negative feeling about the self, maladjusted behavior, or stereotypical endorsement resulting in an individual's experience, perception, or anticipation of negative social reaction on the basis of a health condition" (Stevelink et al., 2012, p. 101).

*Check out **Textbox 5.7** for a definition of social support, along with its role in mitigating stress. Respond to the SJA discussion prompt that follows.*

---

**Textbox 5.7   Different Types of Social Support**

**WPHC Context: Types of Social Support**

Different types of social support have been identified in communication literature. The types and their definitions are provided here:

- **Emotional support**:
  Defined as the "ability to turn to others for comfort and security during times of stress, leading the person to feel that he or she is cared for by others" (Cutrona & Russell, 1990, p. 322).
- **Informational support**:
  Defined as "providing the individual with advice or guidance concerning possible solutions to a problem" (Cutrona & Russell, 1990, p. 322).
- **Tangible/instrumental support**:
  Defined as the provision of tangible aid and service, such as physically providing needed goods and services to recipients (Cutrona & Suhr, 1992).
- **Esteem support**:
  Defined as the messages that help to promote one's skills, abilities, and intrinsic value (Cutrona & Suhr, 1992).
- **Social network support**:
  Defined as the messages that help to enhance one's sense of belonging to a specific group with similar interests or situations (Cutrona & Suhr, 1992).

**SJA Discussion Prompt**

Watch an episode of a television series such as *Midnight Family* (Hispanic medical family drama), *Black-ish*, or *Insecure* (African American TV series).

1. What are some instances of the different types of social support behaviors or communicative messages you can identify among a range of cultural groups?
2. How would you offer social support under similar circumstances?

### Resources

Cutrona, C. E., & Russell, D. W. (1990). Type of social support and specific stress: Toward a theory of optimal matching. In B. R. Sarason, I. G. Sarason, & G. R. Pierce (Eds.), *Social support: An interactional view* (pp. 319–366). Wiley series on personality processes. John Wiley & Sons.

Cutrona, C. E., & Suhr, J. A. (1992). Controllability of stressful events and satisfaction with spouse support behaviors. *Communication Research, 19*, 154–174.

## WORKPLACE ENVIRONMENT, LEADERSHIP, AND WORKER RESILIENCE

An open and welcoming work environment can communicate social support and worker health in significant ways. Haas (2020) examines how supervisory leadership can improve an organization's safety outcomes. Haas found that the communicative support offered by supervisors to employees can bolster the supervisor-employee relationship with positive safety outcomes in high-risk and dynamic work environments. Providing adequate, tailored informational support bolsters learning, job competence, a sense of belonging, and worker resilience (Bakker & Demerouti, 2008). These outcomes support whole person health and well-being. Resilience labor, constructed with transformative identities and identifications, can bolster and sustain organizational involvement and worker resilience (Agarwal & Buzzanell, 2015). Informational support comprises reality confirmation when supervisors indicate that other coworkers are like them and see things the way they do, task appreciation when supervisors acknowledge employees' efforts and express appreciation for their work, and task challenge when supervisors challenge employees' way of thinking about their work to motivate and foster greater creativity and involvement in work. In these and other forms of workplace support, WPHC relationships ask us to be mindful of differences and tailoring communication for whole person health outcomes for all.

*As we conclude* **Chapter 5, Healthcare Relationships***, review* **Textbox 5.8** *for a deeper dive into CBPR and respond to the SJA discussion prompts regarding its role in strengthening community relationships, capacity building, and addressing systemic inequities.*

### Textbox 5.8    Present Challenges and Future Directions Exercise

#### Community-Based Participatory Approaches

Present Challenges and Call for Future Action:

#### WPHC Context

Community-based participatory approach (CBPA)/CBPR is key to health promotion and addressing inequities among socially disadvantaged and marginalized communities. At its heart, CBPA seeks to be responsive to community needs. In CBPA, community members participate as equal decision-makers and contributors in discussions with all stakeholders and partners. The CBPA builds on principles of community as a unit of identity, recognizing its collective strengths and shared resources, facilitating partnership and capacity building of its members throughout the process, disseminating information to community members and participants, eliciting long-term commitment and involvement, and seeking a balance between research and action (Virginia Department of Health, 2022). In doing so, the CBPA engages the community as an active participant in addressing health disparities in socially disadvantaged populations. CBPA can involve a combination of individual, group, and community-level components, draw upon health information technology and social media elements, and support community resilience.

## SJA Discussion Prompt

CBPA/CBPR approaches seek to be community-based rather than simply "community-placed," in other words, to be authentic to community partnerships and collaborations (Minkler, 2005). They center participation, research, and action with a goal to bring about meaningful social change. The challenges arise in identifying issues of concern to the community and creating meaningful partnerships that reflect the equity and balance in collaboration that CBPR approaches highlight. Questions that must be navigated include which partners to include, such as informal and formal community leaders, nongovernmental organizations, researchers, and community members and professionals (Travers & Flicker, 2004). Another challenge is to be sensitive to the concerns of the different communities involved. At its best, CBPR can improve cultural sensitivity and community participation to bring about long-term meaningful change while building capacity and community resilience. What aspect would you consider in implementing your project to meet the goals of CBPR?

1. Will the methods used be sensitive and appropriate to various communities?
2. What training or capacity-building opportunities will you build in?
3. How will you balance scientific rigor and accessibility?
   (Minkler, 2005; Travers & Flicker, 2004)

## Resources

Minkler, M. (2005). Community-based research partnerships: Challenges and opportunities. *Journal of Urban Health: Bulletin of the New York Academy of Medicine, 82*(2), S2. https://doi.org/10.1093/jurban/jti034

Travers, R., & Flicker, S. (2004). Ethical issues in community-based research. In *Urban Health Community-Based Research Series Workshop*. Wellesley, MA.

Virginia Department of Health. (2022). *Community-based participatory approaches*. https://www.vdh.virginia.gov/health-equity/community-based-participatory-approaches/

## References

Agarwal, V., & Buzzanell, P. M. (2015). Communicative reconstruction of resilience labor: Identity/identification in disaster-relief workers. *Journal of Applied Communication Research, 43*(4), 408–428. https://doi.org/10.1080/00909882.2015.1083602

Airhihenbuwa, C. O. (1995). *Health and culture: Beyond the western paradigm*. Sage.

Airhihenbuwa, C. O. (2007). On being comfortable with being uncomfortable: Centering an Africanist vision in our gateway to global health. *Health Education and Behavior*, *34*(1), 31–42. https://doi.org/10.1177/1090198106291377

Alexis, D. A., Kearney, M. D., Williams, J. C., Xu, C., Higginbotham, E. J., & Aysola, J. (2020). Assessment of perceptions of professionalism among faculty, trainees, staff, and students in a large university-based health system. *JAMA Network Open*, *3*(11): e2021452. https://doi.org/10.1001/jamanetworkopen.2020.21452

Alpert, J. M., Morris, B. B., Thomson, M. D., Matin, K., & Brown, R. F. (2019). Identifying how patient portals impact communication in oncology. *Health Communication*, *34*(12), 1395–1403. https://doi.org/10.1080/10410236.2018.1493418

Anders, H., Munthe, C., Törner, M., & Forsander, G. (2016). The counseling, self-care, adherence approach to person-centered care and shared decision making: Moral psychology, executive autonomy, and ethics in multi-dimensional care decisions. *Health Communication*, *31*(8), 964–973. https://doi.org/10.1080/10410236.2015.1025332

Anderson, J. N., Graff, J. C., Krukowski, R. A., Schwartzberg, L., Vidal, G. A., Waters, T. M., ... Graetz, I. (2021). "Nobody will tell you. You've got to ask!": An examination of patient-provider communication needs and preferences among black and white women with early-stage breast cancer. *Health Communication*, *36*(11), 1331–1342. https://doi.org/10.1080/10410236.2020.1751383

Bakker, A. B., & Demerouti, E. (2008). Towards a model of work engagement. *Career Development International*, *13*, 209–223. https://doi.org/10.1108/13620430810870476

Baptiste-Roberts, K., Gary, T. L., Beckles, G. L. A., Gregg, E. W., Owens, M., Porterfield, D., & Engelgau, M. M. (2007). Family history of diabetes, awareness of risk factors, and health behaviors among African Americans. *American Journal of Public Health*, *97*, 907–912. https://doi.org/10.2105/AJPH.2005.077032

Baxter, L. A., Braithwaite, D. O., Golish, T. D., & Olson, L. N. (2002). Contradictions of interaction for wives of elderly husbands with adult dementia. *Journal of Applied Communication Research*, *30*(1), 1–26, https://doi.org/10.1080/00909880216576

Baxter, L. A., & Montgomery, B. M. (1998). A guide to dialectical approaches to studying personal relationships. In B. M. Montgomery & L. A. Baxter (Eds.), *Dialectical approaches to studying personal relationships* (pp. 1–16). Erlbaum.

Buzzanell, P. M. (2010). Resilience: Talking, resisting, and imagining new normalcies into being. *Journal of Communication*, *60*, 1–14. https://doi.org/10.1111/j.1460-2466.2009.01469.x

Buzzanell, P. M., & Harter, L. M. (2006). (De)centering and (re)envisioning the secular hegemony of organizational communication theory and research. *Communication Studies*, *57*, 1–3. https://doi.org/10.1080/10510970500481797

Bylund, C. L., Peterson, E. B., & Cameron, K. A. (2012). A practitioner's guide to interpersonal communication theory: An overview and exploration of selected theories. *Patient Education and Counseling*, *87*, 261–267 https://doi.org/10.1016/j.pec.2011.10.006

Cassel, J. (1976). The contribution of the social environment to host resistance. *American Journal of Epidemiology*, *104*, 107–123. https://doi.org/10.1093/oxfordjournals.aje.a112281

CDC. (2022). Social determinants of health at CDC. Retrieved from https://www.cdc.gov/about/sdoh/index.html

CDC. (2022). *The social-ecological model: A framework for prevention*. Retrieved from https://www.cdc.gov/violenceprevention/about/social-ecologicalmodel.html

Cohen, S., & McKay, G. (1984). Social support, stress, and the buffering hypothesis: A theoretical analysis. *Handbook of Psychology and Health* (Vol. 4, pp. 253–267). Hillsdale, NJ: Earlbaum.

Cohen, S., & Wills, T.A. (1985). Stress, social support, and the buffering hypothesis. *Psychological Bulletin*, *98*(2), 310–357.

Dorrance Hall, E., Ma, M., Azimova, D., Campbell, N., Ellithorpe, M., Plasencia, J., ... Hennessy, M. (2021). The mediating role of family and cultural food beliefs on the relationship between family communication patterns and diet and health issues across racial/ethnic groups. *Health Communication*, *36*(5), 593–605. https://doi.org/10.1080/10410236.2020.1733213

Dutta-Bergman, M. J. (2005a). The relation between health-orientation, provider-patient communica-tion, and satisfaction: An individual-difference approach. *Health Communication, 18*, 291–303. https://doi.org/10.1207/s15327027hc1803_6

Dutta-Bergman, M. J. (2005b). Theory and practice in health communication campaigns: A critical interrogation. *Health Communication, 18*(2), 103–122. https://doi.org/10.1207/s15327027hc1802_1

Dutta, M. J. (2007). Communicating about culture and health: Theorizing culture-centered and cultural sensitivity approaches. *Communication Theory, 17*(3), 304–328.

Ellner, A. L., & Phillips, R. S. (2017). The coming primary care revolution. *Journal of General Internal Medicine, 32*, 380–386. https://doi.org/10.1007/s11606-016-3944-3

Epstein, R. M., & Street, Jr., R. L. (2007). *Patient-centered communication in cancer care: Promoting healing and reducing suffering.* National Cancer Institute, NIH Publication No. 07-6225. Bethesda, MD. Retrieved from https://cancercontrol.cancer.gov/sites/default/files/2020-06/pcc_monograph.pdf

Farrell, A., & Geist-Martin, P. (2005). Communicating social health: Perceptions of wellness at work. *Management Communication Quarterly, 18*(4), 543–592. https://doi.org/10.1177/0893318904273691

Feltwell, A. K., & Rees, C. E. (2004). The information-seeking behaviors of partners of men with pros-tate cancer: A qualitative pilot Study. *Patient Education and Counseling, 54*(2), 179–185. https://doi.org/10.1016/S0738-3991(03)00212-X

Flentje, A., Clark, K. D., Cicero, E., Capriotti, M. R., Lubensky, M. E., Sauceda, J. ... Obedin-Maliver, J. (2021). Minority stress, structural stigma, and physical health among sexual and gender minority individuals: Examining the relative strength of the relationships. *Annals of Behavioral Medicine.* https://doi.org/10.1093/abm/kaab051

Finney-Rutten, L. J., Hesse, B. W., St. Sauver, J. L., Wilson, P., Chawla, N., Hartigan, D. B., ... Arora, N. K. (2016). Health self-efficacy among populations with multiple chronic conditions: The value of patient-centered communication. *Advances in Therapy, 3*, 1440–1451. https://doi.org/10.1007/s12325-016-0369-7

Goffman, E. (1963). *Stigma: Notes on the management of spoiled identity.* Penguin.

Haas, E. J. (2020). The role of supervisory support on workers' health and safety performance. *Health Communication, 35*(3), 364–374. https://doi.org/10.1080/10410236.2018.1563033

Hong, H., & Oh, H. J. (2020). The effects of patient-centered communication: Exploring the mediating role of trust in healthcare providers. *Health Communication, 35*(4), 502–511. https://doi.org/10.1080/10410236.2019.1570427

Hong, S. J., Goodman, M., & Kaphingst, K. A. (2020). Relationships of family history-related factors and causal beliefs to cancer risk perception and mammography screening adherence among medically underserved women. *Journal of Health Communication, 25*(7), 531–542. https://doi.org/10.1080/1081 0730.2020.1788677

House, J. S., Umberson, D., & Landis, K. R. (1988). Structures and processes of social support. *Annual Review of Sociology, 14*, 293 – 318. https://doi.org/10.1146/annurev.so.14.080188.001453

Hovick, S. R. (2014). Understanding family health information seeking: A test of the theory of moti-vated information management. *Journal of Health Communication, 19*, 6–23. https://doi.org/10.1080/10810730.2013.778369

Israel, B. A., Schulz, A. J., Parker, E. A., Becker, A. B., Allen, A. J., Guzman, J. R. (2003). Critical issues in developing and following community based participatory research principles. In Minkler, M., & Wallerstein, N. (Eds.), *Community-based participatory research for health* (pp. 53–76). Jossey-Bass.

Jain, P. (2022). The stereotype content model as an explanation of biased perceptions in a medical inter-action: Implications for patient-provider relationship. *Health Communication, 37*(1), 64–73. https://doi.org/10.1080/10410236.2020.1816311

Kirby, E. L. (2006). "Helping you make room in your life for your needs": When organizations appropri-ate family roles. *Communication Monographs, 73*(4), 474–480. https://doi.org/10.1080/03637750601061208

Krieger, J. L. (2014). Family communication about cancer treatment decision making. *Communication Yearbook, 38*, 279–305. https://doi.org/10.1080/23808985.2014.11679165

Lefkowitz, E. S., & Stoppa, T. M. (2006). Positive sexual communication and socialization in the parent-adolescent context. *New Directions for Child and Adolescent Development*, *112*, 39–55. https://doi.org/10.1002/cd.161

Lincoln, C. E., & Mamiya, L. H. (1990). *The black church in the African American experience*. Duke University Press.

Maertens, J. A., Jimenez-Zambrano, A. M., Albright, K., & Dempsey, A. F. (2017). Using community engagement to develop a web-based intervention for Latinos about the HPV vaccine. *Journal of Health Communication*, *22*(4), 285–293. https://doi.org/10.1080/10810730.2016.1275890

Miller, L. E., & Caughlin, J. P. (2013). "We're going to be survivors": Couples' identity challenges during and after cancer treatment. *Communication Monographs*, *80*, 63–82. https://doi.org/10.1080/03637751.2012.739703

Minuchin, P. (1985). Families and individual development: Provocations from the field of family therapy. *Child Development*, *56*, 289–302.

Nielsen, A., Krasnik, A., Vassard, D., Holm, L. (2015). Use and preference of advice on small children's food: Differences between parents from ethnic minority, ethnic majority, and mixed households. *Journal of Health Communication*, *20*(12), 1397–1405. https://doi.org/10.1080/10810730.2015.1018627

Olaisen, R. H., Schluchter, M. D., Flocke, S. A., Smyth, K. A., Koroukian, S. M., & Strange, K. C. (2020). Assessing the longitudinal impact of physician-patient relationship on functional health. *The Annals of Family Medicine*, *18*(5), 422–429. https://doi.org/10.1370/afm.2554

Palmer-Wackerly, A., Krieger, J. L., & Rhodes, N. D. (2017). The role of healthcare provider and partner decisional support in patients' cancer treatment decision-making satisfaction. *Journal of Health Communication*, *22*(1), 10–19. https://doi.org/10.1080/10810730.2016.1245804

Peterson, J. C. (2010). CBPR in Indian country: Tensions and implications for health communication. *Health Communication*, *25*(1), 50–60. https://doi.org/10.1080/10410230903473524

Peterson Center on Healthcare and KFF. (2022). *How does health spending in the U.S. compare to other countries?*https://www.healthsystemtracker.org/chart-collection/health-spending-u-s-compare-countries-2/#Average%20annual%20growth%20rate%20in%20health%20consumption%20expenditures%20per%20capita%202000%20through%202020,%20U.S.%20dollars,%20PPP%20adjusted%C2%A0

Petronio, S., & Caughlin, J. P. (2006). Communication privacy management theory: Understanding families. In D. O. Braithwaite & L. A. Baxter (Eds.), *Engaging theories in family communication: Multiple perspectives* (pp. 35–49). Sage.

Pulvirenti, M., McMillan, J., Lawn, S. (2014). Empowerment, patient-centered care, and self-management. *Health Expectations*, *17*(3), 303–310. https://doi.org/10.1111/j.1369-7625.2011.00757.x

Ricks-Santi, L. J., Thompson, N., Ewing, A., Harrison, B., Higginbotham, K., Spencer, C., … Frederick, W. (2016). Predictors of self-reported family health history of breast cancer. *Journal of Immigrant and Minority Health*, *18*, 1175–1182. https://doi.org/10.1007/s10903-015-0253-6

Rogers, E. (1995). *Diffusion of innovations* (4th ed.). Free Press.

Rositch, A. F., Atnafou, R., Krakow, M., & D'Souza, G. (2019). A community-based qualitative assessment of knowledge, barriers, and promoters of communicating about family cancer history among African Americans. *Health Communication*, *34*(10), 1192–1201. https://doi.org/10.1080/10410236.2018.1471335

Russell, N., Igras, S., Kuoh, H., Pavin, M., & Wickerstrom, J. (2008). *The active community engagement continuum*. ACQUIRE Project Working Paper. https://pdf.usaid.gov/pdf_docs/Pnadm497.pdf

Singh, S., Evans, N., Williams, M., Sestinas, N., & Baryeh, N. A. K. (2018). Influences of socio-demographic factors and health utilization factors on patient-centered provider communication. *Health Communication*, *33*(7), 917–923. https://doi.org/10.1080/10410236.2017.1322481

Stevelink, S. A. M., Wu, I. C., Voorend, C. G., & van Brakel, W. H. (2012). The psychometric assessment of internalized stigma instruments: A systematic review. *Stigma Research and Action*, *2*, 100–118. https://doi.org/10.54631/SRA.v1i1

Stewart, M. (2001). Towards a global definition of patient-centered care: The patient should be the judge of patient -centered care. *British Medical Journal*, *322*, 444–445.

The Commonwealth Fund. (2021, August 4). *Mirror, mirror 2021: Reflecting poorly: Health care in the U.S. compared to other high-income countries*. https://www.commonwealthfund.org/publications/fund-reports/2021/aug/mirror-mirror-2021-reflecting-poorly

Thompson, T., Seo, J., Griffith, J., Baxter, M., James, A., & Kaphingst, K. A. (2015). The context of collecting family health history: Examining definitions of family and family communication about health among African American women. *Journal of Health Communication, 20*(4), 416–423. https://doi.org/10.1080/10810730.2014.977466

Trivedi, N., Moser, R. P., Breslau, E. S., Chou, W.-Y. S. (2021). Predictors of patient-centered communication among U.S. adults: Analysis of the 2017–2018 Health Information National Trends Survey (HINTS). *Journal of Health Communication, 26*(1), 57–64. https://doi.org/10.1080/10810730.2021.1878400

Valdez, R., Yoon, P. W., Qureshi, N., Green, R. F., & Khoury, M. J. (2010). Family history in public health practice: A genomic tool for disease prevention and health promotion. *Annual Review of Public Health, 31*, 69–87. https://doi.org/10.1146/annurev.publhealth.012809.103621

Wallerstein, N., & Duran, B. (2003). The conceptual, historical and practice roots of community-based participatory research and related participatory traditions. In M. Minkler & N. Wallerstein (Eds.), *Community-based participatory research for health* (1st ed., pp. 27–52). Jossey-Bass.

Wanzer, M. B., Booth-Butterfield, M., & Gruber, K. (2004). Perceptions of health care providers' communication: Relationships between patient-centered communication and satisfaction. *Health Communication, 16*, 363–384. https://doi.org/10.1207/S15327027HC1603_6

Williams, T. T., Pichon, L. C., & Campbell, B. (2015). Sexual health communication within religious African American families. *Health Communication, 30*(4), 328–338. https://doi.org/10.1080/10410236.2013.856743

Wilson, K., Bleasdale, J., Przybyla, S. M. (2021). Provider-patient communication on pre-exposure prophylaxis (PrEP) for HIV prevention: An exploration of healthcare provider challenges. *Health Communication, 36*(13), 1677–1686. https://doi.org/10.1080/10410236.2020.1787927

Yoon, P. W., Scheuner, M. T., & Khoury, M. J. (2003). Research priorities for evaluating family history in the prevention of common chronic diseases. *American Journal of Preventive Medicine, 24*, 128–135. https://doi.org/10.1016/s0749-3797(02)00585-8

Yoon, P. W., Scheuner, M. T., Peterson-Oehlke, K. L., Gwinn, M., Faucett, A., & Khoury, M. J. (2002). Can family history be used as a tool for public health and preventive medicine? *Genetics in Medicine, 4*, 304–310. https://doi.org/10.1097/00125817-200207000-00009

Zhuang, J., Bresnahan, M. J., Yan, X., Zhu, Y., Goldbort, J., & Bogdan-Lovis, E. (2019). Keep doing the good work: Impact of coworker and community support on continuation of breastfeeding. *Health Communication, 34*(11), 1270–1278. https://doi.org/10.1080/10410236.2018.1476802

## Additional Resources

Bartunek, J. M. (2010). Intergroup relationships and quality improvement in healthcare. *BMJ Quality & Safety, 20*(S1). http://dx.doi.org/10.1136/bmjqs.2010.046169

Goold, S. D. (2002). Trust, distrust, and trustworthiness. *Journal of General Internal Medicine, 17*(1), 79–81. https://doi.org/10.1046/j.1525-1497.2002.11132.x

Nundy, S., Kvedar, J. C., & Cella, G. M. (2020, April 6). From one-to-one to one-to-many: Rethinking healthcare relationships in the digital age. *Health Affairs*. https://doi.org/10.1377/forefront.20200320.600000

# Healthcare Systems

---

## Chapter Learning Outcomes

Upon completing **Chapter 6, Healthcare Systems**, the student will be able to apply the WPHC SJA framework to:

1. Identify the system-level sources of structural healthcare inequities and outcomes.
2. Explain community-based care through the Accountable Health Communities model and the lens of the value-based care model.
3. Identify how disparities arise and can be mitigated at the translational research and clinical trial recruitment level.
4. Identify and address health inequities stemming from system-level forces impacting the structure and delivery of health services in primary, secondary, and tertiary care settings.
5. Situate diagnostic, rehabilitative, and palliative care contexts through the lens of the system-level care provided, infrastructure challenges, and racial and ethnic disparities.
6. Identify structural and institutional barriers to health equity in self-care, home healthcare, adult day care centers, and community care settings.
7. Engage in communicative action to support prevention, patient education, and coordination of care ethos.

### Consider the following contexts:

A study including nearly all the infants born to first-time mothers from 2007 to 2016 in California, the state with the most annual births, showed how childbirth is deadlier for Black families even when they're rich. The best medical care for mothers and babies in 2023, the study showed, is still not equally accessible to everyone (Kennedy-Moulton et al., 2022). In Baltimore, Maryland, a 5-mile trip from the Roland Park neighborhood to the Madison East End community yields a 20-year drop in life expectancy (Ames et al., 2011). Death is three times more likely for Black infants in the United States than for White infants if their care is administered by White doctors, according to a study published in *Proceedings of the National*

DOI: 10.4324/9781003214472-8

*Academy of Sciences* (PNAS). However, if Black infants are cared for by Black doctors, their mortality rates drop by up to 58%.

(Picheta, 2020, Aug. 20)

Approximately 13 percent of the total population of the United States has a disability. Yet, more non-Hispanic Black adults and Hispanic adults report having a disability compared to White, non-Hispanic adults (US Census Bureau, 2014). Furthermore, adults with disabilities are almost twice as likely as other adults to report unmet healthcare needs due to problems with the accessibility of a doctor's office or clinic (Internal Revenue Service, 2018). One of the most prominent challenges for individuals with disabilities is overcoming the barriers to enter and navigate healthcare facilities including entrances, hallways, exam rooms, medical equipment, and restrooms. Many healthcare facilities are not architecturally fully accessible, and many lack weight scales and examination tables that are accessible for individuals with disabilities.

(Kraus et al., 2017)

## Chapter Organization

**Chapter 6, Healthcare Systems**, is organized as follows: **First**, in line with the WPHC SJA ethos of health, the chapter lays out the system-level sources of systemic and structural health and healthcare inequities and health-related outcomes. It places these factors within a larger SJ and racial equity frame to contextualize the Affordable Care Act and the Healthy People 2030 initiative. It also places the community in healthcare engagement at a system level and discusses community-based care through the Accountable Health Communities model and the lens of the value-based care model. **Second**, the chapter presents the parameters of primary, secondary, and tertiary care, paying attention to health inequities and disparities stemming from system-level forces impacting the structure and delivery of healthcare services in primary, secondary, and tertiary care settings, focusing on the 2018 Astana Declaration and coordination of care. **Third**, the chapter will cover the contexts of diagnostic, rehabilitative, and palliative care through the lens of the system-level care provided, infrastructure challenges, and racial and ethnic disparities. **Fourth**, the chapter will examine self-care, home care, and community care through the lens of self-care initiatives and interventions, the home healthcare service sector, structural and institutional barriers, community health centers, and adult day care centers. **Fifth**, the chapter will discuss the communicative factors involved in prevention, patient education, and coordination of care through concepts like health behaviors, health promotion, disease prevention, wellness programs, home healthcare, patient-centered care medical home models, and care coordination for chronic condition self-management. Along the way, to highlight the WPHC SJA principles in each section of the chapter, the student will be provided with numerous examples, contexts, statistics, and principles ranging from translational research to primary care, and home healthcare. Students will be encouraged to engage in direct and actionable SJA prompts invoking contexts such as the Americans with Disabilities Act, market-based reforms, and academic health centers. The scholar interview with Dr. Annabella Beju will illustrate her work with mental health care for the displaced and migrant populations. Discussion Questions and Thought Scenarios for Reflection will highlight the challenges of clinical trial recruitment as they lend to system-level disparities. The Present Challenges and Future Directions Exercise will encourage students to consider the system-level challenges underpinning the health outcome inequities and disparities in the context of American Indian and Alaska Native populations and brain health.

## A Systemic WPHC SJA Look at Healthcare Inequities

In the United States, systemic and structural health, and healthcare inequities in health-related outcomes between groups continue to challenge healthcare administrators, policy-makers, and public health professionals. Justice is one of the four pillars of medicine's ethical framework. It seeks to ensure fair distribution of health resources and to be fair when making decisions about who gets what treatment. The Charter on Medical Professionalism encourages physicians to "promote justice in the healthcare system" and to "work actively to eliminate discrimination in healthcare, whether based on race, gender, socioeconomic status, ethnicity, religion, or any other social category" (ABIM Foundation, 2003). Likewise, health centers (e.g., academic health centers, AHCs) have an ethical responsibility to address injustice(s) as they threaten the health of the populations that they serve. Unfortunately, a disconnect exists between the lived experience of populations facing inequity in healthcare and the missions of most healthcare systems.

### SJ and Racial Equity Frame

Communication can play a central role in engaging awareness and advocacy to address health inequities and promote SJ (Rosen et al., 2020). For instance, communication researchers Thompson et al. (2022) illustrate how an opportunity for engaging youth around health and disease that promotes a reframing of SJ and racial equity frame was provided by the COVID-19 pandemic. Their experimental study determined the impact of providing an online adaptation of The Bigger Picture (TBP), a spoken word, arts-based public health literacy campaign and a comparison campaign. The campaign uses outcomes incorporating the culture of health framework concepts such as health-related mindset and expectations, sense of belonging, and civic engagement. The researchers found that TBP participation results in a measurable shift in students' mindsets around structural drivers of health and health inequity and increased plans for future civic engagement. Communication-based research such as this shows how strategies incorporating arts-based messaging and civic engagement can be impactful ways of engaging youth advocates in access and SJ inequities stemming from complex structural and systemic factors.

### Value-Based Care Model

Justice in healthcare systems, professions, and interactions relates to addressing access and societal inequities stemming from SDoH on the health of patients and communities. At a system level, the Affordable Care Act (ACA) supports universal access to affordable healthcare as advocated under Healthy People 2030. The shift to value-based care in healthcare systems underscores an emphasis on the *ethical* imperative to eliminate disparities to achieve justice in health and healthcare. In value-based healthcare, hospitals and health systems are economically incentivized to address the structural and policy-based barriers to address change at the community level that impacts negative health system outcomes (Alberti et al., 2018). Rather than a focus on individuals, the Center for Medicaid and Medicare Innovation Center's

"Accountable Health Communities" model focuses on screening for and development of interventions targeting gaps in meeting social needs that can lower total healthcare costs, reduce inpatient and outpatient healthcare utilization, and improve quality of care (CMS.gov, 2016). In the value-based care model, not-for-profit hospitals (NPHs) are also legally required to identify, prioritize, and address local community health needs on a regular basis. By connecting the tax-exempt status of NPHs with such community-level needs assessments and delivery, the value-based care model goes a major way toward addressing structural inequities.

### Involving the Community

Involving the community in healthcare engagement is a powerful way of reducing the burden on healthcare systems by addressing the patient's needs. A study from the Perelman School of Medicine at the University of Pennsylvania shows that engaging community health workers helps reduce hospitalizations by 65%, a key criterion of value-based care principles. Community health workers' efforts are effective, as they target the SDoH. They help community members with health promotion and disease prevention goals in ways that avoid healthcare system interactions. Lower healthcare utilization relates to keeping healthcare costs low, another key principle of value-based care.

### Community-Based Care

It is important to include community voices in research and program planning of community-based care. Being inclusive brings equity to healthcare outcomes by ensuring that the goals and their implementation are responsive to community needs and voices. It also builds community capacity, ownership, prioritization of initiatives, and ability to sustain efforts to advocate for their own health and well-being.

Community-based health workers like patient navigators help with patient communication, while others use their experiences to help patients with social interactions, planting a

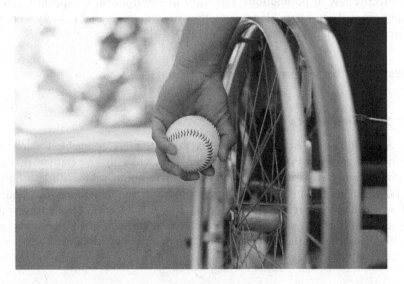

*Figure 6.1* Involving the Community in Engaging Equity.

community garden, and other patient-centered approaches. We now recognize the importance of including community voices in research and program development as supported through translational research. The National Institutes of Health (NIH) supports community-engaged research through its Clinical and Translational Science Award program. There are several barriers to including community voices of marginalized and disadvantaged populations in the research process.

*Review the challenges faced in recruiting diverse and disadvantaged populations in clinical and translational research in* **Textbox 6.1**. *Attempt the SJA prompt.*

---

### Textbox 6.1   Translational Research, Clinical Trial Enrollment, and Tertiary Care Settings

#### WPHC Context

##### Need for Translational Research

Translational research plays an important role in translating scientific research findings into practice-based interventions and policies to eliminate health disparities. Translational research promotes the integration of basic research (i.e., research that looks at advancing theoretical concepts and processes), patient-oriented research, and population-based research into applied practice (Rubio et al., 2010). Thus, it is important that translational research should be conducted in a culturally sensitive manner, include research participants as partners, be responsive to biases by researchers, and promote trust and respect in the research process. Diversity in research participation ensures that such interventions benefit all populations equally (Hong et al., 2021). Examples illustrating the successful inclusion of research participants in translational research include the COVID-19 clinical trials. In these trials, by using representation from communities disproportionately affected by COVID-19, researchers were better able to understand vaccine effectiveness in populations who vary in environmental exposures and other lived experiences. They were able to show that vaccine safety and efficacy were similar across racial and ethnic populations (NIMHHD, 2023).

#### Barriers Faced by Vulnerable Populations

##### Patient-Specific Factors

Poverty, education level, employment status, and age are responsible for low accrual rates with rural patients. Poor clinical trial enrollment of diverse patient populations either in invitation, participation, or motivation by race and ethnicity and other SDoH factors poses a significant barrier to developing and implementing interventions in translational cancer research (Boulware et al., 2022; Hong et al., 2021). Research findings suggest that minority patients with glioma who enrolled in clinical trials lived on average 30 miles closer to the cancer center when compared with minority patients who elected to not enroll in a clinical trial (Loree et al., 2019). Rural patients with cancer are less likely to participate in clinical trials (Gaddy & Gross, 2022). To address this gap, the researchers recommend patient screening combined with carefully targeted outreach toward vulnerable populations be considered. Providing community outreach to rural patients is another avenue for alleviating the impact of these factors. Providing resources such as gas cards to help defray travel costs or linking patients to national support programs offered through the American Cancer Society is another alternative.

## Steps to Address Disparities

### Including Community Sites

The National Cancer Institute (NCI) recognized the need to include community sites to improve cancer care and trial participation in rural areas under the NCI Community Oncology Research Program (NCORP). Structural changes such as the use of central institutional review boards and remote consenting have facilitated rural enrollment. Post-COVID-19 pandemic, the use of telemedicine visits, central imaging review, remote trial site monitoring, and local administration of approved therapies for trial participants have benefited rural trial participant enrollment.

## Telehealth

### Using Telehealth to Optimize Care in Diverse Communities

Optimizing patient outcomes in cancer care depends upon the expertise of the treating physicians, radiology and pathology technicians, and support services like palliative care, social work, and rehabilitation specialists familiar with common syndromes that occur after cancer diagnosis and treatment. Telehealth can help bridge the gap and decrease the burden of treatment for patients experiencing socioeconomic challenges or rural divides. With virtual consultations between surgical oncologists and local surgical teams or telehealth radiology oncology consultations, much of the care can be obtained in conjunction with local providers.

## SJA Prompt

Findings from clinical trial research can provide greater insight into the health behaviors of individuals. Emerging technologies like virtual reality, telemedicine, and mobile apps can provide timely healthcare for patients in their lived settings.

Apple Watch and other wearables on the market provide a wealth of biometric data such as heart rate, heart health indicators such as atrial fibrillation, and cardio fitness notifications. What implications can disparities in clinical trial enrollment and equitable inclusion of participants in research done by Apple Watch, Fitbit, and other mobile technologies to gather and interpret biometric data have on the health of minority and marginalized populations who may suffer from low enrollment in such trials?

## Resources

Boulware, L. E., Corbie, G., Aguilar-Gaxoila, S., Consuelo, H. W., Ruiz, R. Vitale, A., & Egede, L. E. (2022). Combating structural inequities: Diversity, equity, and inclusion in clinical and translational research. *The New England Journal of Medicine*, *386*, 201–203. https://doi.org/10.1056/NEJMp2112233

Gaddy, J. J., & Gross, C. P. (2022). Addressing racial, ethnic, and age disparities in cancer clinical trial enrollment: Time to stop tinkering around the edges. *JAMA Oncology*, *8*(12), 1792–1793. https://doi.org/10.1001/jamaoncol.2022.5006

Hong, Y-R., Tabriz, A. A., & Turner, K. (2021). Racial and ethnic disparities in clinical trial recruitment in the U.S. *American Journal of Preventive Medicine*, *61*(5), E245–E250. https://doi.org/10.1016/amepre.2021.05.007

Loree, J. M., Anand, S., Dasari, A., et al. (2019). Disparity of race reporting and representation in clinical trials leading to cancer drug approvals from 2008 to 2018. *JAMA Oncology*, *5*, e191870. https://doi.org/10.1001/jamaoncol.2019.1870

Mastroianni, A. C., Faden, R., & Federman, D. (Eds.). *Women and health research: Ethical and legal issues of including women in clinical studies—Volume I*. Retrieved January 19, 2022, from www.ncbi.nlm.nih.gov/books/NBK236531

Medicare.gov. (n.d.). *Home health services*. Retrieved on January 19, 2023, from https://www.medicare.gov/coverage/home-health-services

National Academies of the Sciences, Engineering, and Medicine. (2022). *Improving representation in clinical trials and research: Building research equity for women and underrepresented groups*. The National Academies Press. https://doi.org/10.17226/26479. Retrieved January 18, 2022, from https://nap.nationalacademies.org/catalog/26479/improving-representation-in-clinical-trials-and-research-building-research-equity

National Cancer Institute Community Oncology Research Program. Retrieved January 18, 2022, from https://ncorp.cancer.gov/

National Institute on Minority Health and Health Disparities (NIMHHD). *Diversity and inclusion in clinical trials*. Retrieved January 18, 2023, from https://www.nimhd.nih.gov/resources/understanding-health-disparities/diversity-and-inclusion-in-clinical-trials.html

Tucker, C. M., Kang, S., & Williams, J. L. (2019). Translational research to reduce health disparities and promote health equity (Editorial). *Translational Issues in Psychological Science*, *5*(4), 297–301. https://doi.org/10.1037/tps0000215

US Food and Drug Administration. *Clinical trial diversity*. Retrieved January 18, 2023, from https://www.fda.gov/consumers/minority-health-and-health-equity/clinical-trial-diversity

US Department of Health and Human Services Office of Minority Health. *The national CLAS standards*. Retrieved January 18, 2022, from https://minorityhealth.hhs.gov/omh/browse.aspx?lvl=2&lvlid=53

US Food and Drug Administration. *2015–2016 drug trials snapshots summary report*. Retrieved January 19, 2022, from www.fda.gov/media/103160/download

## Primary, Secondary, and Tertiary Care

Primary, secondary, and tertiary care refers to the three tiers of healthcare systems within which care can be classified. Quaternary care is a fourth level of care that is sometimes recognized as a more complex level of tertiary care. It references uncommon, highly specialized, and experimental treatments and procedures. The three tiers represent increasing levels of complexity of healthcare conditions, technical sophistication, and specialization of the treatment setting. Coordination of care between the three levels of care is a primary tenet of

WPHC. The primary care setting is the first point of contact with a healthcare system for a patient, followed by secondary and tertiary care settings. These settings comprise the prevention and evaluation, diagnostics, provision of treatment, and onward referrals to the next level of care.

### Primary Care (PC)

The National Academies of Sciences, Engineering, and Medicine (NASEM) defines PC as the provision of whole person, integrated, accessible, and equitable healthcare by interprofessional teams that are accountable for addressing an individual's health and wellness needs across settings and through sustained relationships with patients, families, and communities. PC is characterized by the "4 Cs" (i.e., first contact that is comprehensive, continuous, and coordinated). Patients often seek PC for diagnosis of a new symptom, or when they come down with a flu or cold or infection; for an injury such as a broken bone or sore muscle, a skin rash, or for a referral and coordination of care among the different levels of care.

#### Primary Care Providers (PCPs)

PCPs are often referred to as the family physician or primary care physician. PC settings are the site for regular screenings, general checkups, patient education, and wellness visits. PCPs may include physicians (including specialties such as OB-GYNs, geriatricians, and pediatricians), nurse practitioners (NPs), and physician assistants (PAs). PC can be provided at the health center or urgent care center or emergency room (ER) for the un- or underinsured. Trust and relationships are central to effective PC. PCPs are the hub connecting patients to resources such as health insurance, telehealth, and digital health interventions for access. To achieve health equity, it is important for PC to be (a) culturally and linguistically appropriate, (b) utilize coordination of care, and (c) engage the community for community-in-practice and system-level decision-making.

*Examine Textbox 6.2 for the relationship between PC settings and health inequities and respond to the SJA prompt that follows.*

---

**Textbox 6.2    PC Settings and Health Inequities**

**WPHC Context**

In populations experiencing **health inequities**, PC offers access to **preventive services** like chronic disease management, vaccinations, and screenings to improve health.

Consider the following markers of inequities:

In 2018, the overall life expectancy of the US population was 78.7 years. When stratified by race, life expectancy was 74.7 for the non-Hispanic Black population, 78.6 years for the non-Hispanic White population, and 81.8 for the Hispanic/ Latin(o/a/x) population (National Center for Health Statistics, 2020). The COVID-19 pandemic amplified and exacerbated these long-standing inequities, resulting in higher cases and death rates among communities of color, rural residents, and other socially vulnerable populations. Peaking in September 2021, rural Americans had a mortality rate due to COVID-19 more than twice the rate of their urban counterparts. The COVID-19 pandemic increased the Black-White gap in life expectancy from around 3.6 years to over 5 years between 2019 and 2020, a difference not observed since 2006 (Andrasfay & Goldman, 2020). SDoH are the primary drivers of health inequities including racism and discrimination, social and economic disadvantages, and built environments.

Primary healthcare (PHC) delivers frontline care. It is best positioned to target the inequities described in the preceding paragraph. It is considered the most inclusive, cost-effective, equitable, and efficient approach to enhancing physical and mental health, as well as social well-being. The PHC approach encompasses integrated health services with an emphasis on PC and essential public health functions (EPHFs), multisectoral policy and action, and empowering people and communities. In this way, PHC is a critical, people-centered, whole-of-society approach to health that reaches underserved populations and ensures no one is left behind.

The 2018 Astana Declaration charted a renewed focus on PHC. Globally, PHC has improved equity and access, healthcare performance, accountability of health systems, and overall health outcomes. The impacts of the COVID-19 pandemic have increased this disparity.

### SJA Prompt

a.   Do you have a PC physician? How often do you avail of PC services?
b.   Studies show that White Americans are more likely than individuals from minority and marginalized populations to visit PC physicians in their community. Can you identify one way in which this disparity can result in health inequities?

### Resource

Andrasfay, T., & Goldman, N. (2020). Reductions in 2020 US life expectancy due to COVID-19 and the disproportionate impact on the Black and Latino populations. *Proceedings of the National Academy of Sciences of the United States of America*, *118*(5), e20147446118. https://doi.org/10.1073/pnas.2014746118

*PC and Health Equity*

PC settings are vital in advancing health equity. The benefits of PC include increased life expectancy and decreased mortality. Research shows that people living in rural counties with less than 1 physician per 3,500 residents had a shorter life expectancy than people living in counties above that threshold. Structural components that make PC equitable include policies such as expanding the PC net, including equity and social needs in quality assessment and measurement, revising PC's fee-for-service payment paradigm, and making telehealth services responsive to diverse cultural and linguistic needs (Mudrick et al., 2012). Furthermore, structural changes involve encouraging Black, Latino, and Native Americans to enter the medical fields. Racial and ethnic underrepresentation of these specific groups means that patients of those racial and ethnic backgrounds are less likely to find providers who share their race (Salsberg et al., 2021). Health inequities are exacerbated when Black and Native Americans facing housing discrimination are also less likely to live in areas that are well served by PC settings.

*Examine Textbox 6.3 for a look at the shared principles of PC. Respond to the SJA prompt that follows.*

---

### Textbox 6.3   Shared Principles of PC

#### WPHC Context

The **PC Collaborative** has promoted the Shared Principles of PC, which characterize advanced PC as person- and family-centered, continuous, comprehensive and equitable, team-based and collaborative, coordinated and integrated, and accessible and high value.

Over 350 organizations have signed on to these Shared Principles.

The Institute of Management (IOM) report assessing the differences in the kinds and quality of healthcare received by US racial and ethnic minorities and nonminorities finds the following:

- Disparities in healthcare exist and are associated with worse health outcomes.
- Healthcare disparities occur in the context of broader inequality.
- There are many sources across health systems, providers, patients, and managers that contribute to disparities.
- Bias, stereotyping, prejudice, and clinical uncertainty contribute to disparities.
- Racial and ethnic minority patients are more likely to refuse treatment.

#### SJA Prompt

How can family-centered PC be mindful of cultural values, diversity of lifestyle choices, and knowledge and expertise that families of different racial and ethnic backgrounds bring to the physician-patient relationship?

#### Resources

American Medical Association (AMA). (2023). *Health disparities physician resources.* Retrieved January 16, 2023, from https://www.ama-assn.org/delivering-care/patient-support-advocacy/reducing-disparities-healthcare

Primary Care Collaborative. (2022, May). *Primary care: A key lever to advance health equity.* Retrieved January 13, 2023, from https://www.pcpcc.org/sites/default/files/resources/PCC-NCPC%20Health%20Equity%20Report.pdf

Smedley, B. D., Stith, A. Y., & Nelson, A. R. (Eds., IOM). (2023). *Unequal treatment: Confronting racial and ethnic disparities in health care.* National Academies Press. Retrieved January 16, 2023, from https://nap.nationalacademies.org/read/12875/chapter/1

*PC and Continuity of Care*

PC settings are centered on continuity of care and provide the foundational relationship that supports patients through their healthcare spectrum, from preventative services to the management of chronic conditions. PC settings provide high-value services like screenings for cervical, breast, and colorectal cancers, diabetes care, vaccinations, and blood pressure monitoring. PC is the major source of care for the overall population. Most of the populations experiencing health inequities (e.g., poverty, people of color, uninsured patients) receive their care from PC settings while only about 30.5% of adults without any markers of social disadvantage receive their care from a family physician (Ferrer, 2007).

## Secondary Care (SC)

SC refers to the healthcare services received by the patient after their visit with the PC physician. SC includes visits with specialists and the support provided for patients who have been referred to them for expert care. SC health professionals typically do not have initial contact with patients as in PC. Patients will typically access SC on the referral of their PCP. For instance, a PCP may refer their patient to an endocrinologist, rheumatologist, or urologist. Hospital-based settings, acute care settings, and clinics are often sites for SC services. These services can include planned operations, specialist clinics (e.g., oncology, cardiology, neurology, or renal clinics), or rehabilitation services like physiotherapy. SC specialists may include psychiatrists, cardiologists, obstetricians, dermatologists, pediatricians, and gynecologists.

*SC Settings*

SC services address the needs of patients who have been diagnosed with complex health conditions that require the services of a specialist beyond the PC setting. Patients in SC settings will meet with a specialist who has deeper knowledge and expertise in their condition. Examples of SC settings include services like cancer treatment, or a follow-up visit with a neurologist to interpret an MRI scan. They can also include specialist attendance in childbirth, medical imaging (radiology) services, and care within an intensive care unit (ICU). SC services include allied health professionals such as physical therapists, respiratory therapists, occupational therapists, speech therapists, and dietitians.

SC AND COORDINATION OF CARE

A key tenet of WPHC is the coordination of care for chronic conditions and other patients with multiple comorbidities who are being treated by a team of specialists. In an ideal setting, the SC specialists work with the PC team to ensure everyone knows what others are recommending. Sustained focus toward identifying, addressing, and eliminating disparities at the SC level involves addressing challenges in enhancing the diversity of healthcare professionals (e.g., in specialized domains like neuro-oncology), combating structural racism, and encouraging the recruitment of racial/ethnic minorities and underserved populations.

SC AND HEALTH INEQUITIES

Research shows that optimal patient outcomes can be achieved when treating physicians, the SC team (e.g., neuroradiology and neuropathology), and support services all coordinate patient care in complex health domains. However, even with the presence of specialist providers, patient access to specialized and multidisciplinary care remains limited and excludes marginalized communities disproportionately. Such disparities result in increased morbidity and mortality for patients from backgrounds with various elements of diversity.

### Tertiary Care (TC)

TC refers to care that is more specialized than SC. TC can also often occur over a longer period. It involves advanced and complex diagnostics, procedures, and treatments performed by medical specialists in state-of-the-art facilities. Referrals for TC may come from both PC and SC health professionals. TC is often provided as an inpatient-based service. Often, for a patient to receive TC, they may have to travel to a specialized TC center. For geographically disadvantaged patients, this may result in delayed diagnosis and treatment and an increase in the cost of healthcare treatment. Examples of TC include specialist cancer management, neurosurgery, cardiac surgery, neurosurgery, transplant services, plastic surgery, burn treatment, specialized intensive care units, advanced neonatology services, palliative, and other complex medical and surgical interventions.

### Barriers to TC

TC services are often not available at local or regional hospitals. It is important for the PC setting provider to maintain continuity of care for patients in TC who are managing multiple or complex chronic conditions. The lack of access to TC impacts minority and disadvantaged populations disproportionately. For example, rural women experience poorer health outcomes and have less access to healthcare than urban women. The disparity in obstetric and reproductive health outcomes can be attributed to the limited number of women's health providers and TC centers.

*Review **Textbox 6.4** for a deeper look at how PC, SC, and TC impact minority and marginalized populations with the case of the Americans with Disabilities Act. Attempt the SJA prompt that follows.*

---

**Textbox 6.4    Americans with Disabilities Act (ADA)—Compliant Primary, Secondary, and Tertiary Healthcare Settings**

**WPHC Context**

The ADA of 1990 is the federal civil rights law that prohibits discrimination against individuals with disabilities in everyday activities. Section 1557 of the ACA prohibits any healthcare clinician that receives funding from the federal government to refuse to treat an individual or discriminate against an individual based on disability. Section 504 of the Rehabilitation Act of 1973 prohibits discrimination on the basis of disability by any programs or activities receiving federal financial assistance. Section 504 prohibits discrimination by any facilities receiving reimbursement from Medicare or Medicaid.

The ADA requires the following from healthcare organizations:

- Provide equal services to individuals with disabilities.
- Make reasonable accommodations in policies and practices to provide equal access.
- Provide auxiliary aids and services when necessary to provide effective communication.
- Provide resources for physicians and practices to ensure their healthcare practice is a safe, accessible, and compliant establishment for patients with disabilities to receive personal, high-quality care.

Information about the ADA:

- ADA Standards for Accessible Design. https://www.ada.gov/
- ADA checklist for existing facilities https://www.ada.gov/
- ADA checklist: Healthcare facilities and service providers—Ensuring access to services and facilities by patients who are blind, deaf-blind, or visually impaired. https://www.ada.gov/
- American Foundation for the Blind. https://www.afb.org/
- Access to medical care for individuals with mobility disabilities. https://www.ada.gov/

### SJA Action Prompt

Some actions primary, secondary, and tertiary healthcare facilities can take include taking an inventory of physical barriers, such as steps, stairs, narrow doorways or hallways, heavy doors, and nonadjustable exam tables or chairs.
Visit a PC, SC, or TC in your community:

1. Is the parking accessible and adequate for individuals with disabilities?
2. What are potential risks for individuals with disabilities, such as chairs with wheels on hard surfaces that may be difficult to get in and out of?
3. Is a wheelchair and scooter-accessible ramp installed?
4. Are there proper accommodations for vision-impaired patients such as large-text or audio versions of forms and paperwork?
5. For hearing-impaired patients, are paper and pen or computer for communication available? If the patient needs or prefers it, can the services of an interpreter be proved for patients who prefer or whose disability necessitates it?
6. How can providers be proactive with patients to help give a patient with a disability a comfortable, safe, and proper evaluation and visit?
7. How can members of a healthcare team, including physicians and other staff, be properly trained to provide care in an accessible manner such that they are able to operate special equipment, assist with transfers and positioning of patients with disabilities, communicate clearly and ask appropriate questions, and interact with patients with disabilities without bias, labels, stereotypes, or insensitivity?

### Resources

American Medical Association (AMA). (2018). *Ensuring access to care for patients with disabilities: Strategies for ensuring a safe, accessible, and ADA compliant practice.* Retrieved January 16, 2023, from https://www.ama-assn.org/sites/ama-assn.org/files/corp/media-browser/public/publichealth/disability-ada.pdf

### Addressing Barriers to PC, SC, and TC

Access to healthcare is complicated by barriers including patient SDoH factors and delivery of care. Obstetric and gynecologic health services, including family planning, are limited in many nonmetropolitan areas. Regional organization of perinatal services has been an important strategy for improving outcomes for underserved women and their infants in rural communities (ACOG, 2021). For instance, Wyoming is a state with no TC centers for pregnant women or infants and few pediatric specialists. To address this barrier, Wyoming recently started approving out-of-state healthcare providers and facilities as state Medicaid providers, allowing the state to reimburse transport to and care and delivery in an out-of-state subspecialty hospital when medically necessary (Wyoming Department of Health, 2023).

## Diagnostic, Rehabilitative, and Palliative Care

### Diagnostic Care (DC)

DC refers to the treatment or investigation of a health issue. It focuses on the diagnosis of the existing symptoms or risk factors of the patient. Where preventive care helps to detect healthcare problems before symptoms develop, DC focuses on diagnosing or treating the symptom. Most healthcare plans cover preventive care at no cost, while payment in the form of a deductible, a copay, or coinsurance is usually associated with DC. Preventive care visits are also known as well-care visits, annual physical exams, or annual wellness visits. An example of preventative care is the case of diabetes screening. When a blood glucose test is used to check for problems with the patient's blood sugar control, even though they may not have any symptoms, that is preventive care. However, as an example of DC, if the patient has diabetes, the doctor will regularly check the patient's blood sugar with an A1C test. The A1C test is a diagnostic test. Likewise, taking medication to treat high cholesterol is DC. Diagnosis or treatment for health conditions, laboratory tests and X-rays, and procedures (e.g., removing skin tags) are examples of DC.

### Rehabilitative Care (RC)

RC or rehabilitation services are healthcare services that help patients keep, get back, or improve skills and functioning for daily living that have been lost or impaired due to sickness, injury, or disability (Healthcare.gov, 2022). These services may include physical and occupational therapy, speech-language therapy, and psychiatric rehabilitation services in a variety of inpatient and/or outpatient settings. The goal of RC is to improve the patient's daily life and functioning. The abilities may be physical, mental and/or cognitive (e.g., thinking and learning). Other settings for RC include major surgery; severe infections; developmental disabilities; stroke; side effects from medical treatments, such as from cancer treatments; and chronic pain, such as back and neck pain.

Rehabilitation focuses on helping the patient achieve independence in their day-to-day activities. RC can vary depending on the cause of the problem, its scope, and impact. For instance, an active person who has had a heart attack may go through cardiac rehabilitation to try to return to exercising. Or, someone with lung disease may receive pulmonary rehabilitation to be able to breathe better and improve their quality of life (MedlinePlus.gov, 2022). Early access to RC through integration in PHC can help optimize outcomes, mitigate disability, and improve people's ability to live independent lives. The WHO's recent launch of the Rehabilitation 2030 Call for Action emphasizes the importance of strengthening the goals of rehabilitation within the health system and specifically within PHC.

## Palliative Care

Palliative care is specialized medical care for people living with serious illnesses, such as cancer, dementia, Parkinson's disease, chronic obstructive pulmonary disease, or heart failure (NIA, 2022). Patients in palliative care may receive medical care for their symptoms, or palliative care, along with treatment intended to cure their serious illness. It is distinct from DC in its focus on enhancing a person's current care by focusing on quality of life for the patient and their family. Palliative care is often given along with curative treatment. A palliative care team is multidisciplinary and comprises palliative care specialist doctors and nurses, social workers, nutritionists, and chaplains. In order to address physician burnout, Omillion-Hodges and Swords (2016) illustrate how mindful communication practices can be used individually or in concert, by sole practitioners or within interdisciplinary teams, and by new and seasoned physicians in various palliative care settings.

## Palliative Care Settings

Palliative care settings include hospitals, nursing homes, outpatient palliative care clinics, and other specialized clinics, including home care. For instance, a patient receiving cancer treatment who develops anemia may benefit from palliative care by management of anemia to relieve the fatigue and related symptoms and continue her curative chemotherapy treatment (National Institute of Aging (NIA), 2022).

Palliative care can transition into comfort care or hospice care if the curative treatment is no longer working, or it is believed the patient is likely to die within six months. With hospice care, the focus shifts to providing comprehensive care, comfort, and quality of life for a person who is approaching the end of life. It can be offered in-home, hospital-, or hospice-center settings. At the heart of the SJA approach to ensuring care for the underserved is the need for physicians, collectively and individually, to be agents of social change. Omillion-Hodges and Swords (2017) capture how storytelling helped in the management of the tensions straddling the living-dying dialectic and the practicing-advocating dialectic that palliative care providers experience in their practice within traditional biomedical models that privilege curative treatment and biosocial models of medicine that privilege holistic care for patients.

### Equity Challenges in Palliative Care

Researchers Davis et al. (2019) study communication and discourse within a Pediatric Palliative Care Team (PPCT) in a children's hospital. Using the concepts of spatiality and temporality, smooth and striated spaces, space and time biases, and Foucault's concept of heterotopian space, or places with multiple layers of meaning, they examine end-of-life care in the context of compassionate communication and the end of life. They draw out the notion of care and cure, life and death, hopelessness and hope, separation and connection as shared by team members, patients, and family members. Such research highlights how physicians have a moral obligation to see how structural influences on care like poverty, lack of insurance, and other determinants of health impact advocacy for care (List, 2011). Physicians who treat patients without insurance and who cannot pay often do based on benevolence, rather than on systemic injustice experienced by the receiver. Benevolence reflects attention on fixing short-term needs rather than on addressing systemic inequities that create an environment in which disparities arise. SJA asks physicians to advance professional values in patient care as delivered in a range of settings, and as communication researchers Ragan and colleagues note, by incorporating a holistic and patient-centered approach, whereby vulnerable patients (e.g., the elderly) are seen as active agents of and guide the interpretation, management, and creation of the meaning of their own health and illness in an active manner (Ragan, Wittenberg, & Hall, 2003).

## DOMAINS OF DISPARITIES IN PALLIATIVE CARE

Racial and ethnic disparities in palliative care include the domains of pain management, satisfaction, and communication. In a survey of bereaved family members, surrogates of African Americans reported being less satisfied with the quality of end-of-life care and more often reported concerns about provider communication. Provider communication in palliative care includes the extent to which providers listen and share information. Disparities in these instances were greater in discordant patient-provider relationships. Such communication disparities result in disparities in end-of-life care. In a prospective study of cancer patients, researchers found that the end-of-life discussions between physicians and their African American patients were less likely to result in care consistent with patient preferences as compared with White patients. Research has also documented the challenges faced by minorities in accessing pain medicines. African Americans, Hispanics, and Asian patients are also less knowledgeable about advance directives and less likely to complete them. Minority older adults evidence lower rates of hospice use compared with Whites across diagnoses, geographic areas, and settings of care.

## ADDRESSING DISPARITIES IN PALLIATIVE CARE

Disparities in palliative care have been attributed to numerous factors. Racial and ethnic differences, spiritual and religious beliefs (for African Americans), mistrust of the healthcare system, and less positive attitude toward disclosure of terminal illness (in African Americans compared to Asians and Hispanics). Organizational barriers to the use of palliative care by racial and ethnic minorities are exacerbated by a lack of minority staff, interpreters, and community outreach to diverse communities. Development of culturally competent hospice educational materials, videos to improve health literacy, and patient navigation to address disparities in care for African Americans and Latinos have the potential to reduce disparities.

## Self-Care, Home Care, and Community Care

### Self-Care

The WHO (2021) defines self-care as the ability of individuals, families, and communities to promote their own health, prevent disease, maintain health, and cope with illness and disability with or without the support of a health worker. This definition recognizes individuals as active agents empowered to manage their own healthcare in health promotion, disease prevention and control, self-medication, providing care to dependent persons, and rehabilitation and palliative care. Self-care has seen significant interest in the face of the pandemic disruptions to healthcare services and the burden on disadvantaged populations.

### SJ Advantages of Self-Care

Self-care has the potential to alleviate pressure on healthcare providers while empowering individuals to take control of their own health. In addition, self-care has the potential to offer preventive services in an equitable, accessible, and person-centered manner. Communication researchers studying the impact of self-care during times of crisis find that stressful events and SJ intertwine with issues such as racial unrest, disasters around the world, and the need to make loved ones and patients feel valued and appreciated in the ambit of self-care (Beach, 2021). For those who are disadvantaged, self-care options offer a way to access quality health information, services, and products, in a nonstigmatizing and discriminatory manner. When connected with digital platforms, self-care options can be incorporated into the education of health workers for maximum scale and reach.

### SJ and Self-Care Initiatives and Interventions

Self-care initiatives span the range of sexual and reproductive health, noncommunicable diseases, and mental health. Many community-based and nonprofit organizations provide underserved and underrepresented populations with services that range from HIV testing and prevention to chronic care management support in partnership with a healthcare provider. Self-care interventions are tools to support self-care. Self-care interventions include evidence-based, quality drugs, diagnostics, and/or digital products that can be provided fully or partially outside of formal health services and can be used with or without healthcare professionals. To be effective, it is important to ensure that the interventions and products are evidence based, regulated, and of approved quality; that health information provided is verified and legitimate; and that the self-management of conditions is supported by access to health workers and health facilities for guidance or management of side effects. In addition, the products recommended should be affordable. A third piece is ensuring an enabling environment in which self-care interventions can be made available and implemented. The elements of such an environment can include education, justice and social services sectors, and qualified social workers.

### Examples of Self-Care Products and Settings

Examples of self-care products include pregnancy tests, condoms, HPV and STI self-sampling, HIV self-tests, COVID-19 tests, self-monitoring of blood pressure and blood glucose levels. Self-care interventions have the advantage of being convenient and low-cost. The pandemic experience highlighted many of the self-care interventions that helped individuals successfully navigate a health risk through personal self-care actions such as wearing masks and physical distancing at a time when healthcare services were overburdened. Oftentimes, self-care options are often chosen because they fit with an individual's lifestyle or schedule. At other times, a self-care option can offer healthcare services that may not otherwise be accessible or present in an individual's environment. Self-care activities include managing healthy weight, getting daily physical activity, getting quality sleep, healthy eating, and managing stress, among other behavioral actions.

## Home Care

Home care or home healthcare (HHC) is a unique healthcare service. In HHC, care is delivered in patients' homes rather than in a centralized physical location (e.g., doctor's office, hospital, nursing home; American Academy of Home Care Medicine, 2023). HHC is usually less expensive and more convenient than PC, SC, or TC (SNF, Medicare.gov, 2023). The utilization of home health services is predicted to rise as care shifts from healthcare facilities to home-based settings. Examples of HHC services include wound care for pressure sores or a surgical wound, patient and caregiver education, monitoring serious illness and unstable health status, and intravenous or nutrition therapy. The goal of HHC is to help patients get better, regain independence, become self-sufficient, or slow decline (Medicare.gov, 2023). A doctor's order is required to start HHC.

*Review **Textbox 6.5** for a detailed look at the HHC service sector. Attempt the SJA prompt that follows.*

---

### Textbox 6.5   HHC Service Sector Outlook

#### WPHC Context

- Employment of home health and personal care aides is projected to grow 25% from 2021 to 2031, much faster than the average for all occupations.
- The need for companionship, personalized in-home care, and group care homes is expected to grow. More than one-third of adults aged 45 years and older struggle with loneliness, making companionship services a high priority for care agencies, particularly with COVID-19 (CDC).
- Remote patient monitoring (RPM) has increased in popularity because of COVID-19 healthcare shortages. RPM allows for real-time data, monitoring, and treatment adjustment when controlling symptoms and disease advancement.
- The US HHC services market is projected to grow from $94.17 billion in 2022 to $153.19 billion by 2029.
- The nursing care segment is projected to lead the HHC market by type.
- The growing geriatric population with chronic ailments will lead the demand for home health services in the United States. In particular, demand for respiratory therapy services and infusion therapy services at home is projected to increase.

#### SJA Prompt

Women of color, particularly Asian, Latinx, and Black women, are overrepresented in home health aide jobs. About one-fifth of Latinx and Black women employed as home health aides live in poverty (Goubert et al., 2021).

a.  Given the shift to home-based, noninstitutional care for the aging US population, what implications will this disparity in earnings and market demand have on the economic well-being of women of color who work as home health aides and their families?
b.  Speak to a home health aide. What challenges do they encounter to their well-being? Identify one way you can work to address these challenges.

**Resources**

Bureau of Labor Statistics, US Department of Labor. (2022, September 8). *Occupational outlook handbook. Home health and personal care aides*. Retrieved January 19, 2023, from https://www. bls.gov/ooh/healthcare/home-health-aides-and-personal-care-aides.htm

Fortune Business Insights. Healthcare IT. US. *Home Healthcare Services Market*. Retrieved January 19, 2023, from https://www.fortunebusinessinsights.com/u-s-home-healthcareservices-market-105568

Goubert, A., Cai, J. Y., & Appelbaum, E. (2021, October 27). Home health care: Latinx and Black women are overrepresented, but all women face heightened risk of poverty. *CEPR*. Retrieved April 30, 2023, from https://cepr.net/home-healthcare-latinx-and-black-women-are-overrepresented-but-all-women-face-heightened-risk-of-poverty/

## Home Healthcare

Home health is a large and growing segment of the Medicare program. Medicare Part A and Medicare Part B cover services such as part-time skilled nursing care, medical social services, physical therapy, and medical supplies for use at home. These services are coordinated by a Medicare-certified home healthcare agency (Medicare.gov, 2023).

## SJ Challenges to Home Healthcare

Recent studies how access to consistent in-home services is challenging for beneficiaries of color due to several factors including communication of inaccurate information regarding the benefit to patients by providers and home health agencies, the provision of fewer hours of home health aide services than the benefit allows the law, and the financial strain of securing home health services and supports (The Commonwealth Fund, 2023). The study also found that Medicare beneficiaries are more likely to rely on unpaid informal caregivers than White beneficiaries. This also places an additional financial burden on unpaid informal caregivers such as family or friends. These factors highlight the importance of addressing the concentration of racial and ethnic minority groups into segregated neighborhoods as a legacy of structural racism.

## STRUCTURAL RACISM

One of the consequences of structural racism is the greater exposure to stressors and poorer services and diminished neighborhood resources to minorities, marginalized, and disadvantaged populations. The growing population of Americans over 65 is Medicare-eligible, meaning that they all have or will have health insurance coverage that includes home healthcare benefits. Structurally, Medicare reimbursements have shifted in favor of the value-based care model, which supports improved patient outcomes while controlling costs. With its cost advantages compared with hospital-based care, home healthcare is becoming a popular treatment modality.

*Review* **Textbox 6.6** *for information on how market-based reforms shape disparities through access to care. Attempt the SJA prompt that follows.*

**Textbox 6.6    Market-Based Reforms and Disparities in Access to Care**

**WPHC Context**

**Market-based reforms** such as the Home Health Value-Based Purchasing (HHVBP) initiative and Home Health compare five-star ratings. As the HHVBP data source and measures that follow indicate, these programs are "colorblind" market-based reforms intended to improve quality of care. However, similar programs have been shown to exacerbate health disparities in home health and other settings. For example, after the introduction of five-star ratings in nursing homes, high-quality facilities selectively admitted more profitable residents while avoiding Medicaid residents, exacerbating existing socioeconomic disparities in the use of high-quality facilities.

**SJA Prompt**

Although public reporting can mitigate inequities, these policies can inadvertently exacerbate disparities in high-quality home health agency use for marginalized groups (Fashaw-Walters et al., 2023). What is one way local interventions can raise awareness of five-star quality ratings among marginalized populations facing an increasing health inequity gap?

**Resources**

Centers for Medicare & Medicaid Services. (2023, January 18). *Expanded Home Health Value-Based Purchasing Model (HHVBP)*. Retrieved January 19, 2023, from https://innovation.cms. gov/innovation-models/expanded-home-health-value-based-purchasing-model#:~:text=The %20Expanded%20Home%20Health%20Value,require%20an%20emergency%20room%20visit

Fashaw-Walters, S. A., Rahman, M., Gee, G., More, V., Rivera-Hernandez, M., Ford, C., & Thomas, K. S. (2023). Potentially more out-of-reach: Public reporting exacerbates inequities in home health access. *The Milbank Quarterly*, https://doi.org/10.1111/1468-0009.12616

## RESIDENTIAL SEGREGATION

In their study, Fashaw-Walters and colleagues identify the adverse consequences of low-quality home care (2022). Patients who receive home care from high-quality home health agencies experience fewer negative outcomes (e.g., hospitalizations, emergency department (ED) use, and poorer functional improvement) than patients receiving services from low-quality agencies. Policies that dismantle structural and institutional barriers related to residential segregation are central to addressing these inequities. Fashaw-Walters and colleagues conducted regression analyses on administrative data from 2016 to examine individual- and neighborhood-level racial, ethnic, and socioeconomic factors associated with the use of high-quality home health agencies. Researchers find disparities among race, ethnic, and income factors in the use of home health services. The study finds structural and institutional barriers of racism. These factors intersect along the lines of residential segregation, ethnic, and socioeconomic inequities. About 40%–77% of the disparities in high-quality home health use were attributable to neighborhood-level factors, suggesting that racial, ethnic, and socioeconomic inequities in access to high-quality home healthcare are pervasive.

Review **Textbox 6.7** *for a look at structural factors impacting HHC. Attempt the SJA prompt that follows.*

---

### Textbox 6.7   Structural Factors Impacting HHC

#### WPHC Context

**Value-based healthcare** is a healthcare delivery model in which providers (e.g., hospitals, physicians, home health aides) are paid based on patient health outcomes. Value-based care agreements reward providers for improvement in patient health, reduction in the effects and incidence of chronic disease, and improvement in quality of life in an evidence-based manner. In a fee-for-service or capitated approach, providers are paid based on the amount of healthcare services they deliver. The value in value-based healthcare compares health outcomes against the cost of delivering the outcomes (NEJM, 2017).

#### SJA Prompt

How can community partnerships strengthen value-based care and help eliminate healthcare disparities for members of marginalized and vulnerable populations in PC?

#### Resources

New England Journal of Medicine. (2017, January 1). *Innovations in care delivery: What is value-based healthcare?* Retrieved January 19, 2023, from https://catalyst.nejm.org/doi/full/10.1056/CAT.17.0558

---

INCOME-LEVEL DISPARITIES

Home health patients residing in neighborhoods with higher proportions of Black and low-income older residents had a lower probability of high-quality agency use. Likewise low-income patients had a lower probability of high-quality agency use. These disparities pose a barrier to accessing high-quality home health agency services for vulnerable Medicare home health patients. Data suggests that the key driver of this inequity is location, with prior research showing that providers are less likely to serve predominantly Black, Hispanic, and disadvantaged neighborhoods. Some of the recommendations to ensure equitable access and aging for older adults included making high-quality home health services available for disadvantaged and marginalized populations. However, Fashaw-Walters and colleagues find that even when Black, Hispanic, and lower-income home health patients reside in neighborhoods with a greater number of high-quality home health agencies, the disparities in access to high-quality agencies persist. Such disparities may reflect the effects of interpersonal racism and discrimination by home health agencies and nurses against racial and ethnic minority home health patients. They may also be exacerbated by the findings that healthcare providers are less likely to serve predominantly Black, Hispanic, or disadvantaged neighborhoods.

## Community-Based Care (CBC)

CBC is care provided to vulnerable populations focusing on support in the community including people experiencing homelessness, agricultural workers, residents of public housing, and the Nation's veterans. Community health centers (CHCs) are the largest source of comprehensive PC for medically underserved communities and populations (Kaiser Family Foundation (KFF), 2017). CHCs have a major impact on patient-centered care and in promoting access to care in vulnerable or medically underserved populations (Health, 2023).

### Structural Organization of CBC

CHCs are a part of the federally qualified health center (FQHC) umbrella. FQHCs are government-funded networks of care providers that include CHCs, migrant health centers, health centers for the homeless, and public housing PCPs (Federally Qualified Health Center, 2022). CHCs operate on funds allocated by the ACA for patients with no other options for affordable care (e.g., those who cannot afford private health insurance (HealthCare.gov)). Often, CHCs can replace home care and offer a welcoming and trusting source of healthcare. CHCs are affordable safety net clinics and are the largest providers of PC to the most vulnerable and medically underserved communities in the United States. CHCs can be found in both urban and rural communities that have high poverty rates or low numbers of private or nonprofit health systems and hospitals. Health centers also integrate access to pharmacy, mental health, substance abuse, and oral health services in areas where economic, geographic, or cultural barriers limit access to affordable healthcare services (HRSA, 2023).

Review **Textbox 6.8** for **Dr. Anabella Maria Beju's** scholar interview and a look at migrant health challenges.

---

**TEXTBOX 6.8    Equity in Mental Healthcare for the Displaced**

**Dr. Anabella Maria Beju**
*Lucian Blaga University of Sibiu, Romania*

*Men live in a community by virtue of the things which they have in common; and communication is the way in which they come to possess things in common.*

(John Dewey)

The current political context and the rising figures of forcibly displaced people bring to the fore once again the urgency to address mental healthcare and aid in a lasting sustainable manner. While the concerted efforts to ensure emergency mental health interventions and psychosocial support for refugees cannot be questioned, policies and programs continue to gravitate around biomedical aspects, remaining largely ignorant to the increasingly complex mélange of factors and forces that shape mental health and well-being or the lack thereof.

This call for awareness and action builds on previous scholarly efforts to challenge the limits and to question the dominant biomedical rehabilitative paradigm as the "regime of truth" and as the most appropriate response for refugees (Fennig & Denov, 2019).

Alternatively, I argue that a more comprehensive approach ultimately aiming to remove *unfreedoms* and to create *capabilities* and *real freedom of agency* (Sen, 2000) has the potential not only to ensure more efficient care and aid but to achieve meaningful change in mental well-being equity for the displaced and by proxy for the entire population. An intersectionality-centered critical discursive approach that understands mental health as a social-discursive construction (Foucault, 1965) inseparably linked to the broader sociocultural and historical context and the power of language to create meaning and social practice is highly illuminating for translating this vision into operational mental health frameworks.

First, it enables the distinction between the biological condition and the intricate psychosocial and cultural web of meanings that shape multiple intersecting identities and subjective experiences (Hogan, 2016, Wodak, 2020, Volkan, 2019). Second, it unmasks and challenges ideological stakes, structural dominance, power relations, and inequalities reproduced by mutually reinforcing stigma-laden discourses on migration and mental health, contributing to both systemic and everyday exclusionary practices. In so doing, a critical discursive perspective does not only shed light on the subtle mechanisms of limiting freedoms, but it equally highlights avenues of undoing mental health inequity. Notably, mental health policy frameworks and programs that prioritize inclusive mental health communication and literacy, and address discursively constructed privileges or burdens hold promise for flourishing lives of the displaced and all people as well as more resilient multicultural communities.

## Resources

Fennig, M., & Denov, M. (2019). Regime of truth: Rethinking the dominance of the bio-medical model in mental health social work with refugee youth. *The British Journal of Social Work*, *49*(2), 300–317.

Foucault, M. (1965). *Madness and civilization; a history of insanity in the age of reason*. Pantheon Books.

Hogan, N. (2016). "We're all mad here" – Power and identity in the modern era of mental illness. *Intersect: The Stanford Journal of Science, Technology, and Society*, *10*(1). https://ojs.stanford. edu/ojs/index.php/intersect/article/view/899

Sen, A. K. 2000 (1999). *Development as freedom*. Anchor Books

Volkan, V. D. (2019). Mourning, large-group identity, and the refugee experience. In Wenzel, T., & Drozdek, B. (Eds.), *An uncertain\ safety* (pp. 23–35). Springer. https://doi.org/10.1007/ 978-3-319-72914-5_2

Wodak, R. (2020). *The politics of fear: The shameless normalization of far-right discourse*. Sage.

*Adult Day Care Centers*

As a form of CBC, adult day care centers provide a wide range of social and support services in a group setting. Examples of adult day care centers include churches and community centers. They provide care for people who need supervision and help with activities of daily living (e.g., patients with dementia) while primary caregivers are at work or need respite. The services offered by adult day care centers range from basic nonmedical care to advanced medical services. For example, a registered nurse may be available for on-site health services, medical assessment and monitoring, and to help with medication management. Adult day care is not covered by Medicare, but some costs may be covered by Medicaid and other insurers.

*Examine **Textbox 6.9** for the CBC actions that can be taken by academic health centers to promote health equity and justice. Respond to the SJA prompt that follows.*

---

**Textbox 6.9    CBC Actions for Academic Health Centers to Promote Health Equity and Justice**

How can CBC inform clinical care? Clinicians can:

- Devote less focus to biological determinants and more to SDoH.
- Incorporate home visits.
- Be more involved with the community and understand community needs.
- Look at each patient as an individual.

How can CBC inform medical education? Medical training can include learning about the following:

- The challenges and social circumstances community members face.
- Navigating culturally diverse situations.
- The traditions of certain communities.

**SJA Prompt**

Write three questions that clinicians can use to learn about their patients' social and lived circumstances. What language and content factors were you mindful of when drafting your statements?

**Resource**

Alberti, P. M., Sutton, K. M., Cooper, L. A., Lane, W. G., Stephens, S., & Gourdine, M. A. (2018). Communities, social justice, and academic health centers. *Academic Medicine*, *93*(1), 20–24. https://doi.org/10.1097/ACM.0000000000001678

---

*Program of All-Inclusive Care for the Elderly (PACE)*

PACE is a type of comprehensive adult day care model, funded by the Centers for Medicare and Medicaid Services (CMS), for frail older adults 55 or older, who require a nursing-home level of care (National PACE Association, 2023). PACE allows an older person to spend their day at the program and get medical care while caregivers are at work. The goal of PACE is to keep participants in the community for as long as it is medically, socially, and financially feasible. Research suggests that the PACE model is associated with improved health outcomes including fewer hospitalizations and ED room visits, fewer unmet needs, and better caregiver support. In addition, it reduces the burden on family and informal caregivers, which allows them to keep their jobs while caring for themselves and their families. PACE uses a team of healthcare providers who know the patient and caregivers well, and who can provide complete care for the patient in a variety of settings such as in the home or in the hospital, in an alternative living situation, or in a nursing home. It also allows for adult day care, respite care, transportation, medication coverage, rehabilitation, hearing aids, eyeglasses, and other benefits.

Review **Textbox 6.10** *for a deeper look at CHCs. Attempt the SJA prompt that follows.*

---

**Textbox 6.10   CHC**

**WPHC Context**

In 2015, 1,375 CHCs provided care to 24.3 million patients, including 1 in 12 US residents and nearly 1 in 6 Medicaid enrollees.
Almost three-quarters of all CHC patients had income below the poverty level.
Seventy-six percent of CHC patients were insured (49% through Medicaid), up from 65% in 2013 (before ACA).
CHCs report increased numbers of insured patients who are unable to pay their deductibles and cost-sharing.

**SJA Prompt**

• Make a list of three health disparities that are present in your community. Which populations do they affect the most? How can the CHCs in your community address these disparities?

**Resource**

Kaiser Family Foundation (KFF). (2023). *Community health centers: Recent growth and the role of the ACA.* Retrieved January 19, 2023, from https://www.kff.org/medicaid/issuebrief/community-health-centers-recent-growth-and-the-role-of-the-aca/

---

The need for community-based long-term services and supports (LTSS) among older rural adults is acute and growing. The percentage of older adults who rely on PACE services in rural communities is nearly double that of PACE organizations in other areas. Disparities arise for patients in rural areas because of challenges in accessing and benefiting from the care provided by PACE programs. Telehealth and expanded coverage for vulnerable populations (e.g., veterans) can help address equity gaps in CBC.

## Communication in Prevention and Coordination of Care

### Communication in Prevention

Health promotion and disease prevention programs have the goal of keeping and maintaining health. Their goal is to engage and empower individuals and communities to choose healthy behaviors and make changes that reduce the risk of developing chronic diseases and comorbidities. Health promotion covers a "wide range of social and environmental interventions that are designed to benefit and protect individual people's health and quality of life by addressing and preventing the root causes of ill health, not just focusing on treatment and cure" (WHO, 2016). Disease prevention focuses on specific efforts aimed at reducing the development and severity of chronic diseases and other morbidities. Wellness programs comprise the active decisions made by an individual that contribute to positive health behaviors and outcomes. Communication is central to all the activities that comprise health promotion, disease prevention, and wellness programs.

### SJ Impact of Communication Initiatives

Communication can help raise awareness about healthy behaviors for individuals. Examples of communication include public service announcements, health fairs, mass media campaigns, newsletters, education that empowers behavior change, and actions through increased knowledge. Health education communication strategies can include courses, trainings, and support groups. Making systematic changes to the policy, systems, and environment through improved laws, rules, and regulations, functional components (e.g., systems), and economic, social, and physical environment. These initiatives and strategies encourage people to construct a healthy living environment.

### SJ Impact of Prevention Communication with Providers

Communication with healthcare providers is an important facet of patient education in minority and disadvantaged populations. For example, heart disease is the leading cause of death among women. Yet, almost 44% of women were unaware of this, with the highest percentages of unawareness among Blacks and Latinas. A key reason for the lack of knowledge reported by women included a lack of physician conversations about heart health, and, in some cases, misdiagnosed symptoms of heart disease as panic, stress, or even hypochondria (Wenger et al., 2022).

### PATIENT-LEVEL FACTORS

Health disparities are closely related to patient education. Preventable health and socioeconomic differences not only manifest as shorter lives and poorer health; they also impose substantial economic costs on our health system and society. One study estimate that eliminating race-based health inequities would have reduced direct medical costs by $230 billion and indirect costs by more than $1 trillion between 2003 and 2006. A recent report from Citigroup found if racial gaps in social drivers of health like wages, education, housing, and investment for Black people were closed 20 years ago, $16 trillion could have been added to the US economy (Peterson & Mann, 2020, September). Structural influences such as accountable care organizations (ACOs) assign accountability to providers who are encouraged to tailor care by integrating quality metrics of success and improving quality while cutting costs (Beebe & Schmitt, 2011).

### IMPACT OF SYSTEM-LEVEL FACTORS

In the home healthcare setting, for example, people have multiple comorbidities and require attention to patient safety measures at home (Blaney-Koen & Dickey, 2008). These include being knowledgeable about the supplies and equipment needed, factors that contribute to the risk of falls, and addressing respiratory illness and air quality challenges. The steps required to achieve these such as talking with the healthcare team to ensure all the supplies are available, refilling medicines, checking the house for health hazards, eliminating smoke, and replacing filters are often the responsibility of the patient.

## COMMUNITY-BASED FACTORS

Achieving quality health outcomes in healthcare settings requires engaging patients to make good decisions about their health and healthcare. Effective utilization of healthcare systems requires techniques and knowledge with which most patients, particularly those that are disadvantaged and marginalized, are unfamiliar. Assuming responsibility for shared decision-making places an assumption of an educated patient. Thus, patient-centered care medical home models (PCM) place an emphasis on educated patients who actively share responsibility in shared decision-making for assuming self-management and personal responsibilities (Pelzman 2020). For example, although diabetes self-management education (DSME) programs have been in existence for almost 20 years, and their reimbursement avenues are available, their utilization by people living in underserved areas is still inadequate. Community health workers, dietitians, health-club personnel, and certified diabetes educators (CDEs) are among the expanded diabetes education team members involved in supporting patient education and self-management responsibility across the lifetime (Beebe & Schmitt, 2011).

*Review **Textbox 6.11** for the example of disparities in neuro-oncology settings and coordination of care. Attempt the SJA prompt that follows.*

---

**Textbox 6.11    Discussion Questions/Thought Scenarios for Reflection**

**Coordination of Care and Disparities in Neuro-Oncology Settings**

*WPHC Context*

As researchers Porter et al. (2021) note, although clinical trials represent the highest standard and quality of care in medicine, the inclusion of underrepresented and underserved groups lags behind majority racial and ethnic groups. On average, only 3%–5% of US patients with cancer get an opportunity to participate in clinical trials. Of these enrolled patients, men with European ancestry comprise an overwhelming majority. The disparities in clinical trial enrollment represent a major therapeutic challenge for the general population. Provider education of implicit bias and health literacy, increasing clinical trial enrollment for minorities, offering opportunities to the underserved to participate through telemedicine, and opportunities for improving access to high-quality specialized care offer possible ways to address the disparities at the SC. For instance, in the field of neuro-oncology, sources of disparities include patient, provider, and systemic factors. Research shows that in the instance of malignant gliomas, for example, minority patients present with greater premorbid illness, have longer symptoms of disease with delayed presentation, experience less information transfer during patient-provider encounters, have greater perioperative surgical morbidity, have less molecular

---

tumor subclassification, and experience greater delays in starting chemoradiation when compared with nonminority patients (National Brain Tumor Society (NBTS), 2022).

**Glioblastoma** is the most common malignant primary brain tumor and affects over 12,000 cases projected annually in the United States. Sociodemographic factors such as age, gender, race, and socioeconomic status affect provider treatment decisions for glioblastoma. Many elderly patients often receive no treatment or significantly less than the standard of care. Researchers Dressler et al. (2018) find that the strongest determinant of treatment was age; however, other factors such as race, gender, histology, primary site location, education, and insurance status also influenced the likelihood and modality of treatment receipt with females and Hispanics 10% less likely to receive standard therapy.

## SJA Discussion Question

1. What are some ways provider education can address the disparity in oncology settings?
2. How can CHCs provide support to disadvantaged and vulnerable populations in this context?

## Resources

Dressler, E. V., Liu, M., Garcia, C. R., Dolecek, T. A., Pittman, T., Huang, B., & Villano, J. L. (2018). Patterns and disparities of care in glioblastoma. *Neuro-Oncology Practice*, 6(1), 37–46. https://doi.org/10.1093/nop/npy014
National Brain Tumor Society (NBTS). Retrieved January 18, 2022, from https://braintumor.org/
National Brain Tumor Society (NBTS). *Personalized support and navigation program*. (n.d.) https://braintumor.org/brain-tumor-information/personalized-support-and-navigation-program

### Coordination of Care

Coordination of care or care coordination is a key healthcare quality criterion. According to the Agency of Healthcare Research and Quality (AHRQ, 2018), care coordination involves deliberately organizing patient care activities and sharing information among all the participants concerned with a patient's care to achieve safer and more effective care. Care coordination supports patient-centered and accessible care that is in alignment with SJ principles. The IOM identified care coordination as central to improving care effectiveness, safety, and efficiency.

### Challenges to Care Coordination

A recent National Healthcare Quality and Disparities Reports (NHQD), 2023) finding suggests that five out of nine care coordination measures have shown improvement, but one-third have shown worsening trends. Among domains of care coordination improved were communication with patients at hospital discharge, timely initiation of HHC services, and fewer home healthcare patients needing hospital admission. Challenges to care coordination remained in domains including effective utilization of PC, home care, or ambulatory care and disregard of patients' preferences during hospital discharge.

## COMMUNICATION AND CARE COORDINATION

Communication is central to successful care coordination. The main goal of care coordination is to meet the patient's needs and preferences in the delivery of high-quality, high-value healthcare. This means that the patient's needs and preferences are known and communicated at the right time to the right people in the patient's care team and that this information is used to guide the delivery of safe, appropriate, and effective care. Examples of care coordination activities include establishing accountability and agreeing upon responsibility among members of the care team, communicating knowledge, helping with the transition of care, assessing patient needs and goals, creating a proactive care plan, timely monitoring and follow-up, supporting patients' self-management goals, linking to community resources, and working to align resources with patient and population needs.

## PATIENT-, PROVIDER-, AND SYSTEM-LEVEL CONCERNS IN CARE COORDINATION

For the **patient**, it is important that all their information, needs, and preferences are communicated across the healthcare team, sites, and systems. For **providers**, care coordination means being patient-centered and family-centered in their processes, alignment of information-sharing, and transition between systems to be able to support their patients' needs, provide referrals and transfer information among healthcare entities, and manage accountability among interprofessional team members (e.g., doctors, nurses, social workers, managers, clinical staff). At the **system level**, care coordination means being an *ACO* that responsibly integrates personnel, information, and patient resources required for optimal patient care between and among participants.

The preceding description illustrates how care coordination plays an important role in bringing together all the healthcare personnel involved in the delivery of patient care.

In conclusion, **Chapter 6, Healthcare Systems**, has discussed how WPHC SJA involves myriad healthcare processes and settings. For example, chronic condition management may involve integration of medication management, use of health information technology, and coordination of activities with the patient-centered home; bridging healthcare systems and processes among and between PC sites and specialty sites; ensuring education and awareness of patients who are partners in decision-making about care processes, including referrals from PC to a specialist, how to make appointments, and what to do after seeing a specialist; specialists who are in the loop with the care team regarding reasons for the referral and have adequate information on tests that have already been done; primary care physicians who receive information about what happened in a referral visit; and referral staff who are able to coordinate different processes and lost information (AHRQ, 2018). The smooth functioning of all processes at the system level is essential for the delivery of SJ healthcare.

*Review **Textbox 6.12**, Subjective Cognitive Decline (SCD) in American Indian and Alaska Native (AI/AN) Populations: The Potential of CBC, and attempt the SJA prompt that follows.*

**Textbox 6.12   Present Challenges and Future Directions Exercise**

**Subjective Cognitive Decline (SCD) in American Indian and Alaska Native (AI/AN) Populations: The Potential of CBC**

*WPHC Context*

Between 2014 and 2060, the number of AI/AN aged 65 and older living with memory loss is projected to grow over five times. In 2015–2017, one of every six AI/AN adults aged 45 and older reported experiencing SCD (CDC, 2022). Nearly two-thirds of those with SCDs had to give up some day-to-day activities. The impact of dementia is multi-generational. Family members and friends feel the impact and may often serve as informal caregivers too. The CDC's Healthy Brain Initiative's (HBI) *Road Map for Indian Country* suggested eight strategies that embrace community strengths. These are:

1. Work with community members to understand brain health, early warning signs of dementia, and benefits of early detection and diagnosis for persons with dementia and their caregivers.
2. Encourage community members to use effective interventions, best practices, and traditional wellness practices to protect brain health, address cognitive decline, and support persons with dementia and their caregivers.
3. Provide information and tools to help older adults with dementia and their caregivers anticipate and respond to challenges that typically arise during dementia.
4. Promote engagement among tribal leaders in dementia issues by offering information and education on the basics of cognitive health and impairment, the impact of dementia on caregivers and communities, and the role of public health approaches in addressing this priority problem.
5. Support collection and use of local data on dementia and caregiving in AI/AN communities to plan programs and approaches.
6. Promote the inclusion of healthcare quality measures that address both cognitive assessments and the delivery of care to AI/ANs with dementia.
7. Educate healthcare and aging services professionals in Indian Country about the signs and symptoms of dementia and about caregiving for persons with dementia.
8. Educate healthcare and aging services professionals on the best ways to support families and caregivers of older adults with dementia.

*SJA Prompt*

Examine the eight strategies for embracing community strengths to address brain health in AI/AN populations. Strategies to improve brain health need to reflect cultural differences across populations and eliminate systemic barriers, the prevalence of discriminatory attitudes in the healthcare system, and social exclusion.

i. Among AI/AN communities, elders are highly valued for their knowledge, wisdom, and contributions. Because Alzheimer's Disease-Related Dementia's (ADRD) largely affects people who are older, it is critical that conversations about ADRD within

AI/AN communities respect cultural norms while simultaneously balancing health and safety (Olivari et al., 2022). Moreover, stigma, fear, and lack of knowledge of ADRD can lead to delayed or missed diagnoses.

Design a community initiative that would bring people together from a CBPR perspective in addressing any one of the strategies.

ii. Discrimination when seeking care for ADRD is a significant problem. Half of African American, 42% of AI/AN, and 33% of Hispanic persons reported experiencing discrimination when seeking healthcare (Alzheimer's Association, 2021). They were less likely than their White counterparts to feel listened to, treated with courtesy and respect, and receive the same quality of service. Over 85% of individuals in these three disproportionately affected groups feel it is important that providers understand their racial or ethnic background when providing care for a person with ADRD, while only about half have access to a provider who does understand (Alzheimer's Association, 2022).

How can technology help sustain a sense of community?

## Resources

Alzheimer's Association. (2022). *Alzheimer's disease facts and figures*. Retrieved January 19, 2023, from https://www.alz.org/media/Documents/alzheimers-fawcts-and-figures.pdf

CDC. (2022, June 21). *Road map for Indian Country*. https://www.cdc.gov/aging/healthybrain/indian-country-roadmap.html

Olivari, B. S., Jeffers, E. M., Tang, K. W., & McGuire, L. C. (2022). Improving brain health for populations disproportionately affected by Alzheimer's Disease and related dementias *Clinical Gerontologist*, https://doi.org/10.1080/07317115.2022.2043977

## References

*ABIM Foundation*. (2003). The Physician Charter. Retrieved from https://abimfoundation.org/what-we-do/physician-charter

Agency for Healthcare Research & Quality (AHRQ). (2018, August). *Care coordination*. Rockville, MD. Retrieved https://www.ahrq.gov/ncepcr/care/coordination.html

Alberti, P. M., Sutton, K. M., Cooper, L. A., Lane, W. G., Stephens, S., & Gourdine, M. A. (2018). Communities, social justice, and academic health centers. *Academic Medicine*, 93(1), 20–24. https://doi.org/10.1097/ACM.0000000000001678

American Academy of Home Care Medicine. Retrieved January 19, 2023, from https://www.aahcm.org/

American College of Obstetrician and Gynecologists (ACOG). (2021). *Health disparities in rural women. Committee on Health Care for Underserved Women, Number 586*. Retrieved January 18, 2023, from https://www.acog.org/clinical/clinical-guidance/committee-opinion/articles/2014/02/health-disparities-in-rural-women

Ames, A., Evans, M., Fox, L., Milam, A., Petteway, R., & Rutledge, R. (2011). Neighborhood health profile: Greater Roland Park/Poplar Hill. Baltimore City Health Department. Retrieved from https://health.baltimorecity.gov/sites/default/files/22%20Greater%20Roland%20Park.pdf

Beach, W. A. (2021). Caring for health in times of crisis. *Health Communication*, 36(14), 2030–2030. https://doi.org/10.1080/10410236.2020.1797332

Beebe, C. A., & Schmitt, S. S. (2011). Engaging patients in education for self-management in account-able care environment. *Clinical Diabetes, 29*(3), 123–126. https://doi.org/10.2337/diaclin.29.3.123

Blaney-Koen, L., & Dickey, N. (2008). Patient education: Safety in the home health care setting. *Journal of Patient Safety, 4*(4), 263 https://doi.org/10.1097/PTS.0b013e31818f38ec

CMS.gov (2016). Accountable Health Communities Model. Retrieved from https://innovation.cms.gov/innovation-models/ahcm

Davis, C. S., Sniderm, M. J., King, L., Shukraft, A., Sonda, J. D., Hicks, L., & Irvin, L. (2019). A time to live and a time to die: Heterotopian spatialities and temporalities in a pediatric palliative care team. *Health Communication, 34*(9), 931–941 https://doi.org/10.1080/10410236.2018.1443262

Fashaw-Walters, S. A., Rahman, M., Gee, G., Mor, V., White, M., & Thomas, K. S. (2022). Out of reach: Inequities in the use of high-quality home health agencies. *Health Affairs, 41*(2). https://doi.org/10.1377/hlthaff.2021.01408

Federally Qualified Health Center. (2022). Retrieved January 19, 2023, from https://www.cms.gov/Outreach-and-Education/Medicare-Learning-Network-MLN/MLNProducts/downloads/fqhcfactsheet.pdf

Ferrer, R. L. (2007). Pursuing equity: Contact with primary care and specialist clinicians by demograph-ics, insurance, and health status. *Annals of Family Medicine, 5*(6), 492–502. https://doi.org/10.1370/afm.74630

Healthcare.gov. (2022). *Rehabilitative/rehabilitation services.* Retrieved January 18, 2023, from https://www.healthcare.gov/glossary/rehabilitative-rehabilitation-services/

Health Resources & Services Administration (HRSA). *What is a health center?* Retrieved January 19, 2023, from https://bphc.hrsa.gov/about-health-centers/what-health-center

Internal Revenue Service. (2018, March 21). *Tax benefits for businesses who have employees with disabili-ties.* Retrieved January 16, 2023, from https://www.irs.gov/businesses/small-businesses-self-employed/tax-benefits-for-businesses-who-have-employees-with-disabilities

Kennedy-Moulton, K., Miller, S., Persson, P., Rossin-Slater, M., Wherry, L., & Aldana, G. (2022). Maternal and infant health mortality: New evidence from linked administrative data. *National Bureau of Economic Research Working Paper Series, 30693* https://doi.org/10.3386/w30693. Retrieved on February 12, 2023, from https://www.nber.org/papers/w30693

Kraus, L., et al. (2017). *Disability statistics annual report.* Institute on Disability. University of New Hampshire.

List, J. M. (2011). Beyond charity: Social justice and health care. *Virtual Mentor, 13*(8), 565–568 https://doi.org/10.1001/virtualmentor.2011.13.8.msoc1-1108. Retrieved January 14, 2023, from https://journalofethics.ama-assn.org/article/beyond-charity-social-justice-and-healthcare/2011-08

Medicare.gov (2023) *What's home health care?* Retrieved on January 19, 2023, from https://www.medicare.gov/what-medicare-covers/whats-home-healthcare

MedlinePlus. (2022). *What is rehabilitation?* Retrieved January 18, 2023, from https://medlineplus.gov/rehabilitation.html

Mudrick, N. R., et al. (2012). Physical accessibility in primary health care settings: Results from California on-site reviews. *Disability Health Journal, 5*(3), 159–167.

*National Center for Health Statistics* (2020). National Vital Statistics Reports, Vol. 69, No. 12. United States Life Tables, 2018. Retrieved from https://www.cdc.gov/nchs/data/nvsr/nvsr69/nvsr69-12-508.pdf

National Healthcare Quality and Disparities Report (NHQDR). Retrieved January 19, 2023, from https://www.ahrq.gov/sites/default/files/wysiwyg/research/findings/nhqrdr/2021qdr-final-es.pdf

National Institute on Aging (NIA). (2022). *End of life: What are palliative care and hospice care?* Re-trieved January 18, 2023, from https://www.nia.nih.gov/health/what-are-palliative-care-and-hospice-care

National PACE Association. (2023). https://www.npaonline.org/

Omillion-Hodges, L. M., & Swords, N. M. (2016). Communication that heals: Mindful communication practices from palliative care leaders. *Health Communication*, *31*(3), 328–335. https://doi.org/10.1080/10410236.2014.953739

Omillion-Hodges, L. M., & Swords, N. M. (2017). The Grim Reaper, Hounds of Hell, and Dr. Death: The role of storytelling for palliative care in competing medical meaning systems. *Health Communication*, *32*(10), 1272–1283. https://doi.org/10.1080/10410236.2016.1219928

Paradise, J., Rosenbaum, S., Markus, A., Sharac, J., Tran, C., Reynolds, D., & Shin, P. (2017, January 18). *Kaiser Family Foundation* (KFF, 2023). Community health centers: Recent growth and the role of the ACA. Retrieved January 19, 2023, from https://www.kff.org/medicaid/issue-brief/community-health-centers-recent-growth-and-the-role-of-the-aca/

Pelzman, R. (2020, June 1). Social justice: Yes, it's a medical issue. *MedPage Today*. Retrieved January 14, 2023, from https://www.medpagetoday.com/opinion/patientcenteredmedicalhome/86795

Peterson, D., & Mann, C. (2020). Closing the racial inequality gaps: The economic cost of Black inequality in the U.S. Citi GPS: Global Perspectives & Solutions. Retrieved January 14, 2023, from https://www.citivelocity.com/citigps/closing-the-racial-inequality-gaps/

Picheta, Rob. (2020, Aug. 20). *Black newborns more likely to die when looked after by White doctors*. CNN Health. Retrieved January 13, 2023, from https://www.cnn.com/2020/08/18/health/black-babies-mortality-rate-doctors-study-wellness-scli-intl/index.html

Porter, A. B., Chukwueke, U. N., Mammoser, A. G., Friday, B., & Hervey-Jumper, S. (2021). Delivering equitable care to underserved neuro-oncology populations. *American Society of Clinical Oncology Educational Book*, *41*, 38–56. Retrieved January 17, 2023, from https://ascopubs.org/doi/full/10.1200/EDBK_320803

Ragan, S. L., Wittenberg, E., & Hall, H. T. (2003). The communication of palliative care for the elderly cancer patient. *Health Communication*, *25*(2), 219–226. https://doi.org/10.1207/S15327027HC1502_9

Rikard, R.V., Thompson, M.S., McKinney, J., & Beauchamp, A. (2016). Examining health literacy disparities in the United States: A third look at the National Assessment of Adult Literacy (NAAL). *BMC Public Health*, *16*, Article Number 975. https://doi.org/10.1186/s12889-016-3621-9

Rosen, S., Mieres, J., & Nash, B. (2020, August 3). Health care is long overdue for a social justice reckoning. *Scientific American*. Retrieved from https://www.scientificamerican.com/article/health-care-is-long-overdue-for-a-social-justice-reckoning/

Rubio, D.M., Schoenbaum, E.E., Lee, L.S., Schteingart, D.E., Marantz, P.R., Anderson, K.E., Platt, L.D., Baez, A., & Esposito, K. (2010). Defining translational research: Implications for training. *Academic Medicine*, *85*(3), 470–475. https://www.doi.org/10.1097/ACM.0b013e3181ccd618

Salsberg, E., Richwine, E., & Westergaard, S. (2021). Estimation and comparison of current and future racial/ethnic representation in the U.S. health care workforce. *JAMA Network Open*, *4*(3), e213789 https://doi.org/10.1001/jamanetworkopen.2021.3789

The Commonwealth Fund. (2023, January 18). *Medicare beneficiaries of color more likely to rely on unpaid informal caregivers for home health*. Retrieved on January 19, 2023, from https://www.commonwealthfund.org/blog/2023/medicare-beneficiaries-color-more-likely-rely-unpaid-informal-caregivers-home-health

Thompson, H. R., Mendelson, J., Zamek, M., Cortez, G., & Schillinger, D. (2022). Impact of an arts-based public health literacy program delivered online to high school students during the COVID-19 pandemic. *Journal of Health Communication*, *27*(7), 520–534. https://doi.org/10.1080/10810730.2022.2131942

United States Census Bureau. (2014). *Mobility is most common disability among older Americans*. Census Bureau Reports.

Wenger, N. K., Lloyd-Jones, D. M., Elkind, M. S. V., Fonarow, G. C., Warner, J. J., Alger, H. M. … Roger, V. L. (2022). Call to action for cardiovascular disease in women: Epidemiology, awareness, access, and delivery of equitable health care: A presidential advisory from the *American Heart Association*. *Circulation*, *145*, e1059–e1071 https://doi.org/10.1161/CIR.0000000000001071

WHO. (2016). *What is health promotion?* Retrieved January 20, 2023, from https://www.who.int/news-room/questions-and-answers/item/health-promotion

WHO. (2021). *WHO guideline on self-care interventions for health and well-being.* Retrieved January 18, 2023, from https://app.magicapp.org/#/guideline/Lr21gL

WHO. (2022, October 1). WHO Technical Brief. Primary health care. AN integrated approach for delivering universal health coverage with a focus on social justice, equity, and solidarity. https://www.who.int/publications/m/item/primary-healthcare.-an-integrated-approach-for-delivering-universal-health-coverage-with-a-focus-on-social-justice--equity--and-solidarity

Wyoming Department of Health. *Maternal and child health services Title V Block Grant. FY 2022 application.* Retrieved January 18, 2023, from https://health.wyo.gov/wp-content/uploads/2021/11/WY_TitleV_PrintVersion_FY22_71363f28-db86-40f0-9d25-db1cdaa84e87.pdf

## Additional Resources

CDC. (n.d.). *National Center for Chronic Disease Prevention and Health Promotion.* Retrieved from https://www.cdc.gov/chronicdisease/index.htm

WHO. (n.d.). *Guideline on self-care interventions for health and well-being, 2022 revision.* Retrieved https://app.magicapp.org/#/guideline/5512

# Health Literacy

## Chapter Learning Outcomes

Upon completing **Chapter 7, Health Literacy**, the student will be able to apply the WPHC SJA framework to:

1. Understand the evolution and meaning of health literacy as a concept.
2. Identify the different types of health literacy and explain their significance from a WPHC and SJA perspective.
3. Apply the concept of health literacy in a range of personal, social, community, and organizational contexts.
4. Engage different audiences in the application of health literacy from a WPHC and SJA perspective.
5. Understand how the cultural construction of health shapes health communication from a WPHC and SJA perspective.
6. Advocate and enact communications and behaviors in a range of contexts that exemplify health literacy principles from a WPHC and SJA perspective.

**Consider how many times you have encountered the following situations over the past year:**

- Researching health insurance for coverage, rates, and in-network providers.
- Searching online for symptoms, treatments, and risks.
- Reading prescription labels and pamphlets to understand dosage instructions, drug interactions, and side effects.
- Explaining your health condition and trying to follow the doctor's instructions.
- Coming across a prescription advertisement in your social media feed and wondering about the drug's side effects versus benefits for your health condition.

In each of these contexts, and in many other everyday tasks related to these contexts, you are applying the knowledge and ability to understand health information in taking care of your health and engaging in a form of health literacy.

DOI: 10.4324/9781003214472-9

Health literacy is important for health promotion and protection, disease prevention, early screening, health monitoring, and maintenance, and policy making. Health literacy skills are needed for dialogue and discussion, reading health information, interpreting charts, making decisions about participating in research studies, and for using medical tools for personal or familial healthcare (e.g., using an oximeter for measuring blood oxygen level), calculating timing or dosage of medicine, or voting on health or environmental issues.

Surprisingly, even people with high literacy skills, or those who are otherwise able to read and write fluently, may be challenged with low health literacy skills in certain situations. Consider, for example, someone who is stressed and sick when they're accessing health information online about their health condition. Such an individual may have struggled with remembering, understanding, and using that information (Network of the National Library of Medicine, NNLM.gov). Evidence suggests that those who are at greater risk for low health literacy are more likely to be male, from a racial or ethnic minority, and have higher religious belief scores (Christy et al., 2017). As minorities account for an increasing proportion of the US population, especially in urban areas, systematic differences in health literacy will only increase health disparities.

Approximately 9 out of 10 adults or 80 million adults in the United States struggle with health literacy (NNLM.gov; Rikard et al., 2016). The importance of health literacy was recognized in the United States from the unexpected findings of the 1992 National Adult Literacy Survey (NALS). The NALS showed that 40–44 million of the 191 million American adults were functionally illiterate, and another 53.5 million adults had marginally better functional literacy skills. This survey also found that self-reported educational attainment, i.e., years of schooling, did not necessarily imply an equivalent level of reading or comprehension. These findings helped draw attention to the functionality of low-literacy adults in the healthcare domain. Thus, the term "health literacy" was originally developed to refer specifically to functional literacy in the healthcare realm (Lee et al., 2004).

The consequences of low health literacy go far beyond the individual. As the US population ages, the number of adults with multiple chronic conditions (e.g., cardiac conditions and their comorbidities) also increases. Being able to engage in complex chronic disease management and self-care is a component of health literacy. People living with chronic conditions often manage comorbidities such as hypertension, diabetes mellitus, and hyperlipidemia. Chronic conditions require a high level of engagement with healthcare providers and nurse practitioners to coordinate medications and manage appointments. People who have low health literacy are unable to successfully interpret health information and have increased hospitalization rates, develop more diseases, and experience higher mortality. Furthermore, individuals with low health literacy are also more likely to use the emergency department of primary care, resulting in overburdening of hospital resources, excess burden of costs on the patient, and fragmented care (Hickey et al., 2019).

WPHC advocates for an inclusive application of the concept of health literacy. The concept of health literacy as covered in this chapter will elucidate its main tenets with a focus on disadvantaged and minority identities and populations. For example, a

WPHC SJA approach will ask providers, health communication practitioners and scholars, and allied healthcare workers to develop and enact an understanding of health literacy that is free from implicit bias, tailored to their needs and gaps in care and awareness, and seeks to build trust with the healthcare system. To illustrate, people who identify as transgender, for example, report psychosocial challenges, discrimination, and lack of understanding in the care they receive from the healthcare system. A WPHC SJA approach will ask that an inclusive understanding of health literacy be integrated across the interdisciplinary teams addressing transgender care, with particular attention being paid to the needs of transgender people, developing knowledge of transgender medicine, and removing false assumptions (Thomson et al., 2019).

A WPHC health literacy framework is important because the gap between access and provision of information and the ability to act on the information and knowledge is often associated with corresponding health disparities. Health literacy illustrates how just the provision of health information in clinical, organizational, or community-based settings is not enough. A WPHC approach highlights how health literacy means very different challenges and opportunities to those who are disadvantaged and marginalized. More importantly, understood from a WPHC approach, the concept of health literacy takes on a complex interpretation (Schaffler et al. 2018). Each racial and ethnic minority, and the individual circumstances of those within these minority populations, will access, understand, and benefit from the conditions for empowerment offered by health literacy in their own unique and specific ways. The framework offered by WPHC is central to providing the lens through which health literacy can both empower and constrain opportunities for health outcomes based on its interpretation and application. Seen through a WPHC lens, the concept of health literacy is closely connected with health equity and health disparities and interwoven with the cultural construction of health.

As discussed in **Chapter 3, A Social Justice Activism Approach to Health**, health disparities capture the systematic health differences between different groups of people that arise from inequities in social, economic, educational, and other SDoH. For instance, minorities, people who are older, have limited education, lower income, and chronic conditions, and those who are non-native English speakers are more likely to have lower health literacy. Given these facts, it is not surprising that low health literacy has been found to be a stronger predictor of poor health than age, income, employment status, education level, and race (American Medical Association, AMA, 1999). Chapter 7 will extend the concept of health literacy through the lens of WPHC and SJA to underscore its significance for ensuring opportunities for improved health outcomes for all communities and individuals alike.

## Chapter Organization

**Chapter 7, Health Literacy**, will provide a comprehensive look at the concept of health literacy from a **WPHC and SJA** framework tracing its early origins to its present-day definition comprising the components of personal health literacy and organizational health literacy.

**First**, the chapter will situate health literacy in cultural contexts, discuss the notion of acculturation as it relates to health literacy, and explain how culturally sensitive and tailored communication is important in health communication settings. **Second**, it will illustrate how acculturation and culturally sensitive communication are important in health communication settings. **Third**, it will define the different forms of health literacy, including functional, textual, numeracy, and digital health literacy, and situate health literacy in health information-seeking and digital contexts. **Fourth**, the chapter will cover applied aspects such as online social support and health literacy in peer-to-peer online health communication including digital health literacy and ehealth literacy, health information seeking, and health misinformation. **Fifth**, it will situate its relevance in addressing challenges such as those posed by health misinformation. Along the way, to highlight the **WPHC SJA principles** in each section of the chapter, the student will be provided with the many facets of its application, ranging from policy, as articulated in Healthy People 2030, health equity principles in inclusive and digital communication, and health literacy domains in everyday contexts, to attributes of health-literate healthcare organizations, inclusive language, how to avoid health misinformation, and health literacy in clinical contexts. The scholar interview with Dr. Susan Morgan will describe vividly her personal experience with disparities in clinical trial recruitment and the importance of translational communication with minorities. The communication scholar interview with Dr. Satarupa Dasgupta will illustrate her work with health activism addressing health disparities among sex trafficking survivors in international settings and intimate partner violence prevention among immigrant communities in the United States. **Seventh**, the chapter will provide multiple opportunities to reflect upon challenges and opportunities for health literacy and to engage with the content using activities, thought prompts, reflections, and discussion questions. Discussion Questions and Thought Scenarios for Reflection will highlight the challenges of peer-to-peer online health information sharing. The Present Challenges and Future Directions Exercise will encourage students to consider the possibility of harm in patient-provider interaction associated with low health literacy and cultural illiteracy.

## Health Literacy

### Defining Health Literacy

Health literacy refers to the application of literacy in combination with other skills and abilities of the individual in a health context. Health literacy includes specific skills in the healthcare context that are required for maintaining one's health, preventing disease, or obtaining treatment and getting well when sick. However, health literacy is more than just the ability to read. An individual with low health literacy may be able to read but may not be able to comprehend the meaning of the information, evaluate it in the context of their own life, or consider how it compares with similar information available from other sources. Clearly, for individuals living with low health literacy, just providing people access to information is not enough; crafting conditions for their empowerment must ensure health equity.

*Read **Textbox 7.1** to get an overview of how **Health Literacy 2030** is different from the earlier version conceptualized in Health Literacy 2010 and Health Literacy 2020. Follow the question prompts in **Textbox 7.1** to consider how Healthy People 2030 furthers the goals of health equity.*

**Textbox 7.1   Health Literacy: Conceptualization and Application Trajectory**

**WPHC Context**

**Healthy People 2030** recognizes an organization's responsibility to address health literacy. One of its overarching goals is to *"[e]liminate health disparities, achieve health equity, and attain health literacy to improve the health and well-being of all."* Read on to identify how health equity is central to the revised definition of health literacy.

**Previous Definition of Health Literacy in Healthy People 2010 and Healthy People 2020**

The degree to which individuals have the capacity to obtain, process, and understand basic health information and services needed to make appropriate health decisions (Ratzan & Parker, 2000).

**Two Components in Revised Definition of Health Literacy in Healthy People 2030**

In achieving the goal of health literacy, Healthy People 2030 recognizes that, in addition to personal health literacy, organizations are also responsible for providing an opportunity for all to attain the highest level of health and be as healthy as possible.

**Revised Definition**

A. **Personal health literacy** is the degree to which individuals can find, understand, and use information and services to inform health-related decisions *and actions for themselves and others.*

B. **Organizational health literacy** is the degree to which organizations enable individuals to find, understand, and use information and services to inform health-related decisions and actions for themselves and others.

The six **Healthy People 2030** objectives developed by the **Health Communication and Health Information Technology Workgroup** include the following:

1. Increase the proportion of adults whose healthcare provider checked their understanding (HC/HIT-01).
2. Decrease the proportion of adults who report poor communication with their healthcare provider (HC/HIT-02).
3. Increase the proportion of adults whose healthcare providers involved them in decisions as much as they wanted (HC/HIT-03).
4. Increase the proportion of people who say their online medical record is easy to understand (HC/HIT-D10).
5. Increase the proportion of adults with limited English proficiency who say their providers explain things clearly (HC/HIT-D11).
6. Increase the health literacy of the population (HC/HIT-R01).

| WPHC Context | SJA Prompt |
|---|---|
| *How the Healthy People 2030 Definition Addresses Health Equity* | *How Can You Apply the Objectives in Healthy People 2030 Definition to Help Attain Health Equity?* |
| Emphasizes people's ability to use health information rather than just understand it | • *What impact does the ability to find, understand, but also then use health information make in an individual's ability to be healthy?* |
| Focuses on the ability to make "well-informed" decisions rather than "appropriate" ones. | • *What is the difference in a health outcome between making a well-informed decision rather than merely an appropriate one?* |
| Acknowledges that organizations have a responsibility to address health literacy. | • *What can organizations do to address health equity?* |
| Incorporates a public health perspective. | • *What kinds of initiatives can help ensure that all population groups living within an area have access to the resources that promote and protect health?* |

## SJA Activity

Imagine you are researching suitable health insurance for yourself. Look at the question prompts in the column on the right in the table in this textbox (CDC, 2020; CDC 2021). Respond to the questions to consider how health literacy makes a difference in this context. Consider how your university (or an organization that you work for) can help support you in your efforts to make the best decision.

As you complete this activity, reflect upon the following:

• What challenges did you face in the process of researching health insurance options available in the market that best meet your needs?
• What implications did this decision make in your life?

## Resources

CDC. (2020, November 30). *Minority health: Paving the road to health equity*. Retrieved January 8, 2023, from https://www.cdc.gov/minorityhealth/publications/health_equity/index.html

CDC. (2021, July 7). *Clear communication: Health literacy*. Retrieved January 8, 2023, from https://www.nih.gov/institutes-nih/nih-office-director/office-communications-public-liaison/clear-communication/health-literacy#:~:text=emphasize%20people's%20ability%20to%20use,responsibility%20to%20address%20health%20literacy

Ratzan, S. C., & Parker, R. M. (2000). Introduction. In C. R. Seldon, M. Zorn, S. C. Ratzan, & R. M. Parker (Eds.), *National library of medicine current bibliographies in medicine: Health literacy*. NLM Pub. No. CBM 2000-1. National Institutes of Health, U.S. Department of Health and Human Services.

Healthy People 2030. Retrieved January 8, 2023, from https://health.gov/healthypeople/priority-areas/health-literacy-healthy-people-2030

*Health Literacy in Clinical Settings*

Healthcare is provided in a range of contexts and to an increasingly diverse patient population. Patient-provider communication can generate or reduce healthcare disparities. Health literacy in clinical settings is associated with a range of skills for both the provider and the patient.

## PATIENT FACTORS

For the patient, health literacy skills include the ability to communicate effectively with healthcare providers, to negotiate the complexity of healthcare settings, and to obtain proper and timely care. These interrelated skills affect patient outcomes. Researchers Pérez-Stable and El-Toukhy (2018) found that patients who were members of racial and ethnic minorities, with limited English proficiency, and low health and digital literacy demonstrated poor patient-clinician communication scores.

## CLINICIAN FACTORS

On the other hand, the researchers found that clinicians who had poor patient-clinician communication scores were less culturally competent, lacked communication skills to facilitate shared decision-making, and often held unconscious biases. The researchers recommend standardized collection of SDoH in the electronic health record (EHR) as an important step in supporting effective patient-provider communication. Including SDoH information in the EHR can help providers with greater knowledge about the living conditions of their patients such as their neighborhoods and education and thus be able to tailor their communication to each individual patient's unique needs and context.

It is important for providers to be trained in communication skills in addition to providing medical advice. A WPHC health literacy framework asks how providers can take steps to be aware of how a patient's culture and language shape how they communicate and make sense of health information. Healthcare providers who are trained in the implications of health literacy can build a patient-provider relationship that eliminates rather than exacerbates health disparities and barriers to access for minority and marginalized populations. For instance, providers can prompt patients to ask questions to help them feel empowered in their health decision-making, take ownership of their health and well-being, and understand their health condition (Rural Health Information Hub, 2021).

## COMMUNITY FACTORS

Estacio (2013) presents an example of a community-based project in a small indigenous community in the Philippines. In this project, the community members adopt an empowerment education model in health literacy. Using the tenets of empowerment education, community members were trained to engage in critical reflection on how health meanings were constructed. They were able to see how their meanings of health reflected their socioeconomic and political environments and their implications for how they made decisions about their health; whose opinions they valued; how they gained a particular form of knowledge of health over another, alternative form (power relations); and how such understandings shaped their individual experiences (subjective experiences). Estacio's study illustrates how health literacy skills should incorporate an awareness of unbalanced power relations and unfair social-economic structures to bring about positive social change in underserved communities. Knowledge that creates conditions by which community members can bring about positive change is the goal of health literacy.

*Consider **Textbox 7.2**. Examine the different instances in which a specific form of health literacy has aided health decision-making. Read the examples of how health literacy can improve your health (abstracted from AHIMA Foundation, 2022). Then respond to the SJA Prompt that follows.*

---

### Textbox 7.2   Health Literacy Domains in Everyday Contexts

#### WPHC Context

| Health Literacy Domain | Type of Literacy |
| --- | --- |
| Parent taking a child's temperature | Functional literacy |
| Worker reading about proper procedures for handling materials | Textual literacy |
| Shopper calculating the difference in salt content on the labels of two brands of canned vegetables | Numeracy literacy |
| Patient reading about dental options | Functional literacy |
| Elder filling out an application for Medicare | Textual literacy |

#### How Can Health Literacy Improve Your Health?

**Chronic obstructive pulmonary disease** (COPD) is a lung disease that can make it harder to breathe. Patients with COPD who had higher digital health literacy were able to tell the difference between high- and low-quality internet sources (Stellefson, et al. 2017). This helped them make better decisions about managing their COPD symptoms. Patients with higher digital health literacy said they had fewer problems with chest tightness, slept better, and had more energy.

Researchers studied veterans with diabetes who were enrolled in an online patient portal. Patients who refilled their medicines online for more than two years had better blood pressure levels than those who didn't.

#### SJA Prompt

Reflect on a health decision you have made recently.

- In what way did you employ health literacy during your decision-making process?
- What form of health literacy did you apply?
- Did you face any challenges in your decision-making process?
- In what way were these challenges have been better addressed through health literacy skills?

#### Resource

AHIMA Foundation. (2022, June 15). *Digital health literacy as a social determinant of health.* Retrieved January 12, 2023, from https://ahimafoundation.org/understanding-the-issues/digital-health-literacy-as-a-social-determinant-of-health/

## Types of Health Literacy

### Literacy

Literacy is defined as a combination of reading, writing, basic mathematics, speech, and comprehension skills (Kirsch, 2001). It includes oral literacy, print literacy, numeracy, and functional literacy. Health literacy is more than the ability to be competent in the different forms of literacy. For example, an individual who is literate can read the newspaper, the Bible, novels, or a manual at work, but may be challenged in figuring out the directions for taking medicine, researching health insurance, or calculating the dosage of a medicine.

### Oral Literacy

Oral literacy comprises the components of speech comprehension. Speech comprehension involves the complex skills of listening and interpreting gestures, expressions, and tone in the context they were employed and making sense of the overall logic and organization of the thought communicated by the speaker. Oral listening skills are employed in the many contexts of provider-patient communication, organizational communication, and public health communication. These contexts may range from evaluating media messages, critically interpreting public service announcements, interacting with healthcare professionals, and communicating one's symptoms to the doctor.

### Print Literacy

Print literacy refers to the ability to read, write, and understand written language that is familiar, and for which one has the required background language (NNLM). Print literacy includes reading or textual literacy. Print literacy includes the ability to decode letters into sounds and pronounce words. However, just being able to decode letters into sounds and pronounce words is not enough. Someone who can read may not be able to understand the meaning of a sentence formed by these words, much less critically evaluate them, and apply them in the context of their life.

### Fluency

Fluency in reading references the accuracy, rate, and appropriate phrasing and intonation of words. Fluent reading has a natural feel and flow to capture the intention behind the written word. People with low or limited print literacy also have difficulty reading fluently and comprehending materials written beyond very simple levels. This can pose a challenge when medication instructions or public health messages are written in a complex manner.

### READABILITY

Reading or text literacy is related to the characteristics of the text being read such as complexity and format. Readability of a text depends on the skills and background knowledge of individual readers, factors in the text, and the purpose for which readers use the materials. The average American's health literacy skills are around seventh- to eighth-grade level, with many people reading below that level (e.g., at a fourth- to sixth-grade level). By comparison,

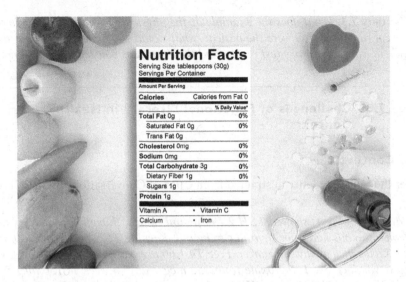

*Figure 7.1* Nutrition Label.

most current health communication material is written at a ninth-grade level or higher (United States Environmental Protection Agency, EPA, 2023).

## Numeracy

When patients use basic calculations (e.g., addition, subtraction, multiplication, division), read medical labels, and try to understand times and days for medication administration, they are drawing upon the numeracy dimension of health literacy. It is also referred to as quantitative literacy. This form of literacy refers to a set of mathematical and advanced problem-solving skills that are necessary to succeed in an increasingly electronic and data-driven healthcare environment (National Association of Secondary School Principals, 2023).

## Functional Literacy

Functional literacy is the use of literacy to perform a particular task. Examples of functional health literacy can be found in everyday contexts of our lives. A website, for example, may serve the function of providing information about how lifestyle choices affect your health. An online patient portal may provide individuals with myriad resources ranging from health management tools to track medical visit history to medication history, discharge summaries, and more (HealthIT.gov). Navigating these contexts requires functional literacy. Researchers Fernández-Gutiérrez and colleagues examine how health literacy impacts functional skills in immigrant populations. Their study underscores the importance of training healthcare providers in health literacy skills for improving immigrant community health (Fernández-Gutiérrez et al. 2018).

The example in **Textbox 7.3** provides the text of a letter sent by a doctor to a patient. The patient had an advanced degree, yet his anxiety was greatly increased as a result of reading the letter. He asked, *"How can I have a recurrence of thyroid cancer if my cancer was removed?"* (see **Textbox 7.3**).

Consider **Textbox 7.3**. *What does the example of the physician's communication in the text of the email reveal to you? If you were the patient, what would you understand about the doctor's interpretation of your laboratory test results and the next steps you should be taking?*

---

### Textbox 7.3  Challenges of Functional Literacy in Health Contexts

**WPHC Context**

Consider the following letter abstracted from Clinical Conversations on the NNLM:

*Dear Mr. Smith,*

*The May thyroid tests showed TSH 2.794 µU/ml, which, though "normal," is too high for someone who has had prior thyroid carcinoma. Keeping TSH between 0.1–0.3 µU/ml minimizes recurrence of thyroid cancer. Free T4 1.60 mg% is a high-normal level.*

*I suggest you increase L-thyroxine from 150 mcg 7 days a week to 150 mcg 5 days a week and 225 mcg (111/22 tablets) Wednesdays and Sundays weekly. Have a repeat TSH, free T4 and total T3 in 8 weeks. I should also on that occasion like you to have a serum plasma metanephrine level.*

*Two weeks after having those tests, please see me for a consultative office visit.*

Sincerely yours,
John Doe, M.D.
Endocrinology

**SJA Discussion Prompt**

1. What are some of the health literacy communication challenges you can identify in the healthcare provider's communication to their patient?
2. Read the NNLM's *Clinical Conversations* program recommendations provided in the URL below. What recommendations would you make to the healthcare provider to address these challenges?
3. From a WPHC SJA perspective, what observations might you make from the conversation based on the identity of the patient? What steps would you recommend be taken and by whom to help address the challenges posed by this situation?

**Resource**

NNLM. *Clinical Conversations*. Retrieved January 12, 2023, from https://www.nnlm.gov/guides/clinical-conversations-training-program Retrieved January 8, 2023, from https://www.ncbi.nlm.nih.gov/books/NBK216035/

---

## A Comprehensive View of Health Literacy

An example of an over-the-counter medication will help illustrate how the different forms of literacy come together under the umbrella of health literacy. The label on a pediatric over-the-counter medicine may provide the parent or caregiver with information ranging from active drug ingredients (for example, in each 5 ml), purpose, warnings, notes on symptoms that may require communication with a doctor prior to use, and dosage calculation directions. Interpreting and acting upon this information effectively often requires complex print, numeracy, and functional literacy skills.

*Try the activity provided in **Textbox 7.4** to see how much of the information you can use in deciding to use the medication, its contraindications, and to calculate the dosage for a 5-year-old child with a cough.*

---

**Textbox 7.4    Assessing Health Literacy: Pediatric Over-the-Counter (OTC) Drug Label**

**WPHC Context**

Visit your local pharmacy and browse the OTC drug labels for common children's cough, cold, and congestion drugs displayed on the aisles (the URL under "Resources" provides the online printer-friendly label; NLM, 2022).

1. What form of literacy will you need to determine if it is safe to give to a 5-year-old child who is also running a fever and taking a fever reducer?
2. Can you identify which active drug is used as a cough suppressant and the active drug for the expectorant?
3. Can you calculate the dosage in milliliters and frequency?
4. What form of literacy did you use to do so?
5. What forms of side effects would you monitor for?
6. Under what conditions would you contact a doctor?

**SJA Prompt**

- How might a non-native speaker of English be challenged to care for their child in this instance?
- What resources might you recommend to overcome the challenges they may face?
- What recommendations might you make from a WPHA and SJA framework to healthcare professionals to revise this information presentation to better address the challenges faced by minorities?

**Resource**

NLM (2022, December 28). *DailyMed*. Retrieved January 25, 2023, from https://dailymed.nlm. nih.gov/dailymed/drugInfo.cfm?setid=b9772292-9eb6-47cf-abb8-007c25478090

---

## Components of Health Literacy

Healthy People 2030 identifies two components of health literacy: personal health literacy and organizational health literacy. Both are important to address gaps in healthcare outcomes and health inequities. This section covers personal health literacy and organizational health literacy, along with describing their application in different factors of literacy (OASH, n.d.).

### Personal Health Literacy

The definition of personal health literacy as given in Textbox 7.1 encourages individuals to make "well-informed" decisions rather than merely "appropriate" ones. There are several examples in research that illustrate how low health literacy is associated with negative health behaviors and outcomes. Hoover et al. (2015) examined the association between health literacy and self-rated physical and mental health, smoking, and perceived stress among 1,467 African American adults in the United States. Their research shows how low health literacy was an independent risk factor for negative behaviors and outcomes. There are different forms of health literacy that fall broadly under the umbrella of personal health literacy based on the specific contexts in which the literacy skills are accessed. These include medical literacy and digital literacy and the closely related ehealth literacy.

#### Medication Literacy

Medication literacy is a form of personal health literacy. Medical literacy references the skills that are required to take medications correctly. Literacy skills employed in taking medication correctly include understanding the concepts of measurement, being able to read and correctly interpret prescription labels, and keeping track of active ingredients in the medicines. Sometimes, literacy skills also involve understanding complex directions from healthcare providers about medicines. These skills often impact those experiencing disparities and inequities disproportionately. Medication literacy can be a challenge for older adults, those with limited vision ability, and those with limited English language skills. Over 4 out of 5 adults over age 65 regularly take a least one prescription medication (American Association of Retired Persons, AARP, 2022).

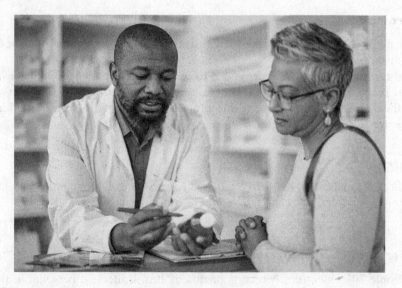

Figure 7.2 Provider with a client.

Consider the situation when a caregiver or a parent with a sick family member or a sick child needs to measure specific dosages of medications following directions included in a prescription label based on their age, weight, or other medications being taken. To complicate matters further, the website of the American Health Information Management Association Foundation (AHIMA) notes that some labels may also have small fonts that pose an additional challenge for those with limited vision, hidden warning signs, and complex drug names. For those with limited English proficiency, language barriers are an additional challenge. Third, keeping track of active ingredients can be challenging (AHIMA, 2023).

## DIGITAL HEALTH LITERACY

Most of the health information accessible today is in a digital format. Consider product websites, websites of organizations providing healthcare information, or insurance websites. Similarly, healthcare services are becoming increasingly digitized. Searching for providers, pharmacies, insurance providers, and researching medication side effects requires an ability to access the internet and navigate the online information environment. The ability to seek, find, understand, and appraise health information form electronic sources and apply the knowledge gained to addressing or solving a health problem is called digital health literacy (Norman & Skinner, 2006). Digital health literacy is also sometimes referred to as ehealth literacy.

Digital health literacy is especially important in online health information seeking. Researchers Yom-Tov and colleagues looked at how people use the internet to learn about type 2 diabetes and understand how health literacy influences this information-seeking behavior (Yom-Tov, et al. 2016). To do this, they analyzed the searches of approximately two million people who queried for diabetes-related information on Microsoft's Bing search engine. The researchers found that overall, the diabetes information-seeking strategies via the internet were similar among adults with limited and adequate health literacy skills. However, the data also revealed that people with limited health literacy take a longer time to read pages that were read quickly by people with adequate health literacy. Although both groups of adults— those with adequate health literacy skills and those with limited health literacy skills— employed similar information-seeking strategies, it was found that people with limited health literacy terminated their information-seeking prematurely. An analysis of the website reading level showed that the reading level required to understand the content corresponded to grade 7 or higher. Because they terminated their information seeking early, they failed to get an equivalent benefit from this information resource compared with users with greater health literacy.

*The table in **Textbox 7.5** lists some ways digital health literacy may be employed in daily circumstances. The center column provides the corresponding barriers to digital health literacy that might challenge disadvantaged and minority populations from benefiting from health information and resources available online. Consider columns one and two in responding to the question posed by the right-most column, "What can providers do?" Then respond to the discussion prompt provided in the textbox and try your hand at the questions from a WPHC and SJA framework.*

**Textbox 7.5    Digital Inequities and Digital Health Literacy in Action**

### WPHC Context

A complex array of health literacy skills are needed for functioning in a variety of health contexts. These skills include reading, writing, mathematics, speaking, listening, using technology, networking, and rhetorical skills associated with requests, advocacy, and complaints. Accessing health information online and being able to apply it in the context of one's life can be especially challenging for those with low health literacy. During the COVID-19 pandemic, researchers found that almost four out of ten older adults were not ready for telehealth visits. Digital inequities are especially pronounced for those with lower household incomes or those living in rural areas (AHIMA Foundation, 2022).

For instance, it can be harder for people to use *technology for health-related tasks* when they:

- Have lower health literacy.
- Don't have access to or experience using a technology device such as a smartphone or a computer.
- Don't have access to high-speed internet.
- Have a disability like not being able to see or hear well.
- Don't have people in their homes who could help them use technology.
- Don't have health technology apps or websites available in their preferred language (AHIMA Foundation, 2022).

### SJA Action Steps

| WPHC Context: Digital Health Literacy in Action | Barriers to Digital Health Literacy SJA Action Step: What Can Healthcare Organizations Do? | Barriers to Digital Health Literacy SJA Action Step: What Can Providers Do? |
| --- | --- | --- |
| Comparing options and enrolling in a health insurance plan on a government website | • Organize community-level numeracy and critical thinking classes to enhance digital and basic literacy skills. | • Have digital health navigators who can help patients get ready for telehealth visits. |
| Sending a private message to your healthcare provider on your patient portal or personal healthcare website | • Ensure technology access and usability.consultants are available to set up patients with the skills and knowledge to use the patient portal and website. | • Ask patients what devices they own and how they usually access the internet. |

| Testing the video and sound for your online therapy appointment | • Provide technology consultants to guide patients with testing and set up of technology. | • Provide technology consultants to guide patients with testing and set up of technology. |
|---|---|---|
| Using a wearable fitness tracker to count your heart rate and steps throughout the day | • Provide free or low-cost wearables to those who may benefit from such tracking to bridge the access gap. | • Work with community groups to make wearable technologies available to those with socioeconomic disparities. |
| Searching online for healthy recipes to prepare for a family member with diabetes | • Provide free training and in-person guidance to help address digital literacy skills. | • Work with local groups or libraries to develop digital literacy training programs. |
| Using a health app or EHR or health organization website in your preferred language | • Ensure the availability of translators for telehealth appointments. | • Make sure your patient portals meet peoples' language and cultural preferences. |
| Facing hearing and vision-related abilities | • Test how accessible your health website is to patients who have disabilities and ensure it is accessible on mobile devices. | • Using closed captioning for telehealth visits to help people with hearing challenges. |

## SJA Discussion Prompt

Studies show that US college students with higher digital health literacy thought it was easier to search for reliable information about COVID-19 online. These students were also more likely to follow COVID-19 safety measures like wearing masks in July 2020. They were also more willing to get the COVID-19 vaccine.

1. What are some initiatives you can implement to increase digital health literacy across all student groups on your campus and community?
2. What are some challenges you are likely to face in implementing your initiative in a way that is fair to all students?
3. What are some potential ways from a WPHC and SJA framework in which you can address those challenges?
4. Which student populations are more vulnerable? Who is more at risk?

## Resource

AHIMA Foundation. (2022). Retrieved January 11, 2023, from https://ahimafoundation.org/understanding-the-issues/digital-health-literacy-as-a-social-determinant-of-health/

eHEALTH LITERACY

The Transactional Model of eHealth Literacy (TMeHL) defines ehealth literacy as "the ability to locate, understand, exchange, and evaluate health information from the Internet in the presence of dynamic contextual factors, and to apply the knowledge gained for the purposes of maintaining or improving health" (Paige et al., 2018, p. 8; see also Chan & Kaufman, 2011). It assesses ehealth literacy as an intrapersonal skillset that enables consumers to negotiate online transactions among diverse sources in the face of adversity such as dexterity limitations and use of jargon.

An important emerging area of focus for health literacy is translational communication or clinical trial communication. Dr. Susan Morgan, a communications professor at the University of Miami, describes how clinical trial communication can have a disproportionate impact on minorities and disadvantaged populations.

*Textbox 7.6, **Scholar Interview** with **Dr. Susan Morgan** gives insight into how her experience with her friend's ovarian cancer illuminated the importance of translational communication for minorities to her.*

---

### TEXTBOX 7.6

#### Dr. Susan Morgan
*Professor, University of Miami, USA*

My interest in clinical trial communication was sparked when my dear friend Heather Macalister was diagnosed with Stage III ovarian cancer. At the time, she was a burlesque dancer in San Francisco and had no health insurance. She soon realized that her best chance to access excellent medical care was to join a clinical trial. I was confident that I could identify a study that she could join because I have a PhD, and I'm comfortable puzzling through even complex medical terminology. I quickly discovered that I was in over my head when I began searching through clinicaltrials.gov, a website that is specifically designed for public access to this information. (I'd encourage everyone to give it a try. Put yourself in the shoes of a newly diagnosed patient or a concerned friend or family member of a cancer patient and see if you think this site meets the information needs of ordinary people.) I felt that I had failed Heather. While she found a wonderful oncologist who identified several successive clinical trials that offered innovative treatments that extended her life, I realized that there are many ways that clinical trials are presented that are not patient-centered, particularly when patients have lower literacy levels or who are overwhelmed with information because of the mental and emotional distress associated with a difficult diagnosis.

After Heather's diagnosis, I began to research the communication issues involved with clinical trial participation decisions, particularly among African American, Black Caribbean, and Hispanic populations, and launched a program of research that addresses these issues. For example, my research team and I developed a decision aid that uses interactive technology to help patients (and members of their support system) figure out whether a clinical trial is a good choice for them based on their circumstances and their personal values. Our research showed that this decision aid, which includes animations to present information in a warm and friendly way, increases knowledge and reduces anxiety compared to standard ways of presenting the same information. We have also created a communication skills training program for clinical research coordinators, research nurses, and other medical staff members who approach patients about participating in clinical trials. There are a number of verbal and nonverbal communication behaviors that doctors and their staff can use to help patients understand what's involved so that patients can provide meaningful informed consent (or informed refusal). Another colleague and I have been working on developing a clinical trial chatbot that can help patients weed through lots of complex terminology to determine whether they are eligible to join a specific study. I've also used my background in health communication to help advise my own academic medical system to develop a clinical trial search tool that is much easier for people to use and understand. By taking a 360-degree multidimensional and multidisciplinary approach to these communication issues, I hope to help members of the public access valuable information about clinical trials—and to support medical science as it pursues new cures and more effective treatments for a wide variety of diseases.

## FUNCTIONAL AND TRANSLATIONAL eHEALTH LITERACY

Functional ehealth literacy references the ability to use the basic features of technology such as the ability to type and read on a screen to access and comprehend health-related content. whereas translational ehealth literacy comprises the highest-level ability to create and carry out an action plan to apply knowledge that is obtained, negotiated, and evaluated for health promotion (Paige et al., 2018). This form of ehealth literacy emphasizes the importance of assessing patients' abilities to produce text messages, communicate with multiple online users, determine their source credibility, and translate knowledge gained from online transactions to offline action.

*Review **Textbox 7.7**. Examine the scenario and respond to the discussion questions that follow. Influencers, especially on social media networks like Instagram and TikTok, can significantly impact minors and those with low health literacy. With the popularity of wellness influencers, the line between healthy eating and the persuasive spread of misinformation and incorrect practices becomes dangerously blurred. Read the thought scenario provided and respond to the discussion questions for reflection that follow.*

---

**Textbox 7.7   Discussion Questions/Thought Scenario for Reflection**

**Peer-to-Peer Online Social Networks: Challenges and Opportunities for Health Literacy**

*WPHC Context*

Researchers Peterson et al. (2019) considered case studies examining health communication in **peer-to-peer health communication networks** online and the impact of health literacy.

---

### Thought Scenario

**Wellness influencers** on Instagram who promote the idea of "clean eating" often focus on the consumption of whole, minimally processed foods. Often, they also emphasize the elimination of entire food groups, such as carbohydrates and fats, food grown by conventional means (e.g., with the use of pesticides), or food that contains artificial ingredients, because they are deemed as dangerous. Although some of the advice dispensed by online influencers may be consistent with scientific evidence (e.g., emphasis on fresh produce), other advice runs counter to evidence-based nutrition guidance and may lead to malnutrition and an unhealthy fixation on food.

The *orthorexia nervosa* disorder is the name of a new disordered eating pattern characterized by a fixation on eating only foods that are considered healthy or pure. Individuals with **lower health literacy** often have trouble *distinguishing between scientifically accurate advice and the more extreme, non-evidence-based views that are sometimes espoused by influencers.*

Misinformation communication on social media by influencers may be easier to accept because of attractive images that accompany the Instagram posts, such as green smoothies and salad bowls, which connote healthfulness, even if the advocated pattern of eating is not healthy overall. Moreover, because influencers have large followings and attractive appearance that reflects a healthful ideal, they can be perceived as authorities on health. Further, social media platforms expose users to content they have previously liked, thus individuals get caught up in an echo chamber of exposure to similar types of behaviors and information, further validating their impression of content legitimacy and normative, healthful behaviors. In addition, Instagram's algorithms prioritize certain content, making it less likely that people will be exposed to contradictory information that might have engendered self-reflection and personal research on the topic.

### SJA Discussion Questions

1. Research has demonstrated the threats that social networks pose to those with low health literacy. What might be some of the opportunities that they present to public health practitioners to adopt health communication strategies that promote healthy behaviors?
2. Blogging communities often form a trusted source of information for their members, who often share personal family stories with family photos, and reveal intimate information that may help people find, process, and understand scientifically complex risk information by making it approachable. Members were also more likely to share the information with others in their social networks. Thus peer-to-peer blogging forums are a promising channel to make information more accessible and boost participant health literacy.

   How can public health information be tailored to those with limited English proficiency and minority communities in ways that will increase the relevance of health-related information and its comprehension and encourage readers to act on its guidance?

### Abstracted From

Peterson, E. B., Gaysynsky, A., Chou, W. -Y. S., & Rising, C. (2019). The role and impact of health literacy on peer-to-peer health communication. *Information Services & Use, 39*(1–2), 37–49. https://doi.org/10.3233/ISU-180039

## Digital Health Disparities

People with low digital health literacy find it harder to use technology for health-related tasks. Digital health literacy is applied in a range of contexts such as accessing an EHR, communicating electronically with the healthcare team, discerning reliable online health information, and using health and wellness apps. Each of these instances of digital health literacy makes the ability to achieve health-related goals easier and increases the likelihood of achieving a positive health outcome. For instance, mobile health apps can help improve health literacy by empowering underserved cancer patients and their caregivers. Mobile health apps often provide easy-to-access features that enhance interactive patient-provider communication and present medical information in an easy-to-understand manner. However, digital health disparities stemming from unequal internet access and low digital health literacy skills mean that disadvantaged populations either do not have equal access to mobile technology or are not familiar with using mobile health applications and cannot understand or comprehend the information in a manner that will lead to actionable knowledge (Kim et al., 2019). Gibbons et al. (2011) study the use of Web 2.0 by racial and ethnic minorities to address health disparities. They recommend several strategies to help health information be presented in a more comprehensible manner, such as identifying approaches and methods to identify strategies for integrating social media into health promotion interventions for health issues that affect members of medically underserved groups.

Review **Textbox 7.8** to understand how inclusive communication is an essential component of health equity.

---

### Textbox 7.8    Health Equity Guiding Principles for Inclusive Communication

#### WPHC Context

Health literacy principles make information clearer. Health equity principles make information more inclusive.

#### SJA Prompt

| Inclusive Communication Guidelines | SJA Action Steps: Achieving Goals of Health Literacy and Health Equity |
|---|---|
| Using a health equity lens | Clear communication can help people access and understand information to act on it, but this is often not enough to encourage action.<br><br>*WPHC and SJA perspective:*<br><br>Work to see how the communication can meet each audience's specific cultural, linguistic, environmental, and historical needs and priorities. |
| Use person-first language | Humanizes the individuals being addressed.<br><br>*WPHC and SJA perspective:*<br><br>What might be some hidden consequences of generalizing identities, personal preferences, and backgrounds for marginalized populations? |

*(Continued)*

| | |
|---|---|
| Avoid unintentional blaming | Address all people inclusively and with respect. |
| | *WPHC and SJA perspective:* |
| | Communication that is mindful that individuals are not blamed for their adverse circumstances. |
| Using preferred terms for populations of focus while recognizing that preferred terms may differ | Accurately and equitably represent all people. |
| | *WPHC and SJA perspective:* |
| | How can healthcare providers be equipped to address their patients using their preferred terms? |
| Looking for ways to be more inclusive in text and images | Use language that identifies the structural conditions as distinct from inherent audience characteristics. |
| | *WPHC and SJA perspective:* |
| | Making visible and acknowledging are powerful modes for being seen. What are some benefits from such communication to healthcare interaction and outcomes? |
| Exploring other resources related to health equity communications | Organizational communication should consider both health equity and health literacy carefully when designing and developing communication. |
| | *WPHC and SJA perspective:* |
| | Consider what might be some implications of poverty, gender, racial discrimination, and lack of education on the ability to access healthcare and healthcare outcomes for groups of people. |

## Organizational Health Literacy

The inclusion of organizational health literacy in the definition of health literacy shows how health literacy is not just an individual responsibility. Health literacy is a balance between individual skills and abilities and their ability to navigate the demands and complexities of the healthcare system and the organizational, social, and media environment. Organizational health literacy is defined as the degree to which organizations equitably enable individuals to find, understand, and use information and services to inform health-related decisions and actions for themselves and others. Organizations, too, in this landscape, have a responsibility to become more health literate and to ensure their communications and initiatives improve health literacy equitably (Parker & Hernandez 2012). The revised definition of health literacy addresses the structural challenges posed by the organizational environment on disadvantaged and minority populations.

*Review* **Textbox 7.9** *to understand the* **Ten Attributes of Health-Literate Healthcare Organizations***. Researchers Palumbo and colleagues systematized their knowledge of digital health literacy in organizations to understand the role of healthcare organizations in delivering health-literate healthcare services in a digital environment (2022). As most organizational information is accessed in online contexts, consider these attributes considering digital health literacy.*

**Textbox 7.9   Ten Attributes of Health-Literate Healthcare Organizations**

## WPHC Context

Several federal healthcare agencies and research organizations have outlined the attributes of a health-literate organization (Agency for Healthcare Research and Quality, AHRQ, 2023; AHRQ, 2020; CDC, 2021; Federal Plain Language Guidelines, 2023; Health Literacy Online, 2016; National Institutes of Health, NIH, 2023; NIH, 2021; NLM, 2020). These attributes include

1. Has leadership that makes health literacy integral to its mission, structure, and operations.
2. Integrates health literacy into planning, evaluation measures, patient safety, and quality improvement.
3. Prepares the workforce to be health literate and monitors progress.
4. Includes populations served in the design, implementation, and evaluation of health information and services.
5. Meets the needs of populations with a range of health literacy skills while avoiding stigmatization.
6. Uses health literacy strategies in interpersonal communications and confirms understanding at all points of contact.
7. Provides easy access to health information and services and navigation assistance.
8. Designs and distributes print, audiovisual, and social media content that is easy to understand and act on.
9. Addresses health literacy in high-risk situations, including care transitions and communications about medicines.
10. Communicates clearly what health plans cover and what individuals will have to pay for services.

## SJA Discussion Prompts

Research the websites of three healthcare organizations.

1. How well do they meet the aforementioned criteria?
2. Which attributes need strengthening from a WPHC and SJA perspective?
3. How can the website communications be more inclusive from a health literacy perspective?

## Helpful Resources

Agency for Healthcare Research and Quality (AHRQ). *Ten attributes of health literate healthcare organizations*. Retrieved January 6, 2023, from URL: https://www.ahrq.gov/health-literacy/publications/ten-attributes.html

AHRQ. (2020). *Be more engaged in your healthcare*. Retrieved January 12, 2023, from https://www.ahrq.gov/questions/be-engaged/index.html

CDC (2021, June 5). *Clear communication index*. Retrieved from https://www.cdc.gov/ccindex/index.html

Federal Plan Language Guidelines. Retrieved January 12, 2023, from https://www.plainlanguage.gov/guidelines/

Health Literacy Online. (2016, June 8). Retrieved from https://health.gov/healthliteracyonline/

NIH. (2021, July 7). Clear and simple. Retrieved January 12, 2023, from https://www.nih.gov/institutes-nih/nih-office-director/office-communications-public-liaison/clear-communication/clear-simple

National Institutes of Health (NIH). *What is health literacy?* Retrieved January 12, 2023, from https://www.nih.gov/institutes-nih/nih-office-director/office-communications-public-liaison/clear-communication/health-literacy

NLM. (2020, March 6). *Understanding medical words tutorial*. https://medlineplus.gov/medwords/medicalwords.html

Healthcare organizations have a responsibility to support the patient's ability to navigate the online healthcare environment and support their ability to co-create, share, and access information (Palumbo et al., 2022). Park and colleagues' study conducted a content analysis of 571 tweets from health-related organizations (Park et al. 2013). They found that nonprofit organizations (NPOs) had more tweets about health literacy than other types of health-related organizations, including health business corporations, educational institutions, and government agencies. Health-related organizational tweets predominantly focused on using simple language rather than complex language.

*Review* **Textbox 7.10**, **Scholar Interview** *with communication researcher* **Dr. Satarupa Dasgupta***.*

## TEXTBOX 7.10   Scholar Interview

### Dr. Satarupa Dasgupta
*Ramapo College of New Jersey*

1. Can you talk a little bit about your scholarship and its intersections with health and disparities, particularly from the perspective of health literacy? What does social justice mean in your work? How do you see health literacy central to the issues of access, empowerment, and voice in diverse health contexts?

   My research focuses on generating health awareness and activism and addressing health disparities among underserved populations. My career trajectory is a bit different from other academics as I have always combined research with practice, and my work has a distinctively applied component. My research lies primarily in health communication program development and implementation, with my experience spanning academia and the not-for-profit sector. My work focuses on HIV/STI intervention development among commercial sex workers, on prevention of sex trafficking and rehabilitation of sex trafficking survivors in international settings, and also on intimate partner violence prevention among immigrant communities in the US. In addition, I serve as a voluntary sexual assault advocate in my state of residence, and

I have worked in the implementation of federally funded and culture-specific victim advocacy programs. In academia, in the not-for-profit sector, and in my work as a voluntary violence advocate, I strive to make the voices of the disenfranchised heard and ensure their social, reproductive, and health rights.

2. How have theory and praxis-centered and engaged social justice activism principles in action in your research and community-centered work?

My scholarship focuses on the role of the community in engendering participatory communication strategies, especially during harm reduction and health promotion initiatives. I believe in community participation that inculcates responsibility, that reinforces community bonds, and that generates a platform for diverse voices to be heard. My work—as an academic, researcher, violence prevention program developer, voluntary advocate, and activist—has allowed me to apply my experiences to my pedagogical practices. Working with vulnerable population members, community members, nonprofit organizations, peer educators, and diverse academic disciplines has reaffirmed the salience of an activist's and a communication practitioner's perspective for me and enabled me to engage with the challenges of inequities in our daily lives and in the classroom.

3. Can you share some thoughts on how your scholarship might address some of the health disparities and inequities we face today? What might be some of the most significant challenges we will need to address? How might your scholarship and work provide a productive avenue for thinking about those challenges and shaping our response to them?

I think interdisciplinarity and intersectionality need to be important components of scholarship that address disparities and inequities. My own research is remarkably interdisciplinary—my projects are collaborative efforts with colleagues in social work, public health, nursing, and psychology. I believe that multisector partnerships involving scholars, researchers, and practitioners that integrate social sciences, health, activism, and human rights represent a critical next step to advance health rights and social justice. Additionally, research which has a commitment to social justice needs to share intersectionality's focus on multiple historically oppressed populations. As I have found through my research, there is intersectionality in marginalization, stigmatization, trauma-response, and support-seeking. Intersectionality is used as a conceptual framework in much of my research since underserved populations often experience and engage with barriers and challenges in their lives through multiple systems of oppression.

4. Can you give an example of how a project from your scholarship that means a lot to you personally illustrates the transformative potential between health communication, health literacy, and empowerment?

A project from my scholarship that means a lot to me personally is my ongoing research that delineates the impact of COVID-19 on support-seeking and service utilization among immigrant victims of intimate partner violence (IPV) living in the US. Previous research suggests that disaster-specific stressors increase IPV victimization and significantly decrease support-seeking by victims. Despite IPV program growth, service gaps remain especially for immigrant and minority women who form a marginalized and vulnerable survivor population in the US. I am a voluntary sexual assault advocate in my state of residence, and I have been affiliated with culture-specific organizations providing support services to immigrant battered women.

Particularly, my experience of volunteering with South Asian IPV victims during the pandemic convinced me of the magnitude of the problem that exists and created a personal investment in the research topic. I hope that the study findings will help to reevaluate existing intervention modalities, explore best practices, and offer recommendations to cater better to the needs of immigrant victims of violence within the context of the pandemic.

### Marginalized Organizational Contexts

Organizational health literacy can be especially important in rural and underserved areas and for minority and marginalized populations. Researchers Nancy Weaver et al. (2012) conduct a needs assessment of rural federally qualified health center clinics. They found low awareness of health literacy and of the challenges posed by low health literacy for minority and disadvantaged patients within the organization, in interstaff communication, and in patient communication. Organizational health literacy emphasizes that healthcare organizations need to address health literacy in their policies and activities to support health literacy-related practices.

Read **Textbox 7.11** to understand what role organizations can play in helping advance the goals of health literacy as they pertain to health equity.

---

**Textbox 7.11   Structural Components for Achieving Health Equity**

**WPHC Context**

**Health equity** is when everyone, regardless of their social, economic, racial, ethnic, or geographic status, has the opportunity to be as healthy as possible (CDC, 2020). Health equity can be achieved when both individual and structural factors, including the organizations, community, and regulatory environments that the individuals belong to, work together toward meeting its goals. Population-level factors, such as the physical, built, social, and policy environments impact health outcomes more than individual-level factors (Office of Disease Prevention and Health Promotion, ODPHP, 2021).

The structural and public health components of health equity include the following four arms:

1. **Programmatic arm**: successful health equity strategies.
2. **Measurement arm**: data practices to support the advancement of health equity.
3. **Policy arm**: laws, regulations, and rules to improve population health.
4. **Infrastructure arm**: organizational structures and functions that support health equity.

**SJA Prompt**

- How does your university address the different arms of health equity?
- Where are the gaps for minority populations?
- Which areas can it improve on?

## Resources

CDC. (2020, November 30). *Minority health. Paving the road to health equity.* Retrieved January 8, 2023, from https://www.cdc.gov/minorityhealth/publications/health_equity/index.html

Office of Disease Prevention and Health Promotion (ODPHP). (2021, October 26). *Health literacy and health equity: Connecting the dots.* Retrieved January 8, 2023, from https://health.gov/news/202110/health-literacy-and-health-equity-connecting-dots

### What Can Organizations Do?

There are specific steps that organizations can take to ensure that the goals of health literacy are met for all employees and stakeholders. To support the goals of health literacy, organizations can ensure that everyone in the community can access the health information they need, provide the health information in plain language and in different languages, provide trainings to health professionals on health literacy best practices, create a database of information about health literacy for health professionals, and review health materials like insurance forms and medication instructions with community members to make sure they understand the information and the actions they need to take (NNLM, 2021).

## Cultural Construction of Health

### Culture

Culture refers to the shared ideas, meanings, and values acquired by individuals as members of society (NLM, 2004). Our group belongings and membership, such as in racial, ethnic, or linguistic groups, shape our identities and culture. Individuals who are members of professional cultures such as medicine and public health communicate using a specific set of language skills that often include complex epidemiological and medical terms (Nutbeam, 2000). Culture shapes our understanding, thinking, and the ways we respond to human experiences and world events. Even as patients make sense of health-related information and meanings of health based on their culture and values, professional medical culture shapes how health communication is crafted and enacted.

*Review Textbox 7.12 to see how words matter, particularly in disadvantaged and minority contexts. Can you think of other disadvantaged communities? In what ways might they be affected? Try your hand at the SJA activity prompts that follow.*

---

### Textbox 7.12   Health Literacy, Health Equity, and Inclusive Language*

#### WPHC Context

The words we choose can help us and those who read and hear them to create a culture of equity for all people. Inclusive language is defined as communication that avoids biases and discriminatory language against groups of people based on their identity (e.g., race, gender, socioeconomic status, sexuality, or ability).

Inclusive language is central to promoting the principles of health literacy in ways that are audience-centered and respectful of all individuals. It helps accomplish the goals of health equity by creating an environment that offers affirmation, celebration, and appreciation of different approaches, styles, perspectives, and experiences, allowing individuals to bring in their whole selves and all their identities.

Inclusive language is characterized by the following:

- Language that includes rather than excludes.
- Language that acknowledges, accepts, and celebrates differences.
- Language that is welcoming to everyone.

| WPHC Context: | SJA Critique: |
|---|---|
| *Terminology Matters: The Words We Choose* | *Inclusive Language and Disadvantaged/Minority Populations** |
| Hard-to-reach communities; underserved communities/people; uninsured | Communities with limited access to [service]; people who are underserved by mental health/behavioral health resources/people who are medically underserved; people who are uninsured |
| Inmates | People who are incarcerated |
| Differently abled/afflicted/hearing impaired | People with disabilities/a disability; people who are deaf or hard of hearing or who are blind; people with an intellectual or developmental disability; people who use a wheelchair or mobility device |
| Drug-users/addicts/drug abusers; alcoholics/persons taking/prescribed medication-assisted treatment (MAT); persons who relapsed/smokers | Persons who use drugs/people who inject drugs; persons with substance use disorder; persons with alcohol use disorder; persons in recovery from substance use/alcohol disorder; persons taking prescribed medications for opioid use disorder (MOUD); people who smoke; people who returned to use |
| Elderly; senior; frail; fragile | Older adults; persons aged (numeric group e.g., 55–64 years); elders (when referencing older adults in a cultural context); elderly or frail elderly (when referring to older adults in a specific clinical context) |
| Blacks, Hispanics, Latinos, Whites, American Indians; Eskimo; Oriental; Afro-American; Caucasian; non-White | Racial groups: Asian persons; Black or African American persons; Native Hawaiian persons; Pacific Islander persons; White persons; People who identify with more than one race |
| | Ethnic groups: Hispanic or Latino persons |
| Rural people; frontier people | People who live in rural/sparsely populated areas; residents/populations of rural areas; rural communities |
| Homosexuals; MSM (men who have sex with men); transgenders/transgendered/transsexual; genetically male/female; gendered pronouns (e.g., he or she/his or her) | LGBTQ (or LGBTQUIA or LGBTQ+), MSM, pansexual, assigned male/female at birth, nonbinary, asexual |

* A sample from a longer list of inclusive terms is provided here by way of illustration.

- **Underserved** relates to limited access to services that are accessible, acceptable, and affordable, including healthcare. This is different from being disproportionately affected.
- **Vulnerable** should not be used when describing people with disabilities.
- **"People with lower socioeconomic status"** (SES) should only be used when SES is defined as, for example, when income, education, or occupation are sued as a measure of SES.
- When possible, be as specific as possible. For instance, **mental health** is a general condition. When referring to people with a mental illness, it is preferable to be as specific as possible about the type of mental illness rather than referring to people with different mental health disorders collectively.
- Consider **racial/ethnic groups** as proper nouns and capitalize (Black, White).
- Use **LGBTQ community** (and not, for example, gay community) to reflect the diversity of the community; consider using "sexual orientation," "gender identity," and "gender expression"; use gender-neutral language (e.g., using actor for both male and female actors); use terms that are inclusive of all gender identities (e.g., parents-to-be).

## SJA Activity

1. How can you change your words to help change our and others' attitudes and reinforce respectful, inclusive behaviors that value a variety of points of view?
   The fitness industry (e.g., Zumba classes, fitness clubs) can often reveal a lack of cultural competence in making assumptions about gender and physical activity, body size, skill level and fitness, age and frailty, fitness level and motivation, diet, and willpower and many other such domains.
2. Examine your local gym's website for the different activities and promotional material they present.
3. How can you make the language and presentation of health and fitness more inclusive of all genders, races, ages, socioeconomic groups, sexualities, body types, and other differences?

## Resources

AHRQ. *Health literacy universal precautions toolkit*. Retrieved January 13, 2023, from https://www.ahrq.gov/health-literacy/improve/precautions/index.html

American Psychological Association (APA). (2023). *Inclusive language guidelines*. Retrieved January 8, 2023, from https://www.apa.org/about/apa/equity-diversity-inclusion/language-guidelines

CDC. *Gateway to health communication: Preferred terms*. Retrieved January 8, 2023, from https://www.cdc.gov/healthcommunication/Preferred_Terms.html

Conscious Style Guide. (2023). *Ethnicity, race + nationality*. Retrieved January 8, 2023, from https://consciousstyleguide.com/ethnicity-race-nationality/

Indian Health Service. *Healthcare communication. Health literacy*. Retrieved January 13, 2023, from https://www.ihs.gov/healthcommunications/health-literacy/

Linguistic Society of America (LSA). (2016, November). *Guidelines for inclusive language*. Retrieved January 8, 2023, from https://www.linguisticsociety.org/resource/guidelines-inclusive-language

National Assembly of State Arts Agencies (NASAA). *Inclusive language guide*. Retrieved January 8, 2023, from https://nasaa-arts.org/nasaa_research/inclusive-language-guide/

Racial Equity Tools. (2020). *Glossary*. Retrieved January 8, 2023, from https://www.racialequitytools.org/glossary

### Acculturation

Acculturation is the ability to assimilate into a given culture. Acculturation comprises a range of factors including English language proficiency, interactions with family and friends, and interactions with neighbors. Researchers Chen and colleagues study acculturation and health literacy among racial and ethnic minorities. Their study examines the relationship between acculturation and health literacy among Chinese speakers in the United States who have limited English proficiency (Chen et al. 2022). Their study finds that higher acculturation in the United States was associated with lower Chinese information appraisal, higher English functional health literacy, and higher English information appraisal.

Petrun Sayers et al. (2021) examined the experiences of vulnerable populations in understanding the materials provided by the Centers for Medicaid and Medicare Services (CMS) through the Coverage to Care (C2C) programs geared toward improving health insurance literacy. They recommend effective acculturation should: (a) highlight the importance of culture-centered materials in building empathy and trust, (b) be translated as appropriate; (c) be disseminated in a way that is responsive to the constraints and preferences of minority populations, (d) employ educational tools in conjunction with individually tailored approaches, and (e) work with local organizations to amplify dissemination.

### Culturally Sensitive Communication

Awareness of culturally sensitive and tailored communication is important in both in-person and online health communication settings and across the healthcare spectrum (Shaw et al., 2009; Whitman & Davis, 2008). In digital health communication, health communication researchers Neuhauser and Kreps (2008) suggest practices that healthcare professionals can follow, including understanding the strengths and weaknesses of online cancer communication for vulnerable groups and supplementing information with oral and tailored communication.

Review **Textbox 7.13** to consider the different contexts of health literacy that may call upon the literacy skills noted.

---

**Textbox 7.13   Health Contexts, Health Inequities, and Digital Health Literacy**

**WPHC Context**

What are some contexts of health literacy referenced in the following contexts?

| Health Contexts | Health Inequities | Digital Health Literacy |
| --- | --- | --- |
| Spotting health misinformation online | **Health misinformation** is a serious threat to public health. It was aggravated during the COVID-19 pandemic. | Health literacy, **data literacy**, misinformation |

(Continued)

| Using your online health information | Accessing **patient portals** for health information and provider communication. | **Accessibility**, critical literacy |
|---|---|---|
| Medication adherence | **Medication adherence** involves understanding measurements, reading, and understanding prescription labels, and keeping track of active ingredients in your medicines. **Medication nonadherence** is not taking your medication correctly as prescribed, such as by taking the wrong dosages, at the wrong times, or for the wrong length of time. IT can be intentional or unintentional. | **Medication literacy**: A type of literacy that includes your ability to review, communicate, and process information about your medicines in a way that helps you make well-informed decisions about the medicines you take and how they affect your health |
| Patient portals in English for racial and ethnic minorities limited English language fluency | **Culturally and linguistically appropriate** patient portals can decrease health inequities. | **Health equity** and access |
| Understanding your medical bill | Understand the **No Surprises Act** (2022). | Health literacy, **numeracy** |

## SJA Prompt

- Learn how to access your patient portal.
- Set up an account with a password to find information about your previous visits, doctor's notes, and lists of your medication and dosages.
- Check that you can send messages to your care teams from your portal.
- What forms of health literacy did you require to complete this process? What forms of health literacy will you require to locate, interpret, share, and engage with health information in a healthcare event? Will an individual with low English language literacy, medication literacy, or data literacy be comfortable negotiating this environment? What steps do you recommend to help bridge health equity concerns with patient portals?

## Helpful Resources

American Health Information Management Association (AHIMA). (2023, February 28). https://ahimafoundation.org/understanding-the-issues/digital-health-literacy-as-a-social-determinant-of-health/

AHIMA. (2023, January 5). https://ahimafoundation.org/understanding-the-issues/tips-to-understand-your-medical-bill/

Consumer Financial Protection Bureau. (2022, April 11). https://www.consumerfinance.gov/about-us/blog/know-your-rights-and-protections-when-it-comes-to-medical-bills-and-collections/

CMS. (2018, April 1). *No Surprises Act*. https://www.cms.gov/nosurprises

U.S. Department of Health & Human Services (HHS). (2022, January 3). https://www.hhs.gov/about/news/2022/01/03/hhs-kicks-off-new-year-with-new-protections-from-surprise-medical-bills.html

U.S. Centers for Medicare & Medicaid Services (CMS). (n.d.) https://www.cms.gov/files/document/nosurpriseactfactsheet-how-do-i-read-my-medical-bill508c.pdf

Wang, P. (2018, April 1). 6 ways to fix mistakes on your medical bills. *Consumer Reports*. https://www.consumerreports.org/medical-billing/ways-to-fix-medical-billing-mistakes/

U.S. Food and Drug Administration. (FDA). (2016, February 16). *Medication adherence*. https://www.fda.gov/drugs/special-features/why-you-need-take-your-medications-prescribed-or-instructed

### Cultural-Linguistic Identity

In the digitally saturated environment, so much health information, whether about pandemics, seasonal infections, chronic conditions, or disease-specific management, is online. Those who are ill-prepared to navigate the digital environment are at a greater disadvantage than ever before. It is important to note that minority cultures encompass a range of racial and ethnic identities, cultural values and beliefs, languages, and educational and socioeconomic characteristics. It is important to tailor the cultural-linguistic identities of each minority culture to how health literacy is understood within that minority culture. For instance, research finds that in first-generation Korean American immigrants, health literacy indirectly influenced health outcomes in the management of type 2 diabetes mellitus through self-care skills and self-efficacy (Kim et al., 2020). The effect of health literacy can often be insidious and act in indirect ways to shape health outcomes (Shahid, et al. 2022).

## Disease Literacy

Cultural factors impact disease literacy in minority populations. Researchers Lopez and colleagues found that inadequate mental health disease literacy, illustrated by a lack of knowledge of mental health disorders in Hispanic women was associated with cultural factors and perpetuated persistent stigma. Stigma, in turn, was a barrier to depression treatment (Lopez et al. 2018). As a result of this stigma, ironically, US-born Hispanics were more likely to have depression compared to Hispanics born in Latin America and were less likely to follow a treatment plan compared to non-Hispanic whites. Thus, as Lopez and colleagues concluded, patient education level predicted mental health literacy for Hispanic women. Minority cultures have their own unique challenges with disease literacy that cannot be painted with a single brush. African immigrants in Norris et al.'s (2022) study had limited disease literacy despite having English proficiency, college education, employment, and connection to a health system. Limited health literacy in their study was associated with decreased use of preventive health services by African immigrants and increased barriers to accessing and utilizing healthcare.

### Health Misinformation

Health literacy in peer-to-peer online health communication is important in navigating a complex online social environment. Peterson and colleagues sought to understand individual beliefs, abilities, and perceived efficacy to navigate online health misinformation to help consumers with different health literacy levels discern the usefulness of health information discovered in peer-to-peer platforms. By understanding health literacy in online social support environments, the researchers sought to facilitate the development of more effective health communication interventions designed for and delivered through online social networks. Researchers Hahn et al. (2015) examined the relationship between health literacy and patient-reported outcomes among underserved Spanish- and English-speaking adults. They found that health literacy was not associated with diabetes self-care, among other things, but was significantly related to social support, diet and medication barriers, and communication with healthcare providers. Increasing health literacy can help facilitate meaning-making and increase the effectiveness of patient-provider communication by reducing the influence of health misinformation.

*Review **Textbox 7.14** to get a sense of the strategies that can be helpful in avoiding the spread of health misinformation. Attempt the SJA activity that follows.*

---

**Textbox 7.14   Strategies to Avoid Health Misinformation**

**WPHC Context**

The US Surgeon General identifies health misinformation as a serious threat to public health. Health misinformation is defined as information related to one's health that is false, inaccurate, or misleading according to the best available evidence at the time (HHS.gov). It has the potential to cause confusion, increase mistrust in expert sources and scientific knowledge, harm people's health, and undermine public health efforts (HHS.gov).

Strategies you can follow to avoid the spread of health misinformation include the following:

1. Learning how to identify and avoid sharing health misinformation.
2. Engaging with your friends and family on the problem of health misinformation.
3. Addressing health misinformation in the community.
4. Identifying and avoiding sharing health misinformation on social media feeds, blogs, online forums, and chat groups by verifying the accuracy of the information and cross-checking with trustworthy and credible sources.
5. If someone in your friend or family has a misperception, engage with them with an open mind using open listening skills, empathy, establishing common ground, asking questions, and providing alternative explanations and sources of information.
6. Working with schools, community groups such as churches and parent-teacher associations, and trusted leaders such as educators and healthcare professionals to develop local strategies against misinformation.

**SJA Activity**

Health misinformation can often spread more quickly than scientific information on social media. One of the ways to combat the spread of health misinformation is to balance sharing, re-sharing, commenting, and engaging with verified content from reliable sources (HealthDay, 2023, March 3). Further, patients need to have equitable access and confidence in accurate, understandable, and relevant information needed to make informed and personally relevant health decisions (HealthDay, 2023, March 3).

The preceding steps are especially important as younger adults, members of racially marginalized groups, individuals with high religiosity and conservative ideologies, and social media users are at increased risk for health misinformation (Nan et al., 2022).

The risk of public health consequences is significant. For example, conspiracy fears of vaccine deniers and other facets play into data revealing that nationally, in 2022, about 35% of all American parents oppose requiring children to be vaccinated for measles, mumps, and rubella before entering school, up from 23% in 2019 (KFF, 2022, December 16).

- How will you spread awareness and information about vaccinations on social media?
- Who will you target?
- How will you combat the sources of medical myths on vaccination side effects?

### Resources

AHIMA. (2022). *Spotting health misinformation online*. Retrieved from https://ahimafoundation. org/understanding-the-issues/spotting-health-misinformation-online/

Department of Health and Human Services (HHS.gov). (n.d.). *Current priorities of the U.S. surgeon general: Health misinformation*. Retrieved March 23, 2023, from https://www.hhs.gov/ surgeongeneral/priorities/health-misinformation/index.html

HealthDay. (2023, March 3). *Dozens of medical groups launch effort to battle health misinformation. U.S. News*. Retrieved March 23, 2023 from https://www.usnews.com/news/health-news/ articles/2023-03-03/dozens-of-medical-groups-launch-effort-to-battle-health-misinformation

KFF. (2022, December 16). *KFF Covid-19 vaccine monitor: December 2022*. Retrieved March 23, 2023 on https://www.kff.org/coronavirus-covid-19/poll-finding/kff-covid-19-vaccine-monitor-december-2022/

Nan, X., Wang, Y., & Their, K. (2022). Why do people believe health misinformation and who is at risk? A systematic review of individual differences in susceptibility to health misinformation. *Social Science & Medicine, 314*, 115398. https://doi.org/10.1016/j.socscimed.2022.115398

NLM. *Evaluating internet health information tutorial*. Retrieved January 12, 2023, from https:// medlineplus.gov/webeval/webeval.html

## Health Information Seeking

Because culture-related beliefs play an important role in what individuals believe are appropriate ways of acting and what they believe, cultural and conceptual knowledge is an important factor in how an individual understands health and illness. Likewise, cultural factors play a key role in who individuals will turn to for health information gathering and decision-making. Social support, such as that from family members, caregivers, and friends, provides an important cultural context for health information seeking. Health communication researchers Manganello and Clayman (2011) examined how health information seeking, trust in sources, and interactions with healthcare providers differed for young adults with lower and higher numeracy. Using a national sample from the Health Information National Trends Survey (HINTS, 2008), they underscore the need to understand how health literacy skills such as numeracy can influence health information-seeking, patient-provider relationships, and, ultimately, health outcomes for young adults.

### Social Capital

Social capital can play an important role in shaping health literacy and health information-seeking behaviors. In a study conducted by interviewing 1,000 residents in person in Seoul, Korea, in 2011, researchers Kim and colleagues found bridging social capital, or the social capital between people who differ based on socioeconomic and other characteristics, contributed to how health literacy impacted health information self-efficacy (Kim et al. 2015). Likewise, they found that bonding social capital, or the social capital between people who are like each other based on socioeconomic and other characteristics, attenuated the relation between health literacy and health information-seeking intention.

In concluding **Chapter 7, Health Literacy**, read through the following example in the Present Challenges and Future Directions Exercise of a provider-patient encounter in a clinical context that had an undesirable outcome. In this instance, the patient was able to access healthcare and obtain a diagnosis and treatment recommendation for her condition. Yet, despite the best intentions of the provider, and despite being able to access care and treatment recommendations, the patient did not survive. What role did health literacy play in this instance?

*Given your knowledge of the challenges and complexities characterizing health literacy for racial-cultural-linguistic minorities, how might the different forms of health literacy play an indirect role in avoiding this outcome in the future?*

---

**Textbox 7.15    Present Challenges and Future Directions Exercise**

**Patient-Provider Communication and Health Literacy in Clinical Contexts**

**WPHC Context**

A 29-year-old African American woman with three days of abdominal pain and fever was brought to a Baltimore emergency department by her family. After a brief evaluation, she was told that she would need an exploratory laparotomy.

She subsequently became agitated and demanded to have her family take her home. When approached by staff, she yelled, "I came here in pain and all you want is to do is an exploratory on me! You will not make me a guinea pig!"

She refused to consent to any procedures and later died of appendicitis.

(Source: NLM, 2004)

**SJA Prompt**

1. What communication advice would you give to the healthcare team to help avoid this negative outcome?

---

2. What is one training initiative you can design to help make the healthcare team aware of health literacy challenges facing the underserved population?
3. How will you address the cultural sensitivity and awareness factors that may inform diverse healthcare contexts, often with significant consequences?

### Resources

NLM. (2004). Committee on health literacy. In L. Nielsen-Bohlman, & D. A. Kindig (Eds.), *What is health literacy? Health literacy: A prescription to end confusion*. National Academies Press. Retrieved January 8, 2023, from https://www.ncbi.nlm.nih.gov/books/NBK216035/

### References

American Association of Retired Persons (AARP). (2022, January 17). *Medication literacy: A helpful concept for understanding medication decision making among older adults*. Retrieved January 12, 2023, from https://www.aarp.org/ppi/info-2022/medication-literacy.html

American Medical Association (AMA). (1999). Health literacy: Report of the council on scientific affairs. *JAMA, 281*, 5552–5557.

Chan, C. V., & Kaufman, D. R. (2011). A framework for characterizing eHealth literacy demands and barriers. *Journal of Medical Internet Research, 13*(4), e94. https://doi.org/10.2196/jmir.1750

Chen, X., Li, M., & Kreps, G. L. (2022). Acculturation and health literacy among Chinese speakers in the USA with limited English proficiency. *Journal of Racial and Ethnic Health Disparities, 9*(2), 489–497. https://doi.org/10.1007/s40615-021-00979-9

Christy, S. M., Gwede, C. K., Sutton, S. K., Chavarria, E., Davis, S. N., Abdulla, R. . . . Meade, C. D. (2017). Health literacy among the medically underserved: The role of demographic factors, social influence, and religious beliefs. *Journal of Health Communication, 22*(11), 923–931. https://doi.org/10.1080/10810730.2017.1377322

Estacio, E. V. (2013). Health literacy and community empowerment: It is more than just reading, writing, and counting. *Journal of Health Psychology, 18*(8), 1056–1068. https://doi.org/10.1177/1359105312470126

Fernández-Gutiérrez, M., Base-Sarmiento, P., Albar-Marín, M. J., Paloma-Castro, O., & Romero-Sánchez, J. M. (2018). Health literacy interventions for immigrant populations: A systematic review. *International Nursing Reviews, 65*(1), 54–64. https://doi.org/10.1111/inr.12373

Gibbons, C. M., Fleisher, L., Slamon, R. E., Bass, S., Kandadai, V., & Beck, R. J. (2011). Exploring the potential of web 2.0 to address health disparities. *Journal of Health Communication, 16*(S1), 77–89 https://doi.org/10.1080/10810730.2011.596916

Hahn, E. A., Burns, J. L., Jacobs, E. A., et al. (2015). Health literacy and patient-reported outcomes: A cross-sectional study of underserved English-and Spanish-speaking patients with type 2 diabetes. *Journal of Health Communication, 20*(suppl), 4–15. https://doi.org/10.1080/10810730.2015.1061071

Hickey, K. T., Creber, R. M. M., Reading, M., Sciacca, R. R., Riga, T. C., Frúlla, A. P., & Casida, J. M. (2019). Low health literacy. *Nurse Practitioner, 43*(8), 49–55. https://doi.org/10.1097/01.NPR.0000541468.54290.49

Hoover, D. S., Vidrine, J. I., Shete, S., Spears, C. A., Cano, M. A., Correa-Fernàndez, V., . . . McNeill, L. H. (2015). Health literacy, smoking, and health indicators in African American adults. *Journal of Health Communication, 20*(S2), 24–33 https://doi.org/10.1080/10810730.2015.1066465

Kim, H., Goldsmith, J. V., Sengupta, S., Mahmood, A., Powell, M. P., Bhatt, J., Change, C. F., & Bhuyan, S. S. (2019). Mobile health application and e-health literacy: Opportunities and concerns for cancer patients and caregivers. *Journal of Cancer Education, 34*(1), 3–8. https://doi.org/10.1007/s13187-017-1293-5

Kim, M. T., Kim, K. B., Ko, J., Murry, N., Xie, B., Radhakrishnan, K., & Han, H. -R. (2020). Health literacy and outcomes of a community-based self-help intervention: A case of Korean Americans with Type 2 diabetes. *Nursing Research, 69*(3), 210–218. https://doi.org/10.1097/NNR.0000000000 000409

Kim, Y.-C., Lim, J. Y., & Park, K. (2015). The effects of health literacy and social capital on health information behavior. *Journal of Health Communication, 20*(9), 1084–1094 https://doi.org/10.1080/108 10730.2015.1018636

Kirsch, I.S. (2001). The framework used in developing and interpreting the International Adult Literacy Survey (IALS). *European Journal of Psychology of Education, 16*(3), 335–361.

Lee, S.-Y. D., Arozullah, A. M., & Cho, Y. I. (2004). Health literacy, social support, and health: A research agenda. *Social Science & Medicine, 1309–1321. https://doi.org/10.1016/S0277-9536(03)00329-0

Lopez, V., Sanchez, K., O Killian, M., & Eghaneyan, B. H. (2018). Depression screening and education: An examination of mental health literacy and stigma in a sample of Hispanic women. *BMC Public Health, 18*(1), 646. https://doi.org/10.1186/s12889-018-5516-4

Manganello, J. A., & Clayman, M. L. (2011). The association of understanding of medical statistics with health information seeking and health provider interaction in a national sample of young adults. *Journal of Health Communication, 16*(S3), 163–176. https://doi.org/10.1080/10810730.2011.604704

National Association of Secondary School Principals. (2023). Retrieved January 10, 2023, from https://www.nassp.org/

*Network of the National Library of Medicine.* (2021). An introduction to health literacy. What is health literacy? Retrieved from https://www.nnlm.gov/guides/intro-health-literacy

Neuhauser, L., & Kreps, G. L. (2008). Online cancer communication: Meeting the literacy, cultural, and linguistic needs of diverse audiences. *Patient Education and Counseling, 71*(3), 365–377. https://doi.org/10.1016/j.pec.2008.02.015

Norris, N. S., Nnaji, C., & Sarkis, M. (2022). "Was test designed for Africans?": Health literacy and African immigrants. *Journal of Racial and Ethnic Health Disparities, 9*(1), 315–324. https://doi.org/10.1007/s40615-020-00959

Norman, C.D., & Skinner, H.A. (2006). eHealth literacy: Essential skills for consumer health in a networked world. *Journal of Medical Internet Research, 8*(2), e9. https://doi.org/10.2196/jmir.8.2.e9

Nutbeam, D. (2000). Health literacy as a public health goal: A challenge for contemporary health education and communication strategies into the 21st century. *Health Promotion International, 15*(3), 259–267 https://doi.org/10.1093/heapro/15.3.259

OASH. (n.d.). Healthy People 2030. *Health literacy in Healthy People 2030.* Retrieved January 8, 2023, from https://health.gov/healthypeople/priority-areas/health-literacy-healthy-people-2030

Paige, S. R., Stellefson, M., Krieger, J. L., Anderson-Lewis, C., Cheong, J., & Stopka, C. (2018). The transactional model of electronic health (eHealth) literacy. *Journal of Medical Internet Research, 20*(10), e10175. https://doi.org/10.2196/10175

Palumbo, R., Capolupo, N., & Adinolfi, P. (2022). Addressing health literacy in the digital domain: Insights from a literature review. *Kybernetes, 51*(13), 82–97. https://doi.org/10.1108/K-07-2021-0547

Park, H., Rodgers, S., & Stemmle, J. (2013). Analyzing health organizations' use of Twitter for promoting health literacy. *Journal of Health Communication, 18*(4), 410–425. https://doi.org/10.1080/10810730.2012.72795

Parker, R. M., & Hernandez, M (2012). What makes an organization health literate? *Journal of Health Communication, 17*(5), 624–627. https://doi.org/10.1080/10810730.2012.685806

Pérez-Stable, E. J., & El-Toukhy, S. (2018). Communicating with diverse patients: How patient and clinician factors affect disparities. *Patient Education and Counseling, 101*(12), 2186–2194. https://doi.org/10.1016/j.pec.2018.08.021

Petrun Sayers, E. L., Bouskill, K. E., Concannn, T. W., & Martin, L. T. (2021). Creating culture-centered health and health insurance literacy resources: Lessons learned from Haitian Creole, Mandarin, Native American, and Vietnamese communities. *Journal of Communication in Healthcare, 14*(4), 312–323 https://doi.org/10.1080/17538068.2021.1930814

Rural Health Information Hub. (2021). *Rural health literacy toolkit*. Retrieved January 13, 2023, from https://www.ruralhealthinfo.org/toolkits/health-literacy

Schaffler, J., Leung, K. Tremblay et al., (2018). The effectiveness of self-management interventions for individuals with low health literacy and/or low income: A descriptive systematic review. *Journal of General Internal Medicine, 33*(4), 510–523. https://doi.org/10.1007/s11606-017-4265-x

Shahid, R., Shoker, M., Chu, L. M., Frehlick, R., Ward, H., & Pahwa, P. (2022). Impact of low health literacy on patients' health outcomes: A multicenter cohort study. *BMC Health Services Research, 1148*. https://doi.org/10.1186/s12913-022-08527-9

Shaw, S. J., Huebner, C., Armin, J., Orzech, K., & Vivian, J. (2009). The role of culture in health literacy and chronic disease screening and management. *Journal of Immigrant and Minority Health, 11*(6), 460–467. https://doi.org/10.1007/s10903-008-9135-5

Stellefson, M. L., Shuster, J. J., Chaney, B. H., Paige, S. R., Alber, J. M., Chaney, J. D., & Sriram, P. S. (2017). Web-based health information seeking and eHealth literacy among patients living with chronic obstructive pulmonary disease (COPD). *Health Communication*, 1–15. https://doi.org/10.1080/10410236.2017.1353868

Thomson, R., Starke, P., & Morris, D. (2019). Transgender health literacy 101: Providing whole-person care without assumption (SA501). *Journal of Pain and Symptom Management, 57*(2), P441, https://doi.org/10.1016/j.jpainsymman.2018.12.181

United States Environmental Protection Agency. (2023). *Readability for developing and pretesting concepts, messages, materials, and activities*. Retrieved on May 8, 2023 from https://www.epa.gov/fishtech/readability-developing-and-pretesting-concepts-messages-materials-and-activities

Weaver, N. L., Wray, R. J., Zellin, S., Gautam, K., & Jupka, K. (2012). Advancing organizational health literacy in health care organizations serving high needs populations: A case study. *Journal of Health Communication, 17*(S3), 55–66. https://doi.org/10.1080/10810730.2012.714442

Whitman, M. V., & Davis, J. A. (2008). Implementing cultural and linguistic competence in healthcare management curriculum. *Journal of Health Administration and Education, 25*(2), 109–126.

Yom-Tov, E., Marino, B., Pai, J., Harris, D., & Wolf, M. (2016). The effect of limited health literacy on how Internet users learn about diabetes. *Journal of Health Communication, 21*(10), 1107–1114. https://doi.org/10.1080/10810730.2016.1222033

# Contextualizing Health

## Chapter 8

# Health and the Environment

DOI: 10.4324/9781003214472-11

**Chapter Learning Outcomes**

After completing the chapter, the reader will be able to apply the WPHC and SJA approach to:

1. Understand how knowledge about the environment and its components as a human health issue informs systematic WPHC and SJA-based action.
2. Explain how the impacts of climate change on food and culture impact human migration emergence of novel pathogens, and transmission of infectious diseases.
3. Explain the relationship between human health and food structures, nutrition security, food stability, sustainability, and social capital.
4. Identify how environmental communication, health, and environmental justice SJA can help address the challenges.
5. Identify how the relationship between planetary ecosystem, health, and individual health impacts individual and public health.
6. Design SJA interventions at the individual, local, community-based, and organizational levels.

**Consider the following facts:**

In 2017, 68.5 million people were displaced by extreme weather events, more than at any point in human history. The World Bank forecasts that between Latin America, sub-Saharan Africa, and Southeast Asia, 216 million people are likely to become climate change migrants due to extreme weather by 2050.

(The World Bank, Groundswell Report, 2021, September 13)

349 million people across 79 countries faced acute food insecurity in 2022, up from 287 million in 2021. Along with being the highest at any point in human history, this number represents a staggering rise of 200 million people compared to pre-COVID-19 pandemic levels (World Food Programme, 2023). Many of the people who are food insecure are small farmers whose main livelihood comes from

agriculture. Food insecurity and hunger also affects women most acutely. Finally, a vast majority of those who are affected by food insecurity live in rural areas.

(US Agency for International Development (USAID), 2022)

With our planet's population expected to grow to 9 billion people by 2050, several significant challenges face us with increasing immediacy: How do we nurture and support the food systems that nourish the most socially vulnerable and feed the planet? How do we protect natural resources and consider how we think about sustainable food choices and food security? And, how do we reimagine key considerations about the environment as a vital human health issue?

(USAID, 2022, February 03)

The WPHC SJA approach states that the health of individuals, families, and communities is intertwined with the health of the planet together with the health of its different elements (species diversity, climate change, and food cultures). The WPHC SJA approach considers how communication can create conditions that can empower each of these interconnected components to achieve health-related behavioral changes in long-term sustainable ways (NCCIH, 2023). A WPHC SJA approach requires a holistic view of health that is fundamentally centered on multidimensional and multisystemic care aligned with planetary and environmental health. It centers environmental factors like global warming and its impact on infectious disease transmission, climate change, and extreme weather events and their impact on human health; biodiversity loss and its impact on the living environment of animals and humans; and the consequences of exposure to a deteriorated environment on the health burden of societies (Zhang et al., 2022). Each of these relationships is challenged by multiple changes arising from human development and geopolitical shifts. A deeper challenge arises from the lack of awareness of the connection between human health and the environment. Environmental communication and the environmental justice movements share the SJA components that provide suggestions for action on an individual, community, and organizational level.

## Chapter Organization

**Chapter 8, Health and the Environment**, considers these questions from a WPHC and SJA perspective, paying attention to their inequitable health impacts in local and global contexts. Along with explicating the knowledge framework underlying the complex relationship between the environment, climate change, planetary health, and human health, the chapter will provide resources to support SJA to consider ways of working with advocacy organizations for engaging in local action in the community. Organizationally, **Chapter 8** is laid out as follows: **First**, it will cover the environment from a systems analysis approach and connect its elements with evolving understandings of the environment as a human health issue. It will lay out the adverse health-related impacts of climate change on human migration and their relationship with the increased transmission of infectious diseases. **Second**, it will examine the impacts of climate change on food, culture, and health by covering food insecurity and its relationship with food structures, food system sustainability, environment, and social capital.

It will also look at the emerging concept of nutrition security and its relationship with culturally appropriate and culturally competent nutrition. **Third**, it will look at how environmental communication, health, and environmental justice can help address these challenges. It will also introduce the nascent environmental health and environmental justice movements. **Fourth**, it will look at the relationship between planetary ecosystem health and individual health. It will look at ecosystem health and integrity and the ecological model of public health and conclude with the most recent emergence of ecological models of health promotion. Along the way, communication scholar interviews with Dr. Phaedra Pezzullo and Dr. Danielle Endres will provide insight into WPHC SJA approaches and raise provocative questions highlighting the significance of the issue. Activities, thought prompts, reflection exercises, and discussion questions will help identify the multiple intersections and perspectives that this domain offers and invite action.

## Environment as a Human Health Issue

The term "environment" is used in many contexts. Some people interpret it as the community, neighborhood, or workplace, others with nature, associating it with wilderness, and the elements of a natural landscape. Others take its meaning to be more closely associated with the relationship of the elements within which life exists such as rural and urban areas, agricultural landscapes, and neighborhood elements. This section will explain the environment as a human health issue and the climate through the lens of climate change, weather events, and their relationship with infectious diseases, social vulnerability, mass migration, and global disparities.

### Environment

Broadly, the term environment refers to habitats, the composition of habitats and their resources, and their interrelationships with each other. In fact, the environment can be all the above elements that comprise the space within which human activity occurs. These elements are interrelated and may include air, water, land, or soil quality, pollution, species diversity, temperature, and weather systems. Thinking about the environment as an interrelated system of interacting components is characteristic of a systems analysis approach. According to the systems analysis approach, the "earth system" comprising the natural, biotic, and abiotic components, along with human activity, and all the elements discussed earlier, interact with each other and affect each other. Their interaction ultimately underlies the expression of complex global environmental issues such as climate change. Climate and its closely associated concept, the weather, are covered next to explain the relationship between climate change and human health. In a later section, this chapter will consider the environment and human health through the lens of ecology and ecosystems.

### Climate

Climate is the average weather in a place over a period of many years or the long-term weather pattern in a particular area. The term "climate" can reference the elements of weather such as the average of precipitation, temperature, humidity, sunshine, and wind over a long period of time in a particular place. The term weather, on the other hand, references changes over a short period of time, such as a few hours, or from hour-to-hour, day-to-day, month-to-month, or year-to-year. Weather includes facets such as cloud cover, rain, shine, temperature, humidity, precipitation, cloudiness, visibility, wind, and atmospheric pressure (NASA, 2005).

Human health can be affected by changing climate and its long-term and short-term impacts. Because of all the different ways this relationship between the climate can influence human health, and to understand the nature of these climate change global processes and changes better, the US Global Change Research Program (USGCRP, 2022) brings together interdisciplinary perspectives including the physical, biological, and social sciences, to examine their impacts from every angle.

### Climate Change

Climate change in environmental science refers to long-term shifts in temperatures and weather patterns (UN, 2022). The long-term shift may happen through the direct effect of heat and extreme weather events. These events underlying climate change can affect human activity and planetary health, both central components of the WPHC framework.

#### Climate Change and WPHC Impacts

One of the ways is how climate change can affect the relationship of human beings with the environment through changes in biodiversity and the habitat of species and wildlife. Climate change can have negative impacts on food systems and the distribution of vectors such as mosquitoes, ticks, and fleas, that transmit diseases such as dengue or malaria. Climate change can also indirectly affect human health through socioeconomic pathways such as increased poverty, population displacement (e.g., migration through disasters or rising sea levels), and conflict. Natural disasters such as earthquakes and floods are often accompanied by outbreaks of infectious disease. Diarrheal illnesses often spread after a natural disaster that is accompanied by population displacement (Liang & Messenger, 2018).

These diseases can contribute to up to 40% of deaths caused by contaminated food and water, disrupted sewage systems, poor sanitation and hygiene, and crowded living situations.

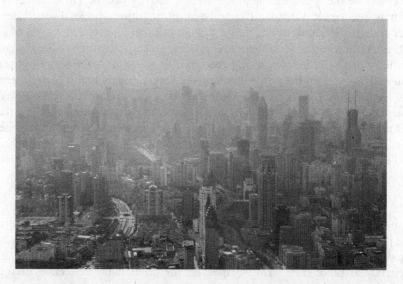

*Figure 8.1* Climate change can indirectly affect human health through socioeconomic pathways such as increased poverty, pollution, and population displacement.

For example, an outbreak of acute gastroenteritis due to Norovirus affected more than 1,000 evacuees and relief workers in a temporary shelter at Reliant Park in Houston, Texas, over a period of 11 days (Liang & Messenger, 2018). Such shifts affect resource-poor, disadvantaged, and vulnerable populations disproportionately by limiting livelihood diversification opportunities and increasing stress and anxiety. Climate change also influences human relationships with other species on Earth by changing habitats and human activity. The global consequences of the COVID-19 pandemic on health, health systems, and economies serve as a reminder that governments, policymakers, and the public should attend to the threat of climate-related changes to infectious disease geographical distribution and burden.

## Mitigating Steps for Climate Change Impacts

Given the complexity of factors that shape the climate, surveillance of infectious diseases and their changing transmission trends is essential. From a WPHC perspective, surveillance helps in guiding the global response to evolving climatic conditions and strengthening health systems to protect vulnerable populations (The Lancet Microbe, 2021). Although vulnerable populations are most at risk for the infectious disease transmission burden due to climate-related changes owing to factors such as pre-existing health conditions and low socioeconomic status, there is little research on how climate change affects resource-poor and low-income global regions. In fact, about 79% of studies on climate and health have focused on how climate change affects high-income and upper-middle-income nations. Greater public awareness and scientific research attending to those vulnerable populations that are most at risk can help identify the threats and propose equitable and sustainable solutions (Manisalidis et al., 2020).

## Climate Change and Human Health Disparities

From a WPHC perspective, climate change affects human health in many ways. The health impacts of climate change and the environment reflect global disparities (Patz et al., 2014). Lower-income nations tend to focus more on food and nutrition; infectious disease; water, sanitation, and hygiene; and maternal and child health. High-income regions tend to focus on hospital admissions, chronic disease, and mortality due to heat, poor air quality, and extreme events. Researchers Berrang-Ford and colleagues note the close association with health concerns of different global regions corresponding to environment elements such as air and water pollution. For instance, they find that respiratory health was a prominent health topic in Asia, while heat stress was one of the top three most frequent topics in Europe, North America, and Oceania. Likewise, vector-borne illnesses like malaria were the top health concern in Africa, while dengue was the top health concern in Latin America and the second most frequent concern in Asia. Research finds that factors such as social vulnerability and greater urban exposure to heat and infectious disease mediate climate-related health impacts. In all such instances, those who are socially vulnerable are also more exposed to the negative impacts of climate change.

## Environment Health Impacts of Climate Change

Climate change has been attributed to the transmission of multiple infectious diseases, either by directly affecting the biosocial features of the pathogens such as their growth, survival, and virulence, or by indirectly supporting transmission through the global reach of their vectors, modification of ecosystems, or their attendant changes in human behavior. The Intergovernmental Panel on Climate Change (IPCC) report states that rising global temperatures have driven "widespread and rapid changes in the atmosphere, ocean, cryosphere, and biosphere." (The IPCC Sixth Assessment Report, n.d.). The health impacts of these widespread changes in environment elements include the spread of a range of diseases with greater intensity or reach. Rising temperatures and increased precipitation, for example, promote infectious diseases ranging from vector-borne diseases such as malaria, dengue, West Nile virus, and leishmaniasis, to enteric infections and diarrhea such as cholera and to parasitic diseases such as schistosomiasis. Climate-related suitability for the transmission of dengue in 2018 had globally increased from 1950 by approximately 8.9%–15% along with a broadened geographical reach in areas where they were not proliferant before. Vectors of tick-borne diseases such as Lyme disease and the encephalitis virus have increased their global spread. Increasingly, the spread of infectious diseases is seen as an important concern regarding the impact of climate change on health.

## WEATHER

Weather events are a major factor responsible for the rapid displacement of vulnerable populations globally. Mass migration can be sudden, as in the case of extreme weather events, or gradual, such as with famine and food shortages. The health impacts of mass migration include infections caused by ectoparasites such as scabies and lice that thrive in areas of human concentration, dense living conditions, and poor hygiene (Kwak et al., 2021). HIV infection and tuberculosis (TB) can also pose a threat to the health of migrants. Crowded conditions, shared living conditions, and limited sanitation characterizing marginalized communities contribute to their spread. Natural disasters can also exacerbate existing health conditions and make them more difficult to control. For instance, highly transmissible conditions, such as TB, become more challenging to treat during natural disasters. Natural disasters hamper vaccination efforts, TB surveillance, antituberculosis therapies, and other elements of TB prevention that minimize prolonged infectivity, drug resistance, relapse, and death.

## Food, Climate, and Culture

Food and nutrition are central to health and well-being in the WPHC framework. Food is an essential component of cultural practices and provides a sense of well-being and connection with nature. The food composition, gathering, and preparation practices within a culture shape the relationship with nature through agricultural practices, customs, and food production norms. Food structures daily life. Food rituals mark the passage of life stages and religious observances (e.g., fasting or eating cake at weddings). Food practices (e.g., preparation) are an important part of family relationships and a communal activity. Gatherings with friends and community often involve food. The food eaten within a community is determined by biological and geographical conditions and cultural norms. The association of food, health, and well-being, thus, goes beyond just its nutrient composition. It also includes relationships, social support, and a sense of connection with the environment. From a WPHC perspective, the health of the environment, in turn, shapes the availability, stability, sustainability, and accessibility of the dietary sources characteristic of different cultures. This section explains how food security, food sustainability, food stability, and cultural practices of food are central to human health from a WPHC perspective. It provides suggestions for an SJA approach toward the inequities and challenges that face the environment and food production and consumption practices.

## Food Security

Recognizing how food and nutrition vary in their impact on health disparities involves recognizing the relationship of local food and diet with geography, cultural factors, access to healthcare, and food security. The complex interaction between food and health is closely associated with the cultural, sensual, and physical aspects of food in people's lives and plays an important role in aiding the overall experience of being well, feeling a sense of connection with the community, and cultivating coherence in social structure. Structuralist approaches show how shared culinary cultures are associated with shared worldviews.

*Review the Mini-Case Study in Textbox 8.1 for a deeper understanding of the relationship between local food resources and food security. The case study provides a look at how Native populations conceptualize the relationship between food and nature. Textbox 8.1 also unpacks the notion of intact cultures and their relationship with local stewardship of natural ecosystems, sustainable diets, and community resilience from a WPHC perspective. It describes how cultural food practices and nutrition-related cultural beliefs are closely intertwined with the delivery of patient-centered care and associated with positive health outcomes such as improved patient adherence.*

---

### Textbox 8.1   Mini-Case Study

### Protecting Local Stewardship of Ecosystems and Sustainable Diets

#### WPHC Context

Research on global food resources and food security has highlighted the shrinking diversity in major food crops and national diets. Our major food supplies and diet are becoming increasingly homogeneous. This narrowing of our diets and food sources has implications beyond human health. For instance, research shows that increased reliance on meat and dairy foods has reduced dietary sustainability and contributed to environmental degradation and biodiversity loss.

In Native populations, healthy and sustainable food systems that support long-term food security draw upon interconnected principles of nature, food, and culture. Intact cultures and diverse ecosystems support resilient and balanced food webs. Intact cultures reference institutions that sustain healthy food and nutrition that supports physical, mental, emotional, and spiritual health and well-being. Making food choices within the local food system maintained by harvesters and farmers with a sense of belonging to the natural lands and forests contributes to the promotion of sustainable diets, health, and nutrition of Indigenous Peoples.

Support for local ecosystems by Indigenous Peoples requires a multisectoral partnership with community leaders, social institutions, local governments, and community members. Researchers Tremblay et al. (2020) examine local food consumption practices in 21 Indigenous communities across northern North America to illuminate "the sustainability and cultural agency inherent in local food systems and the importance of cultural-ecological coupling in an era of accelerating social and environmental change."

Biodiversity loss following the deterioration of natural ecosystems impacts local and Native food cultures. Sustainable diets are those derived from sustainable food systems following sustainable cultures and sustainable ecosystems. In the instance of Indigenous Peoples, commercial retail outlets that dominate as sources of food create a loss of local biodiversity and traditional dietary diversity and promote food insecurity. The disparities result in malnutrition and overconsumption of dietary energy. Overconsumption of empty calories associated with malnutrition is among the major drivers of the global obesity and chronic condition epidemic impacting Indigenous populations. There are multiple challenges facing sustainable food production. These include the erosion of biodiversity of both wild and cultivated species of animals and plants; destruction of forests, water shortages, hydroelectric dam construction; water pollution from domestic and livestock waste; contamination of lands, water, and food species from industrial development; and climate change.

One way to protect natural ecosystems is to support Indigenous stewardship and management of local ecosystems. Small-scale agriculture using organic methods mitigates ecosystem pollution, enhances the connection of the farmer with their land, builds local knowledge, and promotes community resilience. Combined with culturally relevant nutrition education, such practices minimize the risk of nutritional disparities faced by African Americans and Hispanics (e.g., obesity and chronic diseases, including diabetes, hypertension, and cardiovascular disease).

Understanding the role that food plays in a culture helps providers tailor recommendations to ethnic beliefs about health and medicine and align these with minority patients' values (US Department of Agriculture (USDA), 2022). Research shows that awareness of nutrition-related cultural beliefs and practices is important for patient education and for rapport-building with patients in the healthcare setting. For instance, Nemec's study emphasizes how such knowledge can help dietitians design culturally sensitive patient-centered care through individualized nutrition education plans and communicate their advice in ways that improve patient adherence. To illustrate, in traditional Chinese medicine, foods are grouped as hot or cold, applying the *yin/yang* balance principle. In Hispanic culture, cooking and eating homemade traditional foods together as a family is important. In Japanese culture, *Washoku* is a social practice associated with food embodying the Japanese people's spirit. In Indian culture, a lacto-vegetarian diet is commonly followed by the Hindu population, with local variances across different geographical regions of the country. The Middle Eastern diet predominantly consists of both plan and animal protein sources paired with olive oil, rice, eggplant, dates, olives, figs, tomatoes, and herbs and spices (USDA, 2022). Individualized nutrition plans tailored to different cultural values and practices can increase adherence.

### SJA Prompt

Learn about the food practices of a cultural group. How are these practices connected with the food systems? How do changes in the climate threaten or (re)shape food security and Native food practices?

### Resources

Tremblay, R., Landry-Cuerrier, M., & Humphries, M. M. (2020). Culture and the social ecology of local food use by Indigenous communities in northern North America. *Ecology and Society*, *25*(2), 8. https://doi.org/10.5751/ES-11542-250208

USDA. (2022). *Climate change global food security, and the U.S. food system: A scientific assessment*. Retrieved from https://www.usda.gov/sites/default/files/documents/CCFS_RiB.pdf

## Food, Nutrient Groups, and Social Cohesion

The recognition of food as more than just nutrient groups has led some researchers to examine food from different perspectives, including food as relation, food as body and identity, and food as power, along with food as culture, among others (Nordström et al., 2013). For instance, in thinking of food as relation, food can be understood as providing a medium that creates bonds between people through fostering companionship (e.g., the communal notion of "breaking bread") such as through sharing coffee and a meal with friends and neighbors. Food, Nordström and colleagues note, helps us communicate who we are, where we came from, and who we want to become.

## Food-Based Social Inequities

Pandemics such as COVID-19 highlight the inequities and structural racism in the domain of food by showing how Americans who are most likely to be hungry are also at the highest risk of diet-related diseases including obesity, diabetes, heart disease, and many cancers. These systemic food-based inequities are highlighted by the disproportionate burden of diseases. Class-based struggles and those between ethnic groups and nations illustrate dimensions of food as power. Food is also symbolic of gender relations, as illustrated in the traditional female role of feeding the family. Personalized or tailored nutrition approaches help integrate the scientific and cultural bases of food, express individual identity with food, and serve as a form of empowerment.

*Examine **Table 8.1** for a deeper look at the conceptual definitions of food security, social capital, and culture along with their examples and SJA critiques. Attempt the SJA prompt that follows.*

Table 8.1 Concept Definitions and Examples/Critiques

| Concept Definitions Applicable to a WPHC Framework | SJA Examples/Critiques—Food, Culture, Environment |
| --- | --- |
| **Food security:**<br>Food security is defined as the physical, social, and economic access to safe, sufficient, and nutritious food that meets dietary needs and food preferences for an active and healthy lifestyle. | **Food security** exists "when all people at all times have physical, social, and economic access to sufficient, safe, and nutritious food to meet their dietary needs and food preferences for an active and healthy life."<br>Food security affects people through both under- and overconsumption. Food security requires that food be<br>a. **Available,** that it exist in a particular place at a particular time;<br>b. That people can **access** that food through economic or other means;<br>c. That people can **utilize** the food that is available and accessible to them; and<br>d. That each of these components is **stable** over time. Constrictions in any of these components can result in **food insecurity** (USDA.gov). |
| **Social capital of relationships:**<br>A concept that references the different levels of bonding, bridging, and linking between people. | **Bonding social capital** is the strength of individual close relationships, notably family relationships. Bonding social capital is driven by "**homophily**," the desire to affiliate with people of similar backgrounds. Bonding social capital is linked to positive social outcomes.<br>**Bridging social capital** is the accumulation of "weak ties" that stretch further across heterogeneous communities to increase access to resources and opportunities. The resources of these weak ties could be essential in ensuring food security.<br>**Linking social capital** is the vertical connection between individuals and their communities and leaders, or positions at other levels of hierarchies. This type of social capital is essential for bringing higher-level resources back to communities. |
| **Cultural competence:**<br>Refers to the act whereby a healthcare professional develops an awareness of one's existence, sensations, thoughts, and environment without letting these factors have an undue influence on those for whom care is provided. | **Cultural competence** emphasizes the adaptation of care in a manner that is congruent with the client's culture. It is a dynamic, fluid, continuous process whereby an individual, system, or healthcare agency finds meaningful and useful care-delivery strategies based on knowledge of the cultural heritage, attitudes, and behaviors of those to whom they deliver care.<br>**Culturally competent care** is designed to meet the needs of marginalized groups, individuals, and communities of people who have some distinct characteristics that distinguish them from the mainstream.<br>**Cultural competence in care** includes (a) being competent in one's own cultural heritage, (b) respecting and appreciating the values and behaviors of others, and (c) combining self-awareness with insight about others to demonstrate true sensitivity to others. |

**Ethnic group:**
An ethnic group is a group of people whose members have different experiences and backgrounds from the dominant culture by status, background, residence, religion, education, or other factors that functionally unify the group and act collectively on each other.

**Cultural imperialism:**
The practice of extending policies and practices of one organization (usually the dominant one) to disenfranchised and minority groups.

**Culture:**
A learned, patterned behavioral response acquired over time that includes explicit and implicit beliefs, attitudes, values, customs, norms, taboos, arts, habits, and life ways accepted by a community of individuals.

The **COVID-19 pandemic:**
The most recent pandemic illustrated how the issue of food justice is divided along racial/ethnic lines. Morales et al. (2021) conducted a cross-sectional study on household food insecurity during COVID-19 using data from a nationally representative sample of US households indicated that households headed by Blacks, Asians, Hispanics, or other **racial/ethnic minorities** were not significantly more food insecure than White households during the pandemic.
Among **food-insecure** households, Black households are more likely to report that they could not afford to buy more food; Asian households were more likely to face transportation issues when purchasing food; White households were more likely to report that stores did not have the food they wanted.
Finally, **racial/ethnic minorities** were significantly less confident about their household food security for the next four weeks than Whites.

**Proponents** appeal to universal human rights values and standards.
**Opponents** posit that universal standards are a disguise for the dominant culture to destroy or eradicate traditional cultures through worldwide public policy.
The practice of hunting and consumption of wildmeat (e.g., as endorsed by the Convention on Biological Diversity): This example illustrates the support of the practice while balancing it with a "mutualistic understanding of the complexity and nuance regarding the multiple connections that people maintain with wildlife and how these reflect the value orientations shared within the resource constituency" to address cultural imperialism in approaching the complex and dynamic cultural dimensions of human–wildlife relations (van Vliet, 2018).

**Culture** is primarily learned and transmitted within the family and other social organizations, is shared by most of the group, includes an individualized worldview, guides decision-making, and facilitates self-worth and self-esteem.
**Primary characteristics of culture** are attributes that one cannot easily change and determine the degree to which a person adheres to the dominant beliefs and practices of his or her dominant culture. They include nationality, race, color, gender, age, and religious affiliation.
**Secondary characteristics of culture:** These are attributes that one can change more readily and determine the degree to which a person adheres to the dominant beliefs and practices of his or her dominant culture and include facets like education, occupation, socioeconomic status, political beliefs, rural versus urban status, marital status, gender identity, sexual orientation, and reason for migration (e.g., undocumented or immigrant).

*(Continued)*

*Table 8.1* (Continued) Concept Definitions and Examples/Critiques

| Concept Definitions Applicable to a WPHC Framework | SJA Examples/Critiques/Food, Culture, Environment |
| --- | --- |
| **Cultural awareness:**<br><br>Cultural awareness is being knowledgeable about one's own thoughts, feelings, and sensations and having an appreciation of the diversity of others in terms of the objective (material) culture such as the arts, clothing, foods, and other external signs of diversity. | The example of **type 2 diabetes:** Diabetes and its associated complications place an illness burden on patients and carers, which disproportionately affects those from ethnic minority backgrounds.<br>**Diabetic dietary regimens** are disruptive to patients' daily lifestyles and exist in tension with traditional South Asian diets. This may be a result of poorer access to healthy foods for **South Asian patients** or attributable to lower material resources in these groups.In ethnic minorities, family, friends, and life histories play a central role in shaping the understanding of illness and provide a strong source of knowledge and emotional support for those from South Asian backgrounds (Wilson et al., 2012). |
| **Cultural sensitivity:**<br><br>The ability to recognize, understand, and react appropriately to behaviors of persons who belong to a cultural or ethnic group that differs substantially from one's own. | **Culturally sensitive communication** helps to (a) develop an understanding of one's own cultural beliefs, values, attitudes, and practices and those of others; (b) to describe open and sensitivecommunication; and (c) to describe strategies used to collaborate with the patient and family for optimal care.<br>**Lack of culturally sensitive communication** is associated with (a) decreased patient satisfaction, perception, and experience of care and (b) increased risk of miscommunication and cultural disparities that lead to (c) poor adherence to treatment, poor health outcomes, and increased prevalence of adverse events.<br>**Culturally sensitive provider communication** had a direct effect on dietary adherence for African American patients in a study testing the Patient-Centered Culturally Sensitive Healthcare Model (Tucker et al., 2012). |
| **Cultural diversity:**<br><br>Refers to diversity in race, color, ethnicity, national origin, religion, age, gender, sexual orientation, ability/disability, social and economic status or class, education, occupation, religious orientation, marital and parental status, and other related attributes of groups of people in society. | Culture and ethnicity are intertwined with food.**Diversity in dietetics** helps health and nutrition resources be **inclusive.**<br>**Culturally relevant nutrition education** helps patients establish healthy habits that align with their values and traditions. |

**Cultural imposition:**
Intrusively applies the majority cultural view to individuals and families.

**Cultural relativism:**
The belief that behaviors and practices of people should be judged only in the context of their cultural system.

Prescribing a special diet without regard to the client's culture and limiting visitors to immediate family is an example of **cultural imposition.**
WPHC suggests a way to avoid cultural imposition in healthcare is by remaining open and neutral in expressing **cultural values** to encourage patients to communicate their own values openly and without **bias.**

**Proponents** argue that issues such as abortion, euthanasia, female circumcision, and physical punishment in childrearing should be accepted as cultural values without judgment from the outside world.
**Opponents** argue that cultural relativism may undermine the condemnation of human rights violations and that family violence cannot be justified or excused on a cultural basis.

## SJA Prompt

Select any one of the WPHC contexts from the left-hand side of Table 8.1. How is it relevant to the local community you live in? Design one community-led initiative applying the SJA critique in action in your community.

## SJA Resources

Giger, J., Davidhizar, R. E., Purnell, L., Harden, J. T., Phillips, J., & Strickland, O. (2007). American Academy of Nursing expert panel report: Developing cultural competence to eliminate health disparities in ethnic minorities and other vulnerable populations. *Journal of Transcultural Nursing, 18*, 95. https://doi.org/10.1177/1043659606298618

Morales, D. X., Morales, S. A., & Beltran, T. F. (2021). Racial/ethnic disparities in household food insecurity during the COVID-19 pandemic: A nationally representative study. *Journal of Racial and Ethnic Health Disparities, 8*(5), 1300–1314. https://doi.org/10.1007/s40615-020-008927

Tucker, C. M., Marsiske, M., Rice, K. G., Jones, J. D., & Herman, K. C. (2012). Patient-centered culturally sensitive healthcare: Model testing and refinement. *Health Psychology, 30*(3), 342–350. https://doi.org/10.1037/a0022967

van Vliet, N. (2018). "Bushmeat crisis" and "cultural imperialism" in wildlife management? Taking value orientations into account for a more sustainable and culturally acceptable wildmeat sector. *Frontiers in Ecology and Evolution, 6*, 112. https://doi.org/10.3389/fevo.2018.00112

Wilson, C., Alam, R., Latif, S., Knighting, K., Williamson, S., & Beaver, K. (2012). Patient access to healthcare services and optimization of self-management of ethnic minority/populations living with diabetes: A systematic review. *Health and Social Care in the Community, 20*(1), 1–19. https://doi.org/10.1111/j.1365-2524.2011.01017.x

### Food Insecurity

Given the complex relationship between food, culture, and the environment, food-related disparities can have far-reaching effects. Food insecurity is responsible for undernutrition, micronutrient deficiencies, and obesity. As communication scholars Ramadurai and colleagues note, rural food insecurity and rural healthcare issues have often been overlooked in the United States (Ramadurai et al., 2012). Employing the culture-centered approach (Dutta, 2008), they highlight how individual agency and social capital inherent in the rural culture can help community members arrive at creative solutions and coping mechanisms. Local organizations, such as churches, can play an important role in rural contexts to ensure food security through social capital (Paul et al., 2019; see Table 8.1 for definitions).

Keeping the community central can help with incorporating traditional and commercial foods in a manner that is articulated by the members of the community and is responsive to community traditions. Keeping traditional dietary components central as emphasized in the WPHC approach also helps attend to the environmental sustainability and diversity of local species that comprise diverse dietary systems.

*Examine* **Textbox 8.2** *for some examples of dietary components of food systems comprising traditional and commercial foods that utilize local species. Attempt the SJA prompt that follows.*

---

**Textbox 8.2   Traditional and Commercial Food Sources: Dietary Energy from Local Species**

**WPHC Context**

The mix of traditional foods and purchased commercial foods in daily diet is based on seasons and climate, as well as on socioeconomic factors. Both traditional and purchased food contribute to meeting the total individual dietary needs (Kuhnlein, 2014). Local food production and processing are influenced by local traditions and consumption. They have benefits such as the revitalization of rural areas, economic benefits, and positive relationships between the community stakeholders.

An analysis of the dietary components of the food components comprising traditional foods and commercial foods reveals how local species are used in traditional foods. For example, Kuhnlein found that more than 380 local species and varieties were reported to be used by respondents in the Pohnpei culture in the Federated States of Micronesia and the Karen in Western Thailand. There were 35 traditional food species being used in the drought-prone areas of the Maasai, Kenya. The Maasai in Kajaido District consume about 6% of their dietary energy from traditional foods, while the Mand community in Pohnpei consumed about 27% of their dietary energy from traditional foods. Finally, over 90% of dietary energy came from the local food resources of the Peruvian Awajún and the Igbo in Nigeria.

**SJA Action Prompt**

Look at USDA's MyPlate food groups (use the URL provided in the Resources section).

- How many of them are in your diet?
- How many of these comprise your traditional foods?

- .How close are the grocery stores where you can purchase these food choices in your neighborhood? How much will the food choices for the healthy recipes provided here cost in your grocery store?
- How far are the grocery stores from the disadvantaged neighborhoods?

**Resource**

USDA. (2022). *MyPlate*. Retrieved from https://www.myplate.gov/

## Food System Sustainability

Along with the dietary composition of food and its relationship with the community and culture, the food system includes the logistical facets of production, transport, processing, packaging, storage, retail, consumption, loss, and processing of food waste (IPCC, 2021). The WPHC framework considers how all these aspects of the food system are under pressure from nonclimate stressors, such as population and income growth, an overwhelming demand for animal-sourced products, and climate change. To illustrate, Indigenous Peoples use their knowledge of ecosystem biodiversity and cultural practices to harvest and use biodiverse plant and animal foods for family nutrition and health. Kuhnlein's work on food system sustainability for the health and well-being of Indigenous Peoples provides several important insights. For Indigenous Peoples, the connection to land and place is the foundation of culture and health. Thus, the environmental impacts of human activity mean a fundamental shift in the relationship with nature. Food practices are intimately connected with nature and symbolize the close connection between planetary health and human health. Indigenous Peoples' worldview conceptualizes the environment and people as interwoven with diverse and ever-changing relationships between human and nonhuman life and between the animate and inanimate worlds (Tremblay et al., 2020).

*Review* **Textbox 8.3. Dr. Danielle Endres's Scholar Interview** *provides close insight into how the environmental impacts of climate change and the environmental justice movement are intimately connected to the Indigenous People's relationship with planetary systems.*

## TEXTBOX 8.3   Scholar Interview

### Dr. Danielle Endres
*University of Utah*

### Nuclear Decolonization by and for Indigenous Peoples and Nations

As an environmental communication scholar with scholarship that centers energy transitions, the ongoing impacts of climate change, environmental justice, and Indigenous Lands protection movements, my research and teaching inevitably work in the intersections of environment and health. I think about the environment holistically as an ecology that includes humans, more-than-human beings, places, and planetary systems. I also think of the environment, as environmental justice advocates do, as the places where humans live, work, and play. Stated simply: promoting the health of our planet and the communities that share it is a key motivation in my research. Yet, not all of the threats to our environment are equally experienced. Underrepresented, marginalized, colonized, and otherwise oppressed frontline peoples, places, and more-than-human beings disproportionately experience the harms of environmental destruction, toxicity, and pollution. As such, it is impossible for me to think about the health of our planet without bringing a social and environmental justice lens to the work I do. Because environmental destruction is linked with systems of racism, sexism, classism, colonialism, ableism, capitalism, and more, attempting to address environmental problems—like air pollution, toxic waste, or climate change impacts—without attention to justice ensures shallow solutions that fail to address the root causes of the interconnected oppression of people and the environment. Promoting the health of the plant from an environmental justice lens includes centering frontline communities who have the knowledge, skills, and ability to lead the way in creating futures free from human-caused environmental calamity.

For over twenty years, my scholarship has focused on the intersections between nuclear technologies and the health of Indigenous Peoples and nations, particularly within the continent that settlers named North America. There are over 500 different and diverse Native nations that share borders with the United States. Nuclear decolonization is a theory and practice for protecting Indigenous Lands (the entire ecology of human and more-than-human beings in a place) from nuclear technologies. Created by and for Indigenous Peoples and nations, nuclear decolonization is a collection of Indigenous-led efforts to enact sovereignty, survivance, radical resurgence, and futures free from nuclear pollution. Nuclear colonization is an intersecting phenomenon identified by Native advocates that highlights how the systems/structures of (settler) colonialism and nuclearism converge such that Indigenous Peoples and nations on this continent and globally are disproportionately negatively impacted by the harms of nuclear technologies. This includes the preponderance of uranium mining, nuclear weapons production and testing, and proposals for nuclear waste storage causing disparate radioactive consequences for Indigenous Peoples and Lands. Within the context of what settlers named the United States, the federal government's nuclear testing program that conducted over 60 nuclear weapons tests within Bikini Atoll and Enewetak Atoll, homelands of Marshallese people, and almost 1,000 nuclear weapons tests on Western Shoshone and Southern Paiute homelands in what the US federal government named the Nevada Test Site. In addition to the downwinders who got various cancers and other illnesses from exposure to radioactive fallout, nuclear testing also has devastating ecological impacts. Bikini Atoll, for example, is still uninhabitable, meaning that displaced Marshallese people cannot access their homelands. The largest nuclear accident in the continental United States happened in 1978 when there was a uranium mill spill at the United Nuclear Corporation's Church Rock site, resulting in the radioactive contamination of the Rio Puerco, which traveled downstream to the Navajo Nation. Moreover, some of the stories of Diné (Navajo) uranium miners and their families who got sick and died from radiation exposure are archived through an oral history project called *Memories Come to Us in the Rain*. Considering these and other ways that the entire nuclear production process inequitably harms Native peoples and nations, my research has focused specifically on how Indigenous Peoples and nations have enacted nuclear decolonization to prevent high-level nuclear waste from being stored on their Lands, particularly with regard to Western Shoshone and Southern Paiute resistance to the proposed Yucca Mountain site and Skull Valley Goshute resistance to a proposal to temporarily store nuclear waste on their reservation.

One of the things we learn from the intersections of nuclear decolonization and nuclear colonization is the importance of indigenizing environmental justice. Scholars like Dina Gilio-Whitake and Kyle Powys Whyte highlight how settler colonialism is an environmental injustice because it is premised on removing Indigenous Peoples and nations from their Lands and key relationalities with those Lands, Indigenous-led Lands protection and environmental justice movements center Native sovereignty and decolonization as key outcomes, and mainstream environmental justice policies see Indigenous Peoples as racial/ethnic minorities and not nations. While resisting simplistic stereotypes of Native peoples as noble savages, ecological Indians, and the first environmentalists, the diversity of Native peoples and nations have solutions for environmental crises that are grounded in knowledges, spiritualities, practices, and relationships with the more-than-human world. These solutions do not simply maintain the status quo but offer ways of being, knowing, and doing that prioritize planetary health.

As illustrated by Dr. Endres's description of nuclear decolonization and environmental injustices, the culture and identity of Indigenous Peoples are fundamentally connected with planetary health and its environmental impacts. The WPHC approach highlights how different cultural communities understand the ecological connections, sentience, and communication among diverse entities in different ways that respect differences and diversity while maintaining the possibility of communication and codependency. These relationships strengthen the social capital of relationships (see Table 8.1 for definitions). The local environment comprising the social capital is closely connected with WPHC and shapes food security from an SJA perspective by facilitating support from community members, social norms, and shared behaviors.

*Textbox 8.4 provides a closer look at how food insecurity disproportionately impacts disadvantaged communities and how sustainable development including sustainable diets might offer a way forward toward meeting the challenges of food insecurity.*

---

### Textbox 8.4    Present Challenges and Future Directions Exercise

#### Food Insecurity, Sustainable Development, and Sustainable Diets

#### WPHC Present Challenges and Call for Future Action

In the United States, food insecurity affects minority and older populations most severely. Approximately 11% or 15 million households in the United States experience some form of food insecurity. However, as an illustration of inequity in food insecurity, over 18% of Latinx households and 22% of African American households have inadequate access to food. Disparities stemming from marginalization accompanied by attendant social, economic, and environmental conditions have positioned the approximately 400 million Indigenous Peoples globally at serious health risk (Walker et al., 2002). Rural areas are often challenged by the presence of "food deserts" and are more likely to be food insecure in the United States.

According to the UN's Brundtland Commission on Sustainable Development, "sustainable development [meets] the needs of the present without compromising the ability of future generations to meet their own needs."

Sustainable diets have low environmental impacts, that contribute to food and nutrition security and to healthy life for present and future generations. Sustainable diets are protective and respectful of biodiversity and ecosystems, culturally acceptable, accessible, economically fair and affordable, nutritionally adequate, safe and healthy, while optimizing natural and human resources.

Looking to the future, evidence from existing food systems identifies two key areas for sustainable diets that link human health with environmental sustainability (The EAT-*Lancet* Commission 2.0, 2023). These are healthy diets, understood as a flexible dietary pattern that contains a mix of vegetables, fruits, whole grains, legumes, nuts, and unsaturated oils, along with low to moderate amounts of seafood and poultry and no or low amounts of red meat, processed meat, added sugar, refined grains, and starchy vegetables, and (b) sustainable food production, understood as one that addresses the challenges of climate change, biodiversity loss, pollution, and unsustainable changes in water and land use (The Nutrition Source, 2022).

### SJA Action Prompt

Look at "*The Lazy Person's Guide to Saving the World*," which lists some action steps that each of us can take to make an impact in our local communities.

i. How many of these items are you following? What action steps can you add to the list for levels 1, 2, 3, and 4?
ii. The definition of sustainable development connects the notion of ethical consumption in the present with meeting the needs of the future.
iii. What steps can you advocate in your community to help make your community sustainable with respect to food that meets health, cultural, ecosystem, and nutrition integrity?

### Resources

The Nutrition Source. (2022). *Sustainability*. Retrieved from https://www.hsph.harvard.edu/nutritionsource/sustainability/

UN Foundation. (2022). *Academic Impact: Sustainability*. Retrieved from https://www.un.org/en/academicimpact/sustainability

UN. (2022). *The lazy person's guide to saving the world*. Retrieved from https://www.un.org/sustainabledevelopment/takeaction/

Walker, J. L., Bradley, J. L., & Humphrey, T. J. (2002). A closer look at environmental injustice in Indian Country. *Seattle Journal for Social Justice*, *1*(2), 5. Retrieved from https://digitalcommons.law.seattleu.edu/cgi/viewcontent.cgi?article=1234&context=sjsj

Willett, W., Rockström, J., & Loken, B. (2019). Food in the anthropocene: The EAT-Lancet commission on healthy diets from sustainable food systems. *The Lancet Commissions*, *393*(10170), 447–492. https://doi.org/10.1016/S0140-6736(18)31788-4

## Food Stability

The WPHC approach considers how climate- and nonclimate stressors impact the four pillars of food security: food availability, access, utilization, and stability. Food availability references the production of an appropriate quantity of food to feed everyone. Food access implies access to food of appropriate quality and diversity from market-based contexts and the ability to make culturally appropriate food choices. Food utilization references the way food is available and how it serves to meet the nutritional needs of community members. Food stability is related to people's ability to access and use food in a steady way so that no one experiences hunger. Increasing extreme events associated with climate change can disrupt food stability such as through increasing food price spikes. Additionally, inadequate access to culturally specific foods can create cultural stress that affects one's identity and well-being.

*Look at the work of some organizations working to build local food partnerships and strengthen sustainable food approaches in **Textbox 8.5**. Attempt the SJA activity that follows.*

---

**Textbox 8.5    Food Sustainability and Local Food Nonprofit Organizations: Building Local Food Partnerships**

| WPHC Context: Food Sustainability and Local Food Nonprofit Organizations | Website |
| --- | --- |
| Food Recovery Network | https://www.foodrecoverynetwork.org/ |
| The International Food Policy Research Institute (IFPRI) | https://www.ifpri.org/ |
| National Sustainable Agriculture Coalition (NSAC) | https://sustainableagriculture.net/ |
| Groundswell International | https://www.groundswellinternational.org/ |
| The Land Institute | https://landinstitute.org/ |
| The Sustainable Food Trust | https://sustainablefoodtrust.org/ |

**SJA Activity: Learn the Food Partnerships in Your Community**

Visit a local farmer in your region. Find out all you can about the following aspects from a WPHC and SJA approach:

- What do they farm?
- How does their farming practice contribute to the local dietary patterns in your region?
- What challenges do they face in meeting local food needs?
- How does the work of local farmers in your region contribute to food security?
- What kinds of partnerships of local organizations and community groups support the local farmers?
- How can you contribute to building sustainable partnerships and carving healthy food practices that balance local traditions and produce positive economic and environmental impacts?

### Personalized or Culturally Appropriate Nutrition

Personalized nutrition embodies the WPHC approach. As Nordström and colleagues note, personalized or culturally appropriate nutrition provides individuals with dietary advice emphasizing health promotion alongside the individual as part of a social and cultural context. Cultural competence in nutrition guidelines is presented by keeping culture's influence on lifestyle, food choices, and eating patterns to incorporate diverse food cultures with a focus on overall well-being (Nemec, 2020). Culturally competent nutrition strategies incorporate cultural diversity in nutrition education and dietary intervention approaches in ethnocultural communities. Emerging attention to a related concept known as nutrition security highlights how, in addition to food security, it is important to consider wholesome, healthful foods and drinks, and attend to not only the quantity of food but its cultural alignment and ability to nourish (Mozaffarian et al., 2021).

## Environmental Communication, Health, and Environmental Justice

### Environmental Communication

Given the multiple threats to environmental health, it is not surprising that environmental communication has often been described as a "discipline of crisis and care," a description that highlights its critical calling to also "address questions of environmental justice" (Chad, 2019, p. 1087). The field of environmental communication examines the nature of the relationship between the meanings of environment, nature, and human-environment-nature relationship in larger contexts such as the media and science. Central to the WPHC approach from an SJA perspective, this section will expand upon the engaged, deliberative, participatory, and community-based advocacy facet of environmental communication through the lens of its intersection with environmental justice and the communicative facets of campaigns and movements.

These intersections highlight how WPHC concerns such as the COVID-19 pandemic intersect with environmental communication issues, such as the climate change crisis, and the need for climate action awareness. Environmental communication in crisis and care is highlighted through COVID-19 as a critical event associated with reduced media attention to climate change. At the same time, seen as a health crisis, COVID-19 opened new media coverage opportunities for framing environmental and economic dimensions of sustainability (Stoddart et al., 2021). Thus, as a disciple of care, from a WPHC perspective, environmental communication as a field of study is also intimately connected with concerns of environmental health and justice, and human and planetary health and well-being.

*Look at **Table 8.2** for a closer look at the concepts of environmental racism, environmental justice, and environmental inequality, along with their health implications. Attempt the SJA activity that follows.*

Table 8.2 Environment Communication: Equity, Sustainability, and Justice

| WPHC Context: Key Concepts in Environmental Communication | SJA: Health Implications |
| --- | --- |
| **Environmental racism:**<br>Environmental racism is racial discrimination in environmental policymaking, the enforcement of regulations and laws, the deliberate targeting of communities of color for toxic waste facilities, the official sanctioning of the life-threatening presence of poisons and pollutants in our communities, and the history of excluding people of color from leadership of the ecology movements" (p. 278).<br>Environmental racism "refers to any policy, practice, or directive that differentially affects or disadvantages (whether intended or unintended) individuals, groups, or communities based on race or color" (Bullard, 1996). | Environmental racism is considered a specific form of **environmental inequality**.<br><br>**Environmental racism** is:<br><br>a. Connected fundamentally to the inequities that drive health disparities in communities of color.<br>b. Attentive to the implications of differentially distributed environmental hazards that tie closely into health disparities related to systemic racism and discrimination. |
| **Environmental Justice:**<br>"[T]he fair treatment and meaningful involvement of all people regardless of race, color, national origin, or income with respect to the development, implementation, and enforcement of environmental laws, regulations, and policies.<br><br>**Fair treatment** means that no population, due to policy or economic disempowerment, is forced to bear a disproportionate share of the negative human health or environmental impacts of pollution or environmental consequences resulting from industrial, municipal, and commercial operations or the execution of federal, state, local and tribal programs and policies" (EPA, 2022). | **Environmental Justice** emphasizes the principle that "fairness and equity are inherent in society's efforts to protect the health of all citizens from the adverse effects of environmental agents."<br>**Equity:** Can be understood as two types:<br><br>a. **Outcome equity**—requires balanced spatial and temporal distribution of benefits and burdens.<br>b. **Process equity**—requires the application of equitable environmental, health, physical, legal, economic, and political criteria to arrive at environmental policy.<br><br>The **environmental justice movement** has focused on three distinct facets:<br><br>a. **Implementation science**, whereby activists work with scientific professionals to co-produce new knowledge and challenge institutional barriers<br>b. **Precautionary principle**, which shifts the burden of proof on producers of chemicals to show an absence of harm<br>c. **National and international policy** changes to address a broad range of practices such as housing segregation, transportation policies, and energy policies that systematically create environmental inequality (Brulle & Pellow, 2006) |

(Continued)

*Table 8.2* (Continued) Environment Communication: Equity, Sustainability, and Justice

| | |
|---|---|
| **Environmental inequality/ environmental injustice**: <br><br> References a situation in which a specific social group is disproportionately affected by environmental hazards. | **Environmental injustice** is considered an outcome of social processes that requires social change to realize environmental justice. <br><br> **Social determinants of environmental inequality**: <br><br> A concept that argues addressing **social determinants of environmental inequality** can help achieve an ecologically just and sustainable society (Brulle & Pellow, 2006). |

## SJA Prompt

What does environmental racism look like in your community? How is it connected with social determinants of environmental inequality?

## Resources

Brulle, R. J., & Pellow, D. N. (2006). Environmental justice: Human health and environmental inequalities. *Annual Review of Public Health, 27,* 103–124. https://doi.org/10.1146/annurev. publhealth.27.021405.102124

Bullard, R. D. (1996). Symposium; The legacy of American apartheid and environmental racism. *St. John's Journal of Legal Comment, 9,* 445–474.

Kaufman, J. D., & Hajat, A. (2021). Confronting environmental racism. *Environmental Health Perspective, 129*(5). https://ehp.niehs.nih.gov/doi/pdf/10.1289/EHP9511

Northridge, M. E. (1997). Comment: Environmental racism and public health. *American Journal of Public Health, 87*(5), 730–732. https://doi.org/10.2105/ajph.87.5.730

*Environmental Collaboration and Advocacy*

Environmental communication centers on human activity and participation in the environment and social justice. Environmental communication comprises (a) environmental rhetoric and the social-symbolic "construction" of nature, (b) public participation in environmental decision-making, (c) environmental collaboration and conflict resolution, (d) media and environmental journalism, (e) representations of nature in advertising and popular culture, (f) advocacy campaigns and message construction, and (g) science and risk communication (Cox & Pezzullo, 2016). Cox and Pezzullo define environmental communication as "the pragmatic and constitutive vehicle for our understanding of the environment as well as our relationships to the natural world" (2016, p. 16).

*Review* **Textbox 8.6**, *communication* **Scholar Interview** *for* **Dr. Phaedra Pezzullo's** *interpretation of "cruel irony," her research and teaching on environmental justice.*

## TEXTBOX 8.6  Scholar Interview

### Dr. Phaedra Pezzullo
*University of Colorado at Boulder*

1. Can you talk a little bit about your scholarship and its intersections with health and the environment? How do you conceptualize the environment? What does social justice mean in your work? How do you see engagement and advocacy shaping the relationship between health and the environment?

My research focuses on environmental and climate justice, which is grounded in the assumption—that has been proven again and again—that power inequities enable unsustainable patterns, which disproportionately impact people of color and the Global South, as well as rationalize ongoing ecological degradation that threatens us all. On environmental issues, for example, this means that people of color are impacted by toxic pollution more than White people, leading to health inequities on everything from cancer rates to initial COVID rates. Robert Cox and I call this pattern the "cruel irony" of the climate crisis: those who impact the climate the least are impacted first and worst. Improving environmental and climate conditions, then, requires not only sciences of ecology and public health but also addressing systemic injustices—whose voices are heard in decision-making and whose voices are marginalized or dismissed? From this perspective, environmental racism is vital to addressing public health.

I follow the environmental justice movement's broad definition of the environment as where we live, work, play, and pray. The environment is everywhere and includes you and me; it is a dangerous myth to believe we somehow live separately.

Since scientists used to balk at the term "justice," which was imagined as a political term, I did not always identify as doing health research. But, since health inequities are now more accepted as a pattern globally, it's important to appreciate how justice matters to public health, including procedural justice (how we make decisions) and distributive justice (who is impacted by decisions). Some in the movement say if you don't have a seat at the table, you're likely to end up being what's served as a sacrifice on the table. It is important to have those impacted most by decisions involved so that experiential or everyday ways of knowing can help co-create the most effective and meaningful changes.

2. How have theory and praxis centered and engaged social justice activism principles in action in your research?

That's a big question! Praxis, the intersection of theory and embodied practice, is the only way I believe research can be ethical and realized. That means research is not just about products, but relationships. So, for example, this week, I am in dialogue with people in the community I wrote about for my master's thesis (in Warren County, North Carolina, United States), with colleagues on how to support communities engaged in my dissertation (in southern Louisiana, United States), as well as with people I plan to interview on my podcast for my forthcoming book (in Nakuru, Kenya). Relations may go dormant at times, but one's obligations should exceed the research product initially produced. Working with communities, I also deeply believe we need to resist the deficit model of communication in which people falsely assume those impacted the most do not have solutions. For example, last spring, my environmental justice graduate class partnered with the state I live in to co-produce StoryMaps of the communities most impacted by environmental inequities. Each story was required (by me) to begin with what one might love about living in one of those communities: why are they attached and do not move away? And then, also, we try to feature what they think are their biggest challenges and possibilities. The Ute Mountain Ute Tribe, for example, are highlighted for their ongoing traditional land relations, as well as their efforts to address water contamination and intensifying drought conditions. Sometimes, I write for academic audiences, but I also value thinking about how I can make a positive difference for nonacademics with whom I work.

3. Can you share some thoughts on how your scholarship might address some of the climate change and environmental challenges we face today? How do you see their relationship with health evolving in the coming years? What might be some of the most significant challenges we will need to address? How might your scholarship provide a productive avenue for thinking about those challenges and shaping our response to them?

COVID was a mass public health event that I hope has made everyone more aware of how we're interconnected to nonhuman diseases and global flows, as well as how we can make drastic cultural changes if we want to prevent disease and death. It also revealed that we're not all in agreement that we have an obligation to care about everyone; clearly, the wealthy survived COVID quite differently than essential food workers, for example, in fields, factories, transportation, and grocery stores. So, we will need to address inequities in health messaging and access to medical treatment (like vaccines, tests, and masks).

Some of my research is about the movement for a just transition, which is the shift from a fossil fuel-based economy to a renewable one in a way that centers social and environmental justice. COVID reminded us that labor is a major part of health and environmental stories: who has to work and who does not? How [does] labor shift with remote access for some? Mental health issues were exacerbated for many with remote modes of communication, while many of those with physical disabilities found the embracing of remote access to be long overdue. I was on a panel last year with an organizer from Bangladesh who said they are rethinking the agricultural schedule to begin earlier to avoid the hottest part of the day. They showed how farmworkers are less productive—and less safe—in extreme heat to argue for this transition in how we think of the workday.

My own research tries to help make connections between social inequities and unsustainable environmental decision-making, as well as to help build the capacity and platforms of those most marginalized by dominant decision-makers. My forthcoming book, for example, focuses on public debates about plastics. In the Global North, we tend to hear of single-use plastics as an elite concern of White people worried about turtles (which, to be clear, I think we should care about the fate of turtles) focusing on individual consumption, yet in the Global South, plastics have been a life and death issue warranting systemic transformations. Bangladesh was the first nation to ban single-use plastic bags because they were clogging the drainage during floods that have gotten worse due to the climate crisis; further, banning them enabled a local economy for jute bags to become revitalized. Plastics are toxic throughout their life cycle, including extraction, production, transportation, consumption, and disposal. They have been detected in human blood and lungs—all of us are becoming more plastic. Yet, while transnational corporations profit off this cheap material, the health of everyday people and the more-than-human world pay the cost.

4. Can you give an example of how a project from your scholarship that means a lot to you personally illustrates the transformative potential between communication, environment, and health?

Perhaps the most obvious example of how I realized my scholarship could matter is the first time I thought it made a difference, which was with my master's research. Warren County, North Carolina, is known as the symbolic birthplace of the environmental justice movement. In 1982, African American civil rights leader Dr. Benjamin Chavis coined the phrase "environmental racism" during protests against a PCB (polychlorinated biphenyl) landfill. When I went to graduate school in the 1990s, this community was revered in many articles and books for its pivotal role. Imagine my shock then to discover that the landfill was still there. The community was engaging in a process to clean up the landfill with the state, NGOs, and scientists. When it was time to lobby the state government, I suggested the framing for the messages and created a pamphlet that was used by residents. The governor ultimately granted US$2.1 million to detoxify the landfill. My role was small, mostly I listened and learned from them, but it helped me realize that studying stories can have a profound impact in the world outside of books.

*Equity in Environmental Communication*

Environmental communication aims to address equity in WPHC outcomes by envisioning "a community empowered to become advocates for improving communication within health and environmental contexts" (Center for Health and Environmental Communication (CHEC), 2022). Some questions examined by environmental communication scholars include: "how do human agents represent nature/environment?; what accounts for the development and reproduction of dominant systems of representation or discourses of 'environment'; what communicative practices contribute to the interruption, dilution, or transformation of such discourses? and how do local or indigenous cultures understand 'nature' or 'environment'" (Hansen & Cox, 2015, pp. 15–16).

*Look at **Textbox 8.7** for an illustration of the human health impacts of climate change through the lens of climate elements such as air quality and how the presence of particulate matter (PM) affects daily life. Attempt the SJA prompt that follows.*

---

**Textbox 8.7   Healthy Communities and the Human Health Impacts of Climate Change**

**WPHC Context**

Climate change research suggests that New York and Milwaukee may have three times their current average number of days that are hotter than 90 degrees Fahrenheit (Patz et al., 2014). High temperatures are also associated with high ozone days. Adverse health impacts of climate change health-related disorders include respiratory disorders such as asthma and infectious diseases, food insecurity stemming from increased plant diseases and reduced crop yields, mental health disorders such as posttraumatic stress disorder (PTSD), depression, and reduced work capacity increasing air pollution also has a negative impact on climate change, and thus on public and individual health. PM, which are particles of variable but very small diameter, penetrates the respiratory system via inhalation and causes respiratory and cardiovascular diseases. These diseases include reproductive and central nervous system dysfunctions and cancer (Manisalidis et al., 2020).

### SJA Action Prompt: Gathering and Communicating Climate Stories as Advocacy

Climate change is a local, regional, national, and global issue that illustrates how every component must be healthy for the whole to be healthy and resilient. Browse the following resources to see how climate change communication is enacted at local and global levels.

- What are some common themes shared in the local and global stories that stand out to you?

Healthy communities are characterized by strong relationships among members and stakeholders. Talk about climate change issues with members from different segments of your community. These could include diverse neighborhoods, city public health staff working on issues like environmental justice and air quality, farmers, local businesses, healthcare professionals, and community advocates.

- What are the themes that emerge from the stories in your neighborhoods?
- How is climate change impacting your community?
- What steps can your community take to mitigate and adapt to changing climate in your neighborhoods?

### Resources

Center for Climate Change & Health. (2020). Retrieved from https://climatehealthconnect.org/solutions/stories-from-the-field/

The World Bank (WB) (2022). *Stepping up climate action*. Retrieved from https://www.world bank.org/en/what-we-do/climate-stories-project

*Environmental Communication and Climate Change Communication*

Environmental communication includes climate change communication through messages that frame how climate phenomena are understood and how these messages can guide action. It also includes sustainability science, which focuses on the management of human-environment systems to help meet human needs while protecting ecosystem and environmental integrity. Finally, it centers how the environment is depicted in images and visual means to show nature and its relationship with human beings (Hansen & Cox, 2015; Lindenfeld et al., 2012).

Environmental health communication directs attention to environmental concerns and their health consequences. Environmental concerns become an issue of environmental justice when they place an unfair burden on minority and disadvantaged communities. Environmental health communication is thus concerned with (a) empowering vulnerable community members to address environmental and health concerns, and (b) communication that bridges the gap between experts and nonexperts, clients and providers, community members and decision-makers, and between communities (CHEC, 2022).

*Table 8.3 provides some examples of the agencies, organizations, and networks that are working to address environment-related inequities and disparities. Attempt the SJA prompts provided in the right-hand side column.*

*Table 8.3* Environment Justice Activism

| WPHC Context: Agency/Organization/Network | SJA Food for Thought: What Can I Do? |
|---|---|
| **National Institute of Environmental Health Sciences (NIEHS)**:<br>Reducing environmental health disparities and improving health and well-being by addressing the environmental factors that can lead to disease and health disparities when the places where people live, work, learn, and play are burdened by social inequities. | Browse the "Newsletters" section on the NIEHS website (use the URL in the Resources section). You will notice a range of topics from "Women's Health Awareness" to "Global Environmental Health."<br><br>**SJA Prompt**:<br>How can you make a difference in your local community? Try this activity:<br>1. Identify one vulnerable population in your local community.<br>2. Next, do some library research on the health disparities that are faced by the vulnerable population.<br>3. Third, see if you can speak with some of the members of the community and understand their health concerns.<br>4. Fourth, using the research-based knowledge and your community-based knowledge, discuss with your community members some steps that can help address their health challenges.<br>5. Finally, incorporate your work in a newsletter that is tailored to the community, integrate community voices, and disseminate it with the community members. |
| **The Centers of Excellence on Environmental Health Disparities Research (EHD) program**:<br>Focus on understanding and reducing or eliminating environmental health disparities, defined as inequities in population health stemming from disproportionate adverse exposures associated with the physical, chemical, social, and built environments. | **Community engagement**, research, and capacity building are important components for addressing **environmental health disparities**.<br><br>**SJA Prompt**:<br>1. Can you identify neighborhoods in your city that are exposed to dirty water or air, are a "food desert," lack green space in neighborhoods, or are near toxic metals and chemical pollutants?<br>2. Can you document these instances based on social (income, race, ethnicity) or geographic factors characterizing those communities?<br>3. What do the findings from your mini-field research tell you? |
| **US Environmental Protection Agency (EPA)**:<br>Seeks to protect human health and the environment through initiatives such as attending to clean air, land, and water access; reducing environmental risks; access to accurate information; and cleanup of contaminated lands and toxic sites, among others. | **SJA Prompt**:<br>1. Browse the resources under "key topics" on EPA's website.<br>2. Check out the "air quality" tab and enter your zip code (see URL for *AirNow* in the Resources section).<br>3. What is the air quality data where you live like over one week?<br>4. Does it vary by time of day or the weather?<br>5. Try to enter a different zip code, perhaps of a city with a lower or median household income (see under "income and poverty" tab) or race (see under "race and Hispanic origin" tab), based on US census data (see URL in the Resources section).<br>6. Do you notice any differences? |

(Continued)

*Table 8.3* (Continued) Environment Justice Activism

| WPHC Context: Agency/Organization/ Network | SJA Food for Thought: What Can I Do? |
|---|---|
| **The International Environmental Communication Association (IECA):** <br><br> A professional that seeks to foster effective and inspiring communication that alleviates environmental issues and conflicts and solves the problems that cause them. | The IECA offers courses, sponsors conferences, and empowers people to engage in inclusive environmental communication research, practice, arts, and activism that "deal with the diversity of voices that raise concerns about our planet." <br><br> **SJA Prompt:** <br><br> 1. In what ways does the theme emphasize the "need to reconcile the many injustices of the past and present in order to move forward and create narratives about just and sustainable futures" (URL in the Resources section)? |

## Resources

AirNow. Retrieved from https://www.airnow.gov/
The Centers of Excellence on Environmental Health Disparities Research (EHD). Retrieved from https://www.niehs.nih.gov/research/supported/centers/ehd/index.cfm
The International Environmental Communication Association. Retrieved from https://theieca.org/
National Institute of Environmental Health Sciences (NIEHS). Retrieved from https://www.niehs.nih.gov/
US Environmental Protection Agency (EPA). Retrieved from https://www.epa.gov/
US Census Bureau. Retrieved from https://www.census.gov/quickfacts/fact/table/salisburycitymaryland,US/PST045221

### Communities and Environmental Justice

Meaningful change is possible when communities are actively engaged in all stages of the research, dissemination, and evaluation and when community members are engaged in designing locally owned and shared solutions. For instance, Sarah De Los Santos Upton and colleagues illustrate the rhetorical strategies employed by *Familias Unidas*, a community organization in El Paso, Texas, that works to increase awareness around the issues of education, environmental racism, and public health in the borderlands by connecting school closures to coalitional struggles concerning the environment, citizenship, race/ethnicity, language, and class. *Familias Unidas* does this by employing the strategies of *familia*, *communidad*, and *(in)justicia* (de los Santos Upton et al., 2022).

### Environmental Health Politics

Adopting a critical and feminist communication lens, communication scholar Heather Zoller examines the intersection of women's health, the environment, and corporate activism (Zoller, 2016). She looks at how resistance to dominant power relationships can give rise to individual, collective, and covert forms of resistance. Zoller describes how environmental health politics has been shaped by historical and binary constructions of gender that emphasize the woman's primary role as a caretaker of the health of children and family members. Like Upton and colleagues, Zoller also highlights the relationship between economic and racial inequities, noting that women and minorities are more susceptible to exposure to environmental toxins.

[*Look at the organizations provided under Additional Resources. Which SJA communicative tactics employed by the organizations for environmental justice and health can you identify?*]

The goal of creating healthy, sustainable, and equitable communities highlights the relationship of environmental justice with the SDoH, including housing, environment, transportation, and health issues (Birnbaum et al., 2009). Even as SDoH shapes exposure to environmental health risks, the WPHC perspective emphasizes how ecosystem health, ecology, and individual health are intertwined with food availability, produce available at local grocery stores and farmers' markets, and ultimately, with individual health. The next section explains ecosystem health and individual health through the lens of ecological frameworks of health. These models, espoused by the *One Health, One World* concept, are central to human health and health promotion and to food availability and practices.

*Check out the **Mini-Case Study in Textbox 8.8** on the obesity epidemic in people and pets. What can you do to improve the health of your family and friends and the animals with whom you share your life? Attempt the SJA activity that follows.*

---

**Textbox 8.8    Mini-Case Study**

**Obesity in People and Pets: Walking Your Pet for Better Health for People and Their Pets**

*WPHC Context*

In the article "One Health: It's for All of Us" (see URL in the Resources section), the Food and Drug Administration (FDA) describes how the public health epidemic of obesity negatively affects both people and animals. The One Health approach states that the "health of people, animals, and the environment is intertwined" (WHO, 2019). The instance of zoonotic diseases, such as influenza, West Nile virus, rabies, Lyme disease, and emerging coronaviruses are among the zoonotic diseases of most concern in the United States at present (CDC, 2019). One Health centers interconnectedness and interdependency (see URL in the Resources section for the mission statement). It highlights how the health of different species of plants and animals, and the abiotic environment, can negatively affect the health of human beings and vice versa. As an example of this interdependency, the World Small Animal Veterinary Association (WSAVA) One Health Committee looks at the human-animal bond and its benefits to health and comparative medicine.

Obesity is a complex medical condition that affects a variety of species. Over 71% of Americans are overweight or obese. Over 56% of dogs and 60% of cats are overweight or obese. Horses are also at risk for obesity. It involves multiple factors, including genetic and environmental risk factors, physical activity, stress levels, and lifestyle behaviors (Office of the Surgeon General, 2001).

Like people, obese pets are also at risk for concerns related to obesity such as orthopedic problems; laminitis, or founder (in horses); diabetes (in cats); and a host of other conditions. Given the parallels in the causes and management of obesity in humans and pets (healthy diet, calorie restriction, regular exercise), the human-animal bond can be a mutual positive motivator for a healthy lifestyle. Studies show having a pet and engaging in activities like walking a dog can prevent several obesity-related disorders in both the human and the dog (e.g., Westgarth et al., 2014).

Moving away from a human-centric perspective to a two-way approach to **One Health** can benefit humans, animals, plants, and the planet. This case illustrates a central premise of One Health.

### SJA Activity

For this exercise, consider your own pets, or, if you don't have one, then your friends and family members' pets. Alternatively, you could select an image or instance of a family or human-pet relationship from the media such as magazines, a movie, or a TV series.

1. How do you maintain a healthy weight for your pet? For example, your list could include items like a healthy diet, exercise, a loving and stress-free environment, and appropriate climate factors.
2. What kinds of activities do you and your pet share?
3. In what ways does your pet companion support your health? In what ways does your companionship support your pet's health?

### Resources

CDC. (2019, May 6). *8 zoonotic diseases shared between animals and people of most concern in the U.S.: First-ever CDC, USDA, doi collaborative report lists top-priority zoonoses for U.S.* https://www.cdc.gov/media/releases/2019/s0506-zoonotic-diseasesshared.html#:~:text=Salmonellosis,and%20Middle%20East%20respiratory%20syndrome

Food and Drug Administration (FDA). *One health: It's for all of us.* https://www.fda.gov/animal-veterinary/animal-health-literacy/one-health-its-all-us

Office of the Surgeon General (US). (2001). *The surgeon general's call to action to prevent and decrease overweight and obesity.* Rockville, MD. https://www.ncbi.nlm.nih.gov/books/NBK44210/

One Health Initiative. (2022). *Mission statement.* https://onehealthinitiative.com/missionstatement/

One Health Commission. (2022). *What is One Health?* https://www.onehealthcommission.org/en/why_one_health/what_is_one_health/

Westgarth, C., Christley, R. M., & Christian, H. E. (2014). How might we increase physical activity through dog walking?: A comprehensive review of dog walking correlates. *BMC International Journal of Behavioral Nutrition and Physical Activity*, *11*, 83. https://doi.org/10.1186/1479-5868-11-83

World Small Animal Veterinary Association (WSAVA). (2022). *One Health committee.* https://wsava.org/Committees/one-health-committee/

## Ecosystem Health and Individual Health

### Ecosystem Health

An ecosystem is a system consisting of biotic (all the living things) and abiotic (all the nonliving things) components that function together as a unit. Thus, an ecosystem is an ecological community of different populations of organisms that live together in a particular habitat

(National Geographic, 2022). Ecology is the interaction between populations or organisms and the environment and can be examined at the level of an individual, a population, a community, or an ecosystem. At the level of an individual, ecology is concerned with the individual organism's physiology, reproduction, and overall development. At the level of the population, ecology deals primarily with the attributes and factors affecting the population. At the level of the community, ecology examines the interactions between populations and community patterns. At the level of an ecosystem, ecology puts all the aforementioned elements together to understand how the system operates as a unit.

*Textbox 8.9 provides an instance of how human health is related to ecosystem health and the public health risks of biodiversity loss. Attempt the SJA that follows.*

---

### Textbox 8.9   Biodiversity, Ecosystem Health, and a WPHC View of Health

#### WPHC Context

Human health and well-being are dependent upon the clean air and water, food, nutrients, medicines, energy, and the physical, cultural, and spiritual enrichment that access to green spaces, biodiversity, and ecosystems provides. The vision of the 2050 WHO Strategic Plan for Biodiversity states, "Biodiversity is valued, conserved, restored, and wisely used, maintaining ecosystem services, sustaining a healthy planet and delivering benefits essential for all people" (WHO, 2015). The Millennium Ecosystem Assessment (2005) lays out how ecosystem health contributes to human well-being through sustainable ecosystem conditions for human health (Millennium Ecosystem Assessment, 2005). In line with the WPHC perspective, a broader view of health goes beyond a human-only context to health that encompasses other species, ecosystems, and the ecological underpinnings of the drivers and protectors of health risks.

Protecting public health from the risks of biodiversity loss requires health professionals to work collaboratively with interdisciplinary scientists, conservationists, and those engaged in the sustainable management of natural resources. Transformative change deriving from knowledge of these interrelationships can help achieve food security, biodiversity protection, and climate change mitigation goals.

#### SJA Action Prompt: Becoming a Biodiversity and Health Advocate

Here are two of the nine strategies for health and biodiversity promoted in the report:

a.   Promoting the health benefits provided by biodiversity for food security and nutrition, clean air and water, traditional medicine and pharmaceuticals, and mental, physical, cultural, and spiritual well-being.
b.   Educating, engaging, and mobilizing the public and the health sector, including organizations and associations, to serve as advocates for sustainable management of ecosystems, to articulate the linkage between the ecosystem elements and human health, and to highlight the benefits that sustainable ecosystem management provides to the social and economic health of communities.

Consult the WHO report in the Resources section.

- Identify your local biodiversity elements including different plant and animal species, microbes, ecosystems, and human communities.
- What does each contribute to human health and well-being? How are they interdependent upon each other?
- Identify one way that they sustain the health of a vulnerable population in your community.
- Identify key stakeholders from the community who can help make a difference.
- Make a communication plan that informs and persuades one stakeholder group to help act in support of the biodiversity and health goals that you have researched.

## Resources

Millennium Ecosystem Assessment (2005). *Ecosystems and Human Well-being: Synthesis*. Washington, DC: Island Press.

WHO. (2015). *Connecting global priorities: Biodiversity and human health: A state of knowledge review*. https://www.who.int/publications/i/item/connecting-global-priorities-biodiversity-and-human-health

### Ecosystem Integrity

Ecosystem integrity is "the state or condition of an ecosystem that displays the biodiversity characteristic of the reference, such as species composition and community structure, and is fully capable of sustaining normal ecosystem functioning" (Jones, 2013). An ecosystem has ecosystem integrity when it is stable, in equilibrium, and in its "natural" state, with a capacity to cope with human (anthropogenic) interference. Ecosystem health references the link between ecosystems, human activity, and human health.

### Ecological Frameworks of Health

Human health is co-dependent upon ecological factors in a complex relationship with other organisms comprising the ecosystem and the environment (Alice, 2017). Recently, much attention has been paid to how health threats from human-animal-ecosystems interface (HAEI) and zoonotic diseases (zoonoses) pose an increasing risk to public health. Ecological frameworks of health are premised on the assumption that human health and its determinants are interrelated. An ecological public health model attempts to consider these multiple influences on health arising at the intersection of the ecological determinants. The public health framework of eco-epidemiology is grounded in the principle of ecologism emphasizing the complex interactions between human beings, an agent (e.g., domestic animals, poultry, wildlife), and the environment. This principle expands the disease-centric biomedical model to underline the paradigm shift toward "One Health" (Bousfield & Brown, 2011, p. 2).

### MINORITY AND MARGINALIZED POPULATIONS

Attending to ecosystem health as closely associated with human health has benefits for the well-being and health outcomes of minority and marginalized populations. For instance, in their study, Thurston and Vissandjée (2005) discuss how, in combination with gender and culture, the migratory experience is central to the ecological model of health. Reining et al. (2021) find overall beneficial restorative outcomes across all ecosystem types, with greater benefits for women than men with ecosystem quality (e.g., species richness, naturalness, and ecological integrity) having the greatest positive impact on restorative outcomes. Their study furthers the attention to the nuanced relationship between human health and well-being outcomes and exposure to diverse ecosystems.

## ECOLOGICAL MODEL OF HEALTH BEHAVIOR AND PROMOTION

Ecological models of health behavior and promotion build on the premise that behavior is influenced by intrapersonal (biological, psychological)-, interpersonal (social, cultural)-, organizational-, community-, physical-, environmental-, and policy-level factors. Their goal is to help develop comprehensive intervention approaches that systematically target mechanisms of change at each level of influence (Owen & Fisher, 2008). The ecological models of health recognize the importance of attending to social, environmental, and biological factors together in considering their influence on health (Richard et al., 2010). Such models center the ecology in the understanding of the relationship between health and disease.

*As we wrap up* **Chapter 8, Health and the Environment**, *consider the SJA prompt provided in* **Textbox 8.10**. *Consider how your actions can intervene in this complex web of relationships influencing human health from a WPHC perspective.*

---

**Textbox 8.10    Discussion Questions/Thought Scenarios for Reflection**

**Eating Local, Local Food Systems, and Production Supply Chains**

*WPHC Thought Scenario*

Eating local is a popular theme today. Local food systems are foods that are "produced, processed, and retailed within a geographical area" (Kneafsey et al., 2013). The local is the smallest unit used to describe the origin of food, one where the consumer is familiar with the place where the food is produced. Local producers are also more likely to use sustainable and pesticide-free modes of production. Eating local draws upon local food systems and short supply chains. However, although buying local produce can benefit the health of the environment and human health, studies show that local food systems cannot by themselves ensure food security. For instance, research shows that less than one-third of the global population would be capable of meetings its food demand from local crop production.

At the present time, only about 400 million people worldwide live in an area where enough varieties of the food groups are produced locally to sustain the community's existing dietary compositions. The produce at the grocery store sometimes travels more than 1,500 miles to reach local communities, often leading to significant food waste. Buying local can reduce the environmental impact of the food by cutting down on fuel consumption, air pollution, use of shipping facilities, packing facilities, and refrigeration.

### SJA Discussion Question

Decisions regarding navigating the environmental, social, economic, and WPHC impacts of our dietary choices are complex.

   i. How much of your daily dietary composition is locally sourced?
   ii. Do you know the local farms where your grocery store purchases its produce?
   iii. Where do the farmers in your local farmers market come from?
   iv. What proportion of your daily diet is composed of commercial or prepackaged foods and food products?

### Inspirational Example

*Food Recovery Network* mobilizes college volunteers to donate surplus food to surrounding local communities. Check out their website and other nonprofit organizations working in the food sustainability domain in Textbox 8.5.

### Resources

Dutta, M.J. (2008). *Communicating health: A culture-centered approach.* Cambridge, UK: Polity Press.
Kneafsey, M., Venn, L., Schmutz, U. Balázs, B., Trenchard, L., Eyden-Wood, T., … Blackett, M. (2013). Short food supply chains and local food systems in the EU: A state of play of their socio-economic characteristics. In Gomez y Paloma, S., & Santini, F. (Eds.), *Joint Research Center, Institute for Prospective Technological Studies*, Publications Office. https://data.europa.eu/doi/10.2791/88784

### References

Alice, M. L. Li (2017). Ecological determinants of health: Food and environment on human health. *Environmental Science and Pollution Research International, 24*(10), 9002–9015. https://doi.org/10.1007/s11356-015-5707-9
Birnbaum, L. S., Zenick, H., & Branche, C. M. (2009). Environmental justice: A continuing commitment to an evolving concept. *American Journal of Public Health, 99*(Suppl 3), S487–S489. https://doi.org/10.2105/AJPH.2009.179010
Bousfield, B., & Brown, R. (2011). One world one health. *Veterinary Bulletin of Agriculture, Fish Conservation Department Newsletter, 1*(7), 1–12.
Chad, R. (2019). Engaged communication scholarship for environmental justice: A research agenda. *Environmental Communication, 13*(8), 1087–1107. https://doi.org/10.1080/17524032.2019.1591478
Center for Health and Environmental Communication (CHEC). (2022). James Madison University. CHEC: Mission and vision. https://www.jmu.edu/chec/about_chec_mission.shtml
Cox, R., & Pezzullo, P. C. (2016). *Environmental communication and the public sphere.* SAGE Publications.
De Los Santos Upton, S., Tarin, C. A., & Hernández, L. H. (2022). Construyendo Conexiones Para Los Niños: Environmental justice, reproductive feminicidio, and coalitional possibility in the Borderlands. *Health Communication, 37*(9), 1242–1252. https://doi.org/10.1080/10410236.2021.1911386
Hansen, A., & Cox, R. (2015). *The Routledge handbook of environment and communication.* Routledge.

Jones, H. P. (2013). Impact of ecological restoration on ecosystem services. *Encyclopedia of Biodiversity*, 199–208. https://doi.org/10.1016/B978-0-12-384719-5.00326-9

Kuhnlein, H. V. (2014). Food system sustainability for health and well-being of Indigenous Peoples. *Public Health Nutrition*, *18*(3), 2415–2424. https://doi.org/10.1017/S1368980014002961

Kwak, R., Kamal, K., Charrow, A., & Khalifian, S. (2021). Mass migration and climate change: Dermatologic manifestations. *International Journal of Women's Dermatology*, *7*(1), 98–106. https://doi.org/10.1016/j.ijwd.2020.07.014

Liang, S. Y., & Messenger, N. (2018). Infectious diseases after hydrologic disasters. *Emergency Medicine Clinics of North America*, *36*(4), 835–851. https://doi.org/10.1016/j.emc.2018.07.002

Lindenfeld, L. A., Hall, D. M., McGreavy, D. M., Silka, L., & Hart, D. (2012). Creating a place for environmental communication research in sustainability science. *Environmental Communication*, *6*(1), 23–43. https://doi.org/10.1080/17524032.2011.640702

Manisalidis, I., Stavropoulou, E., Stavropoulos, A., & Bezirtzoglou, E. (2020). Environmental and health impacts of air pollution: A review. *Frontiers in Public Health*, *8*(14). https://doi.org/10.3389/fpubh.2020.00014

Millennium Ecosystem Assessment. (2005). https://www.millenniumassessment.org/en/index.html

Mozaffarian, D., Fleischhacker, S., & Andrés, J. R. (2021). Prioritizing nutrition security in the U.S. *JAMA*, *325*(16), 1605–1606. https://doi.org/10.1001/jama.2021.1915

National Aeronautics and Space Agency (NASA). (2005, February 1). NASA–What's the difference between weather and climate? https://www.nasa.gov/mission_pages/noaa-n/climate/climate_weather.html

National Center for Complementary and Integrative Health. (NCCIH). (2023). *NCCIH strategic plan FY 2021–2025*. Retrieved from https://www.nccih.nih.gov/about/nccih-strategic-plan-2021-2025

National Geographic. (2022). *Ecosystem. Encyclopedic Entry*. https://education.nationalgeographic.org/resource/ecosystem

Nemec, K. (2020). Cultural awareness of eating patterns in the healthcare setting. *Clinical Liver Disorders*, *16*(5), 204–207. https://doi.org/10.1002/cld.1019

Nordström, K., Coff, C., Jönsson, H., Nordenfelt, L., & Görman, U. (2013). Food and health: Individual, cultural, or scientific matters? *Genes and Nutrition*, *8*(4), 357–363. https://doi.org/10.1007/s12263-013-03368

Owen, J. F. S. N., & Fisher, E. B. (2008). Ecological models of health behavior. In Glanz, K., & Rimer, B. K. (Eds.), *Health behavior and health education: Theory, research and practice*. https://www.med.upenn.edu/hbhe4/part5-ch20.shtml

Patz, J. A., Frumkin, H., Holloway, T., Vimont, D. J., & Haines, A. (2014). Climate change: Challenges and opportunities for global health. *JAMA*, *312*(15), 1565–1580. https://doi.org/10.1001/jama.2014.13186

Paul, C. J., Paul, J. E., & Anderson, R. S. (2019). The local food environment and food security: The health behavior role of social capital. *International Journal of Environmental Research and Public Health*, *16*(24), 5045. https://doi.org/10.3390/ijerph16245045

Ramadurai, V., Sharf, B. F., & Sharkey, J. R. (2012). Rural food insecurity in the United States as an overlooked site of struggle in health communication. *Health Communication*, *27*(8), 794–805. https://doi.org/10.1080/10410236.2011.647620

Reining, C. E., Lemieux, C. J., & Doherty, S. T. (2021). Linking restorative human health outcomes to protected area ecosystem diversity and integrity. *Journal of Environmental Planning and Management*, *64*(13), 2300–2325. https://doi.org/10.1080/09640568.2020.1857227

Richard, L., Gauvin, L., & Raine, K. (2010). Ecological models revisited: Their uses and evolution in health promotion over two decades. *Annual Review of Public Health*, *32*, 307–326. https://doi.org/10.1146/annurev-publhealth-031210-101141

Stoddart, M. C. J., Ramos, H., Foster, K., & Ylä-Anttila, T. (2021). Competing crises? Media coverage and framing of climate change during the COVID-19 pandemic. *Environmental Communication*. https://doi.org/10.1080/17524032.2021.1969978

The EAT-Lancet Commission 2.0: Securing a just transition to healthy, environmentally sustainable diets for all. (2023). *The Lancet, 402*(10399), 352–354.

The IPCC Sixth Assessment Report. (n.d.) *Climate change 2021: The physical science basis*. https://www.ipcc.ch/report/ar6/wg1/#outreach

IPCC. (2021). *Special report on climate change and land: Chapter 5, Food security*. https://www.ipcc.ch/srccl/chapter/chapter-5/

The Lancet Microbe (2021, September 01). *Editorial. Climate change: Fires, floods, and infectious diseases, 2*(9), E415. https://doi.org/10.1016/S2666-5247(21)00220-2

The World Bank. (2021, September 13). *Climate change could force 216 million people to migrate within their own countries by 2050. Groundswell Part 2: Acting on internal climate migration*. https://www.worldbank.org/en/news/press-release/2021/09/13/climate-change-could-force-216-million-people-to-migrate-within-their-own-countries-by-2050

Thurston, W. E., & Vissandjée, B. (2005). An ecological model for understanding culture as a determinant of women's health. *Critical Public Health, 15*(3), 229–242. https://doi.org/10.1080/09581590500372121

United States Agency for International Development (USAID). (2022, February 03). *Agriculture and food security*. https://www.usaid.gov/what-we-do/agriculture-and-food-security

United States Department of Agriculture (USDA). (2022). *Culture and food*. https://www.nutrition.gov/topics/shopping-cooking-and-meal-planning/culture-and-food

United States Environmental Protection Agency (EPA). (2022). *Environmental justice in your community*. https://www.epa.gov/environmentaljustice/environmental-justice-your-community

United States Global Change Research Program (USGCRP). (2022). *About USGCRP*. https://www.globalchange.gov/about

World Food Program. (2023). *A global food crisis: 2023–another year of extreme jeopardy for those struggling to feed their families*. Retrieved January 20, 2023, from https://www.wfp.org/global-hunger-crisis

World Health Organization (WHO). (2019). *One Health*. https://www.who.int/health-topics/one-health#tab=tab_1

Zhang, R., Tang, X., Liu, J., Visbeck, M., Guo, H., Murray, V. … Zhou, L. (2022). From concept to action: A united, holistic, and One Health approach to respond to the climate change crisis. *Infectious Diseases of Poverty, 11*, 17. https://doi.org/10.1186/s40249-022-00941-9

Zoller, H. (2016). Women's health activism targeting corporate health risks: Women's voices for the Earth. *Women & Language, 39*(1), 97–119.

## SJA Resources

Advocacy and Action Organizations for Social Change
    Learn more about the following organizations. *How can you further the work done in these domains?*

United Nations. (UN). Sustainable Development Goals (SDG). https://www.un.org/sustainable development/

Intersectional Environmentalist. https://www.intersectionalenvironmentalist.com/

Indigenous Environmental Network. https://www.ienearth.org/

350. https://350.org/

RAVEN Trust. https://raventrust.com/

Black Millennials for Flint. https://www.blackmillennials4flint.org/

Center on Race, Poverty, and the CRPE Environment. https://crpe-ej.org/

New Communities Land Trust. https://www.newcommunitiesinc.com/

Teens for Food Justice. https://teensforfoodjustice.org/

Labor Network for Sustainability. https://www.labor4sustainability.org/

The Nuestra Tierra Conservation Project. https://www.nuestra-tierra.org/

Front and Centered. https://frontandcentered.org/about-us/
Sunrise Movement. https://www.sunrisemovement.org/
Karrkad Kanjdji Trust. https://www.kkt.org.au/
Union of Concerned Scientists. https://www.ucsusa.org/
Center for Diversity and the Environment. https://www.cdeinspires.org/
Just Food. https://www.justfood.org/
WE ACT for Environmental Justice. https://www.weact.org/
Louisiana Bucket Brigade. https://labucketbrigade.org/?fbclid=IwAR1mvYKmWeT4C2VHMmX-osvsc
    BFy6NLNYUmcfPgr20MlTi9WwD4MbnYpM5A
Environmental Justice Foundation. https://ejfoundation.org/
Global Green Grants Fund. https://www.greengrants.org/
Community to Community. https://www.foodjustice.org/mission

## Additional Resources

Berrang-Ford, L., Siesma, A. J., Callaghan, M., Minx, J. C., Scheelbeek, P. F. D., & Haddaway, N. R. …
    Dangour, A. D. (2021, August 01). Systematic mapping of global research on climate and health: A
    machine learning review. *The Lancet Planetary Health*, 5(8), E514–E525. https://doi.org/10.1016/
    S2542–5196(21)00179-0

Executive Order 12898—Federal actions to address environmental justice in minority populations
    and low-income populations. (1994). *Federal Register*. 59(32). [FR Citation 59 FR 7629]. https://www.
    epa.gov/laws-regulations/summary-executive-order-12898-federal-actions-address-environmental-
    justice

National Institute of Environmental Health Sciences (NIEHS). (2022). *Environmental health disparities
    and environmental justice*. https://www.niehs.nih.gov/research/supported/translational/justice/index.
    cfm

Wright, K. E., Lucero, J. E., Ferguson, J. K., Granner, M. L., Devereux, P. G., Pearson, J. L., & Crosbie,
    E. (2021). The impact that cultural food security has on identity and well-being in the second-generation
    U.S. American minority college students. *Food Security*, 13, 701–715. https://doi.org/10.1007/s12571-
    020-01140-w

# Technology and Health

DOI: 10.4324/9781003214472-12

## Chapter Learning Outcomes

Upon completing **Chapter 9**, **Technology and Health**, the student should be able to apply the WPHC SJA perspective to:

1. Define telehealth, telemedicine, telecare, and mhealth and identify the distinctions among them.
2. Identify the potential of wearable technologies in improving healthcare outcomes.
3. Describe the different ways the digital divide is evidenced in wearable device usage.
4. Describe how disparities in the implementation of high-risk medical devices are shaped by the process of FDA approval.
5. Identify the data privacy and security concerns influencing adoption in mhealth and wearable devices.
6. Explain how the digital divide is experienced in low-income, rural, and socially vulnerable populations.
7. Understand the significance of technology in healthcare as a super determinant of health.

## Consider the following context:

When Divya Goel, a 35-year-old woman who was deaf and blind in Orlando, Florida, was able to make two telemedicine doctors' appointments during the pandemic, she was both excited and relieved. However, her excitement soon turned to disappointment. Her telemedicine appointments were held without an interpreter. As a result, she was not confident she was able to fully understand the information provided by her doctors. Under federal law, it is the physician's responsibility to provide an interpreter. However, her doctors were not aware of this responsibility. When Goel's doctors told her she would have to get insurance to pay for an interpreter, she herself was not sure of her rights or aware if she was able to ensure her doctors provided an interpreter for their telemedicine calls with her.

(Weber, 2022, March 14)

Despite the availability of impressive technological advancements in healthcare, however, those who are most vulnerable, such as individuals who have a disability, often get left behind or receive subpar healthcare services. The reasons for such disparities are complex. Like Goel's physician, a Health Affairs study found that about 35 percent of physicians in the U.S. reported knowing nothing or little about their legal responsibilities for providing appropriate healthcare technology to meet the needs of their patients who were disabled, while another 71 percent reported an incorrect understanding about who determines reasonable accommodations. Yet another 20 percent of the responding physicians did not know who pays for these accommodations, and about 68 percent felt they were at risk for Americans with Disabilities Act (ADA) lawsuits.

(Iezzoni et al., 2022)

Technology has made great strides in improving quality of life outcomes, particularly for those individuals who have a disability. Telemedicine appointments can bring timely care to those who are unable to travel, are disabled, or located in underserved areas. Rehabilitative technologies, such as robotics, virtual reality, transcranial simulation, digital health, and mhealth, can help restore function in people who have developed a disability due to disease, injury, or aging. Assistive technologies, such as stair lifts, smart hearing aids, video conferencing tools, prostheses, and devices that support memory, can help people with disabilities live independently, care for themselves and their families, access information through computers, work, and participate fully in community life.

However, the data corroborates Goel's experience. Deaf and hard-of-hearing (DHH) American Sign Language (ASL) users experience significant mental health-related disparities compared with non-DHH English speakers. This is complicated by the low public awareness of the challenges faced by DHH ASL users in navigating everyday contexts and technology. In fact, 41% of mental health facilities and 59% of substance use treatment facilities receiving public funds in 2019 reported not providing services in sign language (James et al., 2022). Thus, they are not in compliance with the ACA section 1557, which requires healthcare facilities receiving government funds to provide effective communication access, such as a sign language interpreter, to DHH patients.

The ADA was enacted in 1990. However, in the past few decades since its enactment, people with disabilities continue to experience healthcare disparities. In 2021, at-home Covid-19 tests helped people with the transition to normal activities. However, those who are blind or have limited vision were not able to read the small print on the instructions for at-home Covid-19 tests or see the results that allowed reentry into society during the post-pandemic phase. The American Council of the Blind engaged in litigation with the two dominant medical testing companies, LabCorp and Quest Diagnostics over touch-screen check-in kiosks at their testing locations (Department of Justice, DOJ, 2022). After a Kaiser Health News

(KHN) investigation in 2020 found that government vaccine registration websites were also inaccessible to the blind, the Department of Justice (DOJ) reached agreements with five New York state and local government agencies and settlements with Rite Aid, Hy-Vee, Kroger, and Meijer to ensure accessible registration for vaccination appointments and to correct such issues.

(DOJ, 2021)

## Chapter Organization

**Chapter 9, Technology and Health**, is organized as follows: the **first** section presents an overview of telehealth, telemedicine, telecare, and mhealth with a discussion of the health applications in each domain, their advantages and barriers, and the distinctions between each. This is followed in the **second** section by an in-depth look at the wearables devices industry with particular attention paid to their use by low-income and minority populations, racial biases, and the use of mobile health applications. The second section situates the wearables industry within overall connectivity and mobile trends and the Internet of Things (IoT). The barriers to adoption are covered with a focus on chronic disease management and the integration of artificial intelligence (AI) into wearable devices. Sources of disparities for people of color are presented with particular attention to the implementation of innovative technologies through the FDA approval process. The **third** section covers data privacy and security concerns through a focus on mobile devices, personal health information breeches, and privacy awareness with respect to third-party operators, and associated challenges to the wearables industry. The **fourth** section provides an overview of the digital divide and its implications through the lens of equitable access to telehealth and its adoption in underserved communities, technology as a "super" determinant of health, barriers to telehealth adoption, digitally disconnected neighborhoods, and digital health equity. The WPHC SJA approach is integrated through the chapter with respect to use, application, adoption, and health implications of these domains and their implications for low-income, rural, and socially vulnerable populations. Students are engaged to apply the themes through a range of WPHC prompts and SJA activities such as Project ECHO, telehealthcare options, and Connect2Health. Textboxes, discussion questions, thought scenarios, and present challenges and future directions exercises provide students with actionable information on statistics pertaining to social media, digital divide, and health and themes related to digital disparities and SDoH with SJA prompts encouraging students to think about actionable steps to address disparities. The communication scholar interview with Dr. Sahar Khamis provides cross-cultural insight encouraging students to examine the issue from a global perspective.

## Telehealth, Telemedicine, and mHealth Applications

### Telehealth

Telehealth has been described as the use of electronic information and telecommunications technologies to support long-distance clinical healthcare, patient and professional health-related education, public health, and health administration (Health Resources Services Administration (HRSA), 2023). The integration of care facilitated by telehealth services supports the delivery of WPHC by making it easier to obtain preventive care, manage chronic conditions, and reduce travel time and cost. Telehealth can make it easier for individuals to obtain care without incurring time off from work or having to travel long distances. For those in geographically underserved areas, telehealth can make it possible to obtain hard-to-access care or specialist care. According to the Federal Communications Commission (FCC), telehealth services include a wide variety of remote healthcare services that can be nonclinical in nature. For instance, it can involve services provided by nurses, pharmacists, or social workers. Such services can include the provision of patient health education, social support, provider training, continuing medical education, administrative meetings, medication adherence, and troubleshooting health issues for patients and their caregivers. The technologies used for telehealth typically include the internet, videoconferencing, stored images, streaming media, and wireless communications.

*Telehealth Applications*

Telehealth applications such as remote patient monitoring allow individuals to talk to their healthcare providers over the phone; send and receive messages from their healthcare providers using secure messaging, email, and secure file exchange; and use live video so their healthcare provider can check on them at home. Telehealth applications can help individuals use a device to gather vital signs to help their healthcare provider stay informed on their progress. Examples of telehealth applications in telemedicine include conducting diagnostic tests, monitoring a patient's progress after treatment or therapy, and facilitating access to specialists that are not located in the same place as the patient. From a WPHC perspective, such applications can help individuals receive care in the context of their lived environment and allow for greater nuance and perspective into the healthcare relationship. However, from an SJA perspective, as this chapter shows, the mere availability of technology and its applications is not sufficient for its access and employment by those who might benefit from it.

*Textbox 9.1 lists the physical and infrastructure barriers and psychosocial barriers that face patients seeking a real-time virtual visit. Look at the barriers and see if you can work your way backward to the root causes of these barriers in the social justice framework. Then attempt the SJA prompt provided in the textbox.*

---

**Textbox 9.1    Real-Time Virtual Visits: How Many Barriers Can You Identify?**

**WPHC Context: Real-Time Virtual Visit Tools**

From the following list, see how many telehealth applications you can identify in the market that would be required to make a virtual visit possible. Then think through how the telehealth applications support a WPHC perspective. Why is it important to consider a WPHC perspective in this context?

I. **Physical and Infrastructure Barriers:**
   1. A device with a camera and software that can accommodate streaming video.
   2. A fast internet connection with minimal lag time.
   3. A data plan that will not make a video visit a costly undertaking.
   4. Digital skills needed to make the appointment, launch the visit, adjust the camera and microphone, and troubleshoot basic issues.
   5. A private, well-lit place to conduct the visit.
   6. Broadband infrastructure with affordable high-speed affordable broadband plans.
   7. Private and secure connection.

II. **Psychosocial Barriers**:

1. Trust in the healthcare system.
2. Confidence that their provider can make an accurate diagnosis by telehealth.
3. Confidence that they will not lose their personal relationship with their provider by prioritizing telehealth.
4. Digital literacy.
5. Ability to select providers that share their ethnic or national background.

### SJA Discussion Prompt

1. Given the barriers listed earlier and others you have identified in the previous exercise, how many ways can you list that will support telehealth adoption?
2. What are some ways that systemic physical and trust barriers among marginalized and disadvantaged communities can be addressed?
3. What are some ways that the physical and infrastructure barriers can be addressed?

### Resource

Telehealth Equity Coalition. *Barriers to telehealth adoption*. Retrieved December 30, 2022, from https://www.telehealthequitycoalition.org/barriers-to-telehealth-adoption.html

*Barriers*

Despite their many advantages, telehealth applications face several barriers that hinder their widespread adoption and implementation. These barriers include gaps in regulations in state statutes; legal and policy considerations in the domains of information security, patient privacy, licensing, and insurance reimbursement; and credentialing and liability concerns. The barriers will be addressed at different points in this chapter.

## Telemedicine

The term "telehealth" is often used interchangeably with telemedicine. However, there are subtle differences between the two terms. A telemedicine visit can be described more appropriately like a virtual clinical visit with a healthcare provider. Examples of telemedicine include when a gynecologist schedules an appointment to discuss birth control options with a patient over video conference or an endocrinologist makes a virtual appointment to go over their patient's latest lab results with the patient. In each of these instances, the provider would have employed telemedicine to coordinate the medical visit (Kopf, 2022). According to the HHS, telemedicine lets the healthcare provider care for their patient without an in-person visit, primarily using technology such as the internet and a computer, tablet, or smartphone.

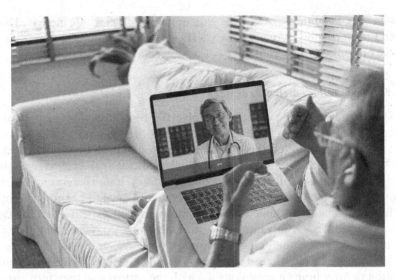

*Figure 9.1* A Telemedicine Appointment Can be Helpful for Seniors.

### Overview

Telemedicine can also be understood as a subset of telehealth. Telemedicine refers specifically to remote clinical services, or the use of technology to deliver medical care from a healthcare provider to a patient in a different or remote location. It emphasizes the use of medical information and how it is exchanged from one site to another using the internet. Telemedicine employs two-way, real-time communication or monitoring to assess and streamline improvements to patients' health. Telemedicine can be classified as real-time telemedicine, remote patient monitoring, and involving "store-and-forward" practices. Examples of telemedicine include digital transmission of medical imaging, remote medical diagnosis and evaluations, and video consultations with specialists. For instance, a mobile app used by your physician to schedule a clinical visit via a video chat, or a secure software system that allows you to send your doctor a picture for a quick diagnosis, or when your doctor remotely monitors your vital signs and activities all constitute different examples of telemedicine in action.

### Real-Time Telemedicine

Real-time telemedicine, or live telemedicine involves the two-way communication between a provider and a patient using internet-based technologies such as video conferencing or phone consultations that facilitate real-time engagement. Remote patient monitoring references the monitoring of a patient's health metrics from their own home. It allows providers the ability to manage chronic and acute conditions without incurring patient travel and increased risk of infection. Remote patient monitoring can involve tracking high blood pressure, weight loss and gain, heart conditions, sleep apnea, asthma, and COPD. Remote patient monitoring can be done through devices used by the patient, including weighing machine scales, pulse oximeters, blood glucose meters, blood pressure monitors, fetal monitors, breathing apparatuses, and heart monitors. Facilitators of remote patient monitoring include increased awareness of telehealth and telemedicine through the COVID-19 public health emergency, greater insurance coverage options, and the availability of advanced medical technologies.

### Store-and-Forward Telemedicine Practices

Store-and-forward telemedicine practices involve the transmission of a patient's recorded health history and clinical data. Such data might comprise lab reports, MRI scans, or X-ray images that are then transmitted through electronic communications systems to healthcare providers. One advantage of store-and-forward telemedicine is the relatively simple technological requirements and ease of setup. A second advantage is its asynchronous nature; unlike live telemedicine, both the provider and the patient do not need to be present simultaneously together. Thus, it can accommodate a range of provider and patient geographical and time availability and schedules. Disadvantages of store-and-forward telemedicine include lack of medical insurance coverage, malpractice insurance coverage, and insufficient patient insurance and teleradiology, a field where a radiology specialist reviews X-rays that were taken at a remote location or after hours and/or consults with the patient and then forwards them back to the referring physician. Other examples of store-and-forward technology include teledermatology or the transmission of digital images of a patient's skin lesion sent to a dermatologist for diagnosis and treatment advice.

### Barriers

Overall, some of the barriers to the adoption of telemedicine in a manner that can serve the medical needs of disadvantaged populations include age, level of education, lack of broadband and digital skills, cost, and poor e-health literacy. These factors are related and often co-occur. For example, older adults may often have poor e-health literacy, or those who lack a higher education degree may be in a socioeconomic position and lack broadband and digital skills. These are discussed further in the section on the digital divide later in this chapter.

## Telecare

A third term, "telecare," is used when the need for virtual healthcare services is emphasized. The FCC describes telecare as care that involves technology that allows consumers to stay safe and independent in their own homes. Telecare has been defined as care offered to patients remotely via telecommunications technology, either through synchronous (live video) or asynchronous means (store-and-forward, remote patient monitoring). Telecare encompasses a broader category of services than telemedicine beyond facilitating remote medical treatment between healthcare providers and patients. Telecare helps expand patient access to care and helps patients manage recovery and well-being at home and monitor risks remotely (e.g., early warning signs). Thus, telecare highlights how care is handled through a range of technology—from telephones to online virtual visits to remote patient monitoring centers.

*Review **Textbox 9.2** for an SJA context to telehealth. Attempt the SJA prompt that follows.*

---

**Textbox 9.2   Digital Disparities, Health Disparities, and SDoH**

**WPHC Context**

The rapid implementation of telehealth programs in rural areas in response to the COVID-19 pandemic holds tremendous potential for addressing rural health disparities. However, as you learned from the barriers to telehealth access in the chapter, overcoming issues in broadband access in rural settings, which limit the reach and effectiveness of telehealth initiatives, must be prioritized before their benefits are fully realized. In addition, other conditions must also be achieved for marginalized and disadvantaged populations to benefit from the promise of telehealth.

The following are some suggestions made by researchers Hirko et al. (2020) to help promote the adoption and access to telehealth by those vulnerable populations who need it the most:

1. Focused evaluation of clinical care outcomes in minority and marginalized populations to integrate their concerns in tailoring the utility of these programs.
2. Ensure sustainability of telehealth programs in rural areas following the COVID-19 pandemic through continuing third-party reimbursement for these services.
3. Continuing research to ensure that the initiatives put in place during COVID-19 do not amplify existing health disparities experienced by those living in rural communities.

**SJA Prompt**

Health equity in telehealth refers to equal access to telehealth services by everyone and especially the underserved communities. Equity in telehealth includes the ability to achieve the goals of digital literacy, technology literacy and access, and evaluation data from minority populations. A lack of equal access to healthcare can lead to consequences such as increased disease and illness severity, higher mortality rates, higher disease rates, higher medical costs, and lack of access to treatment and health insurance (HHS.gov).

Consider the list of underserved communities (HHS.gov) and identify a health equity challenge in telehealth faced by the communities:

1. Low-income Americans
2. Rural Americans
3. People of color
4. Immigrants
5. People who identify as LGBTQ
6. People with disabilities
7. Older patients
8. People with limited knowledge of the English language
9. People with limited digital literacy
10. People who are underinsured or uninsured.

## Resources

Case Western Reserve University School of Medicine. Neighborhood immersion for compassion & empathy. Retrieved December 22, 2022, from https://equityvrtraining.org/neighborhood-immersion-for-compassion-empathy/

FCC. (2019, May 8). *2019 Broadband deployment report*. Retrieved on December 30, 2022 from https://www.fcc.gov/reports-research/reports/broadband-progress-reports/2019-broadband-deployment-report

HHS.gov (2022, June 3). Health equity in telehealth. *Health Resources and Services Administration*. Retrieved March 22, 2023 from https://telehealth.hhs.gov/providers/health-equity-in-telehealth

Hirko, K. A., Kerver, J. M., Ford, S., Szafranski, C., Beckett, J., Kitchen, C., & Wendling, A. L. (2020). Telehealth in response to the COVID-19 pandemic: Implications for rural health disparities. *Journal of the American Medical Informatics Association, 27*(11) 1816–1818. https://doi.org/10.1093/jamia/ocaa156

National Bureau of Economic Research (NBER). (2018, December). Does doctor race affect the health of black men. Retrieved December 22, 2022, from https://www.nber.org/bah/2018no4/does-doctor-race-affect-health-black-men

NCI. (2019). *National Information National Trends Survey*. https://hints.cancer.gov/

National Digital Inclusion Alliance (NDIA). (2020, June). *Limiting broadband investment to rural only discriminates against Black Americans and other communities of color*. Retrieved from https://www.digitalinclusion.org/digital-divide-and-systemic-racism/

NDIA. Retrieved December 30, 2022 from https://www.digitalinclusion.org/

### Monitoring

Social and lifestyle monitoring is a part of telecare. Examples of telecare include consumer-oriented health and fitness apps, sensors, and tools that connect family members or caregivers with consumers, exercise tracking tools, digital medication reminder systems, or early warning and detection technologies. Telecare applications also involve the use of remote monitoring centers to aid the elderly, monitoring for any warning signs of falls or unusual behavior patterns that might be a red flag for intervention. Telecare systems can also monitor the environment such as for a situation when the individual is unconscious and provide the required alerts.

See **Textbox 9.3** *for a summary of the definitions of telehealth, telemedicine, telecare, and mhealth. How many of these have you used?*

---

**Textbox 9.3   Definitions: Telehealth, Telemedicine, Telecare, and mHealth**

### WPHC Context

- **Telehealth**: The use of electronic information and telecommunication technologies to support and promote long-distance clinical healthcare, patient and professional health-related education, public health, and health administration (CDC, 2022).

- **Telemedicine**: Defined by the Federation of State Medical Boards as the practice of medicine using electronic communication, information technology, or other means between a physician in one location and a patient in another location, with or without an intervening healthcare provider.

The WHO defines telehealth as the use of information and communication technologies (ICT) for health.

- **Telecare**: Technology that allows consumers to stay safe and independent in their own homes. For example, telecare may include consumer-oriented health and fitness apps, sensors and tools that connect consumers with family members or other caregivers, exercise tracking tools, digital medication reminder systems, or early warning and detection technologies.
- **mHealth**: The use of mobile and wireless devices (cell phones, tablets, etc.) to support the achievement of health objectives (WHO).

The use of mobile and wireless devices (cell phones, tablets, etc.) to improve health outcomes, healthcare services, and health research (NIH).

## SJA Prompt

Consider your favorite mhealth app (e.g., MyChart, Sleep Cycle, Talkspace, Headspace).

1. What health indicators does it support? Which health objectives does the app support?
2. Now research a version of an app that supports the same health indicators for those who are visually impaired. What choices did you find? What were the strengths and limitations of the choices for the app for the visually impaired compared to yours?
3. What challenges did you face? What implications might such a marketplace for the mhealth domain mean for equity in health outcomes, equity in health research participation, and access to healthcare services for those who are visually impaired?

## Resources

CDC. (2022). *Telehealth and telemedicine: A research anthology of law and policy resources.* https://www.cdc.gov/phlp/publications/topic/anthologies/anthologies-telehealth.html

FCC. *Telehealth, telemedicine, and telecare: What's what?* https://www.fcc.gov/general/telehealth-telemedicine-and-telecare-whats-what

Federation of State Medical Boards (FSMB). Retrieved December 30, 2022, from https://www.fsmb.org/advocacy/telemedicine/

National Institutes of Health. Retrieved December 31, 2022, from https://www.fic.nih.gov/ResearchTopics/Pages/MobileHealth.aspx

WHO. *The Global Health Observatory.* Retrieved December 31, 2022, from https://www.who.int/data/gho/indicator-metadata-registry/imr-details/4774

## mHealth

mHealth falls under the broader category of telehealth. mHealth refers to the specific ways in which mobile technologies are utilized to achieve improved health goals. Given the near ubiquity of mobile technology in the United States, mHealth represents the facet of telehealth that is powered by consumer apps and that often does not involve a clinician. mHealth focuses on user-directed health technology that falls into the fitness and well-being domain, such as through using smartphone apps.

### *Integration of mHealth*

Mobile phone technology has also been incorporated into healthcare monitoring in environments outside the home. Many mobile devices now include GPS tracking, a feature that helps telecare be accessible to more people in different environments. Many systems will also help the person to receive immediate feedback on their environment, health, or situation. Such feedback can help alleviate memory issues and help the person maintain their dignity and independence. In other situations, telecare systems can help to deliver appropriate help from a neighbor, an ambulance, or even the police department to an individual. This facet is mediated via routing through dedicated call centers, which enable easy access to the required telecare services (eVisit, 2022).

Many organizations and agencies are involved in the oversight, development, and implementation of the different facets of the telehealth industry. *A few examples of the organizations and agencies are provided in **Textbox 9.4**. Review the organizations and agencies along with their focus, mission, and vision. Respond to the SJA prompt that follows.*

---

**Textbox 9.4   Digital Health Organizations and Agencies: Focus, Mission, and Vision**

**WPHC Context**

- **The National Consortium of Telehealth Resource Centers**:
  A collaborative of 12 regional and 2 national Telehealth Resource Centers, committed to implementing telehealth programs for rural and underserved communities. Their mission is to provide timely and accurate information on telehealth across the nation.
- **Agency for Healthcare Research and Quality (AHRQ)**:
  Research on the benefits of telehealth through its Digital Healthcare Research Program and Effective Healthcare Program.
- **Telehealth Equity Coalition (TEC)**:
  Focused on equity, inclusion, representation, accountability, collaboration, and innovation, the mission of TEC is to improve access to quality and affordable healthcare by increasing the adoption of telehealth, especially among those communities that have been left out or left behind.

---

- **Trusted Connectivity Alliance (TCA)**:
  Mission: To collectively define requirements and provide deliverables of a strategic, technical, and marketing nature that enable all stakeholders in a connected society to benefit from the most stringent secure connectivity solutions that leverage expertise in tamper-proof, end-to-end security.

## SJA Prompt

Based on your overview of the organizations and agencies that work in the domain of digital health:

1. What are some gaps in the focus areas for the rural underserved populations?
2. What are some gaps in the care of the economically disadvantaged and housing-insecure population?

## Resources

Agency for Healthcare Research and Quality. Telehealth. Retrieved December 31, 2022, from https://www.ahrq.gov/topics/telehealth.html

The National Consortium of Telehealth Resource Centers. (n.d.). Retrieved from https://tele healthresourcecenter.org/

Telehealth Equity Coalition. Retrieved December 31, 2022, from https://www.telehealthequity coalition.org/index.html

Trusted Connectivity Alliance. Retrieved December 31, 2022, from https://trustedconnectivity alliance.org/wearable-devices/

### Wearable Industry

Wearable electronics are defined as devices that can be worn (or mated) with human skin to monitor an individual's activities continuously, without interrupting or limiting the user's motions (Gao et al., 2016). The potential of wearable technology in chronic condition monitoring, therapy delivery, rehabilitation, diagnostics, and activity tracking is enabled by continuous data tracking and its ability to offer immediate healthcare interventions. The increasing digitization of healthcare has led to the increasing popularity of wearables and their contribution to healthcare decision-making (Blanton, 2021). Market expansion factors are enabled by the rise of lifestyle-associated diseases (e.g., hypertension), growing demand for home healthcare, and the need to improve patient outcomes. As Textbox 9.5 shows, the wearable industry has grown rapidly in the past few years. In 2019, data shows a fifth of adults in the United States used a wearable device to help them achieve their health goals (McCarthy, 2019).

*Textbox 9.5 provides a brief snapshot of some salient trends in the wearable devices industry market growth statistics. Given this data, attempt the SJA prompt that follows.*

**Textbox 9.5   Trends in Wearable Devices Industry Market
Growth Statistics**

## WPHC Context

- 2019: 42% of US adults used digital wearables to track at least one health parameter
- 2020: 54% of US adults used digital wearables to track at least one health parameter
- 2021: $18.9 billion: estimated wearable market devices market
- 2022: 320 million consumer health and wellness wearables are shipped worldwide
- 2024: The number of wearables is projected to reach 440 million
- 2027: $60.6 billion: estimated wearable market devices market

## SJA Prompt

- ChatGPT and AI technologies made a splash in the first two months of 2023. What are some disadvantages of AI in healthcare technologies that may adversely impact minority and marginalized populations?

## Resources

Deloitte. *Accelerating the adoption of connected health.* Retrieved December 31, 2022, from https://www2.deloitte.com/content/dam/Deloitte/us/Documents/life-sciences-healthcare/us-dchs-connected-health.pdf

ScienceSoft. Retrieved December 31, 2022, from https://www.scnsoft.com/healthcare/medical-devices/wearable

*Digital Health Monitoring*

Consider the data on one popular wearable for digital health monitoring, the smartwatch. Deloitte's 2021 Connectivity and Mobile Trends survey found that 39% of respondents owned a smartwatch. This number is expected to grow. In fact, wearable technology was named the top fitness trend for 2022 by the American College of Sports Medicine (2021, December 30). According to consumer research data, 320 million consumer health and wellness wearable devices will ship worldwide in 2022 (Deloitte Global, 2021). As healthcare providers become comfortable with the use of digital health devices, by 2024, that number is predicted to reach nearly 440 million units.

Smartwatches and wearable medical devices such as smart patches help people monitor their health. In 2020, during COVID-19, smartwatches were used to measure blood oxygen saturation (SpO2). Smartwatches have supported people in their fitness goals of losing weight and monitoring their health in more widespread and deeper ways than before. These include popular features such as counting steps, calories, sitting and sleep time, and blood pressure and respiratory rate (ACSM, 2021). According to Deloitte's research, in 2021, smartwatches were used to monitor heart health, sleep quality, and chronic conditions. Advances in sensors and AI help detect and manage chronic health conditions. From monitoring their running pace, new hardware, software, and apps have turned smartwatches into a device akin to personalized health clinics. For instance, heart rate monitors are now standard on smartwatches and have FDA approval for detecting abnormalities such as atrial fibrillation, a major cause of stroke.

Review Textbox 9.6 for an overview of the WPHC context of wearable devices. Respond to the impact of wearable device ownership, access, and usage on the digital health of people of color and marginalized populations.

---

**Textbox 9.6   Telehealth Care Options**

**WPHC Context**

**Telehealth services** include an array of care options and domains. These include the following:

- Lab test or X-ray results
- Mental health treatment, including online therapy, counseling, and medication management
- Recurring conditions like migraines or urinary tract infections
- Skin conditions
- Prescription management
- Urgent care issues like colds, coughs, and stomachaches
- Postsurgical follow-up
- Treatment and follow-up appointments for attention deficit disorder (ADD) and attention deficit hyperactivity disorder (ADHD)
- Physical therapy and occupational therapy
- Remote monitoring services that help you track your health goals and manage chronic conditions like diabetes, high blood pressure, and high cholesterol

Information that patients can send their healthcare provider using telehealth:

- Weight, blood pressure, blood sugar, or vital information
- Images of a wound, eye, or skin condition
- A diary or document of symptoms
- Medical records that may be filed with another provider, such as X-rays

**Healthcare providers can send patients information** to manage health at home:

- Notifications or reminders to do rehabilitation exercises or take medication
- New suggestions for improving diet, mobility, or stress management
- Detailed instructions on how to continue care at home
- Encouragement to stick with a treatment plan

### Benefits of Telehealth

- Virtual visits ensure patients get healthcare wherever they are located—at home, at work, or even in their car.
- Virtual visits cut down on travel, time off from work, and the need for childcare.
- Virtual healthcare tools can shorten the wait for an appointment.
- Increased access to specialists who are located far away from the patient's hometown.

### SJA Prompts

- Given our discussion on the causes of disparities in healthcare outcomes through the increasing popularity of wearable devices, what are some steps you can take to address the health inequity for people of color and economically disadvantaged populations?

  Design a community-based initiative that can address some of the infrastructure and cultural causes of healthcare disparities stemming from wearable device access and usage for minorities and marginalized populations. Keep the following questions in mind as you design your community-based digital health initiative:

- What would such a community-based initiative look like for one disadvantaged population in your town?
- Which population would it benefit?
- What health risk factors impact that population?
- What healthcare domain would it target?
- How might it improve health outcomes?

### Resource

Telehealth.HHS.Gov (2022). *What is telehealth?* https://telehealth.hhs.gov/patients/understanding-telehealth/#:~:text=Benefits%20of%20telehealth-,What%20does%20telehealth%20mean%3F,computer%2C%20tablet%2C%20or%20smartphone

### Factors Facilitating Adoption of Wearable Devices

There are several factors impacting the increased adoption of wearable devices. Wearables provide objective data that can help inform patient-provider decision-making and enhance the quality of clinical encounters. Infrastructural factors such as the diffusion of the IoT, for instance, shape the adoption and integration of medical wearables in everyday life. IoT is defined as the network of physical objects that are supported by embedded technology for data communication and sensors to interact with both internal and external objects states and the environment (LeHong & Velosa, 2014). As the IoT evolves and becomes more sophisticated in connecting smart devices over the cloud, data accessibility over time and space will increase. Contextual factors, such as the COVID-19 pandemic, were also key factors in increasing the diffusion and adoption of wearables by increasing demand for remote monitoring and care delivery. Other factors include the rising number of geriatric populations, prevalence of chronic diseases that require consistent monitoring for better outcomes, focus on personalized patient care, and technological advancements in wearable devices. In this context, the wearable industry is well-positioned to provide more fine-grained and nuanced health information on users through the continuous collection, analysis, and transmission of personal health data in real time (Haghi et al., 2014).

### Potential for Racial and Ethnic Bias in Wearable Industry

Wearable device ownership by itself is not enough to increase the likelihood of improved health outcomes with health equity. People of color, for instance, are at a unique disadvantage with medical-grade wearables and their ability to track and monitor their own health data. The ability of smartwatches to track heart rates in people of color has been questioned. As wearable device usage expands into monitoring cardiovascular indications such as ambulatory blood pressure measurement, heart failure detection, and drug monitoring, the lack of representation of people of color and minority populations has the potential to increase health disparities and negative health outcomes in these populations (Zinzuwadia & Singh, 2022). There are some notable shortcomings in this line of research. For instance, Bent and colleagues' study examining the role of skin tone on inaccurate readings in consumer and medical-grade wearables (e.g., Empatica E4+; Apple Watch 4; Fitbit Charge 2; Garmin Vivosmart 3; Xiaomi Miband; Biovotion Everion) has been critiqued for their small sample size and use of the Fitzpatrick Skin Type Scale, which has a substantial literature of racial biases and weak correlation with skin color (Colvonen, 2021). Yet, the concern is indicative of a bias built into the device hardware. Such shortcomings can have serious health implications for minorities, people of color, low-income Americans, and global populations.

### Disparities and mHealth Technologies

Wearable devices and digital technologies are generally not used widely in low-income and minority populations. The most cited barriers that affect their widespread use among these populations are cost and education. This gap is further exacerbated by the exclusion of these populations from ongoing research studies. A lack of representation of minorities and low-income groups in research on the technology evolution and implementation means that the needs of people of color, people from rural communities, and populations with low digital literacy continue to be left behind in their access and utilization (Zinzuwadia & Singh, 2022). In 2021, for example, the FDA warned that at-home, digitally connected pulse oximeters might not recognize severe hypoxemia in people of color (Bent et al., 2020).

*Textbox 9.7 provides some key data on Americans' use of social media for health advice and to track their health metrics for better health outcomes. Read on to see how economically disadvantaged low-income Americans fare in the domain of ownership of digital devices. What might be some of the health implications of such disparities? Respond to the SJA prompt provided.*

**Textbox 9.7 Social Media, Digital Divide, and Health**

**WPHC Context**

The Pew Research Center 2010 survey on internet use found that many people use online resources to compare their options (Vogels, 2021). Social media is a particularly influential source for people looking for advice from friends, family, and experts. People turn to social media for collective knowledge on health and wearable devices to use to track their health metrics. Wearable devices are popular because people believe the ability to track their own health metrics can equip them to make better choices and have better health outcomes.

The Pew Internet Project survey found that, among e-patients living with chronic disease, about

- 37% have read someone else's commentary or experience about health or medical issues on an online news group, website, or blog;
- 25% have consulted rankings or reviews online of hospitals or other medical facilities;
- 25% have consulted rankings or reviews online of doctors or other providers;
- 22% have signed up to receive updates about health or medical issues;
- 13% have listened to a podcast about health or medical issues; and
- 57% of e-patients living with chronic disease have done at least one of the aforementioned activities.

**Digital Divide**

Even as broadband adoption and smartphone ownership has grown rapidly for all Americans, including those less well-off financially, the digital lives of Americans with lower and higher incomes remain different in significant ways.

For instance:

- 24% of adults with household incomes below $30,000 a year say they don't own a smartphone; and
- about four-in-ten adults with lower incomes do not have home broadband services or a desktop or laptop computer.

By comparison, of Americans with higher household incomes (e.g., $100,000 or more a year):

- 63% report having home broadband services, a smartphone, a desktop, or laptop and tablet, compared with 23% of those living in lower-income households, and
- 13% of adults with household incomes below $30,000 a year do not have access to any of these technologies at home, while only 1% of adults from households making $100,000 or more a year report a similar lack of access.

**SJA Discussion Prompt**

Research shows smartphone ownership is associated with the ability to obtain medical care, suggesting that the ability to use smartphone technology may play a role in increasing healthcare access (Oshima et al., 2021). This becomes important in the management of chronic diseases and major illnesses, such as cancer, that have the potential to amplify health engagement.

- What are some steps that can be taken by healthcare providers and organizations to reach patient populations with limited digital access so that these patients are not further disadvantaged in the realm of telehealth?

**Resources**

Oshima, S. M., Tait, S. D., Thomas, S. M., Fayanju, O. M., Ingraham, K., Barrett, N. J., & Hwang, E. S. (2021). Association of smartphone ownership and internet use with markers of health literacy and access: Cross-sectional survey study of perspectives from Project PLACE. *Journal of Medical internet Research, 23*(6):e24947 https://doi.org/10.2196/24947

Vogels, E. A. (2021, June 2021). *Digital divide persists even as Americans with lower incomes make gains in tech adoption.* Retrieved January 11, 2023, from https://www.pewresearch.org/fact-tank/2021/06/22/digital-divide-persists-even-as-americans-with-lower-incomes-make-gains-in-tech-adoption/

### Barriers to Wearable Device Adoption

The barriers to wearable adoption include data privacy and security concerns, power consumption optimization, wearability in design, and reducing the risk of data loss (Haghi et al., 2014). For a device to be easily managed for long-term monitoring without interruption, minimizing power loss is important. Power loss is correlated with several factors including the number of parameters that are observed, efficient code programming, good data packing, encryption, and compression. Wearability design considerations include adapting to the lifestyle and limitations of users, such as vulnerable elderly users managing chronic conditions. Thus, their design should ensure they are easy to wear, easy to carry, and comfortable. Wearables are designed to be light, small, and well-structured, with power consumption needs that allow them to be used for a long time. Finally, for reducing data loss, several factors need to be considered. Data is often collected by a microcontroller and transmitted to a smartphone or cloud storage. This process includes the possibility of disconnection and data loss. To reduce the risk of data loss for safe health monitoring, several options such as temporary data saving (buffering) in the microcontroller providing a large memory are employed (Haghi et al., 2014).

### Disparities Stemming from Research and FDA Approval Process

The implementation of a high-risk medical device or drug therapy in general requires validation in a representative population. For many wearables, the validation studies were done in homogeneous samples that were not externally validated in representative populations.

The FDA 510(k) clearance process paves the way for FDA approval for most wearable devices. This process only requires equivalent safety and efficacy to products that are already available. Digital technology companies have marketed their products as wellness tools with low risk and circumvented the traditional approval process. As wearable device studies have not generally conducted studies examining equity requirements, the gap in equity and utilization in meeting their needs is likely to continue (Zinzuwadia & Singh, 2022). Chronic disease management increasingly relies on the coordination of information between telemedicine, sensor technology, and AI. Research on incorporating AI into wearable devices has produced positive results in arrhythmia detection and physical fitness. This means that the lack of diversity in study populations translates into poorly generalizable models of AI.

The Apple Heart Study had 419, 297 participants and was the most comprehensive study into the accuracy of irregular pulse detection algorithms in the general population (Apple Heart Study, 2020). Its high positive predictive value of an initial irregular pulse notification for subsequent electrocardiogram-confirmed atrial fibrillation allowed for FDA clearance of the feature. However, the requirement to own an Apple product biased the study with a young, wealthy, and technology-proficient population. This translates into disparities by age and people of color. For instance, a 2022 clinical validation of atrial fibrillation detection with an Apple Watch in a population with a mean age of 76 years found a discrepancy in sensitivity—reporting it to be 50%, much lower than the 96% reported by Apple (Ford et al., 2022). As other companies (e.g., Fitbit and Samsung) obtain similar FDA clearance for passive arrhythmia monitoring, such studies highlight how equity issues persist as wearable device use continues. One way of addressing this disparity gap suggested by researchers Zinzuwadia and Singh is to make wearable devices available at community centers such as pharmacies and shops in an affordable manner to create representative study populations.

## Data Privacy and Security

Mobile health and wearable devices provide new and exciting ways for patients and individuals to take control of and participate in their own healthcare. Commercial devices available in the market provide biometric and medical parameter measurement. Technologies such as wearables require simple and secure connectivity that provides secure and private transmission of medical data.

### Steps to Ensure Secure Connectivity in Health and Behavioral Data

The usage of the data from wearables is subject to the rules and regulations established by the FCC (2022) and the Federal Trade Commission (FTC) in the United States (and to the California Consumer Privacy Act in California; California Consumer Privacy Act (CCPA), 2022; FCC, n.d.; FTC, 2022). Medical devices are subject to a higher level of oversight and privacy laws. In a clinical context, an individual's health data is generally well protected. However, the health and behavioral data of users shared through a phone app or wearable device, such as running heart rate or resting heart rate, is not protected to the same extent as that of medical-grade devices. Moreover, the Terms of Service that consumers consent to prior to their usage are challenging to understand. Even with greater digital literacy, interpreting how and in what context the company protects or shares private information is challenging. These challenges underscore the inability of users to give informed consent (Lamensch, 2021).

### Challenges Facing the Wearable Industry

In 2015, personal health information breaches affected 113 million individuals, underscoring how susceptible the health data of users in the wearable industry was to third-party operators (Office of the National Coordinator for Health Information Technology, 2016). Health information is 50 times more profitable for hackers than other individual identifiers like social security numbers (HealthIT.gov., 2022). Wearable devices collect user data regardless of time, place, and occasion, and upload data to the cloud, which makes wearable devices, such as those from Fitbit, Xiaomi, Huawei, Jawbone, and other manufacturers, vulnerable to security attacks and data leakage (Jiang & Shi, 2021).

Increasing user privacy awareness can help mitigate the challenges affecting data security and privacy protection of healthcare wearable devices. Most wearable device users are not knowledgeable about the privacy risks that their data are exposed to or how these data are protected once collected (Cilliers, 2020). Alongside, the Department of Homeland Security (DHS, 2022) states wearable technology should include several technical, logistic, and security requirements, including

- Having flexible and/or stand-alone connectivity with stand-alone connectivity being a key consideration;
- Protecting the privacy of the sensitive, high-value user data they collate, store, and transmit;
- Protecting the integrity and accuracy of user data that is stored and transmitted;
- ensuring the integrity and authenticity of the software/firmware through malware protection;
- Ensuring end-user convenience and flexibility by allowing them to manage mobile subscriptions across multiple devices; and
- Providing ways to protect stored data in case the device is lost or stolen.

Review *Textbox 9.8 for the WPHC context concerning the steps you can take to secure wearable healthcare devices against the privacy and security threats that they are vulnerable to. Respond to the SJA prompt that follows.*

---

**Textbox 9.8   Securing Wearable Healthcare Devices: What Can You Do?**

**WPHC Context**

Consider the following recommendations to consumers to ensure that they apply appropriate cyber hygiene practices on mobile devices such as their smartphone devices (DHS, 2022).

- Use the passcode lock on smartphones, smartwatches, and other devices.
- Protect a smartphone from viruses and malicious software, or malware.
- Use caution when downloading apps.
- Delete apps that are not needed.

- Check the privacy setting on any apps that collect personal data and limit what gets shared.
- Limit location permissions.
- Apply caution when using social network accounts to sign into apps.
- Keep software/firmware updated on your phone, mobile apps, and wearable health-care devices.
- Avoid storing sensitive information like passwords on a mobile device.
- Beware of "shoulder surfers" or other social engineering tactics.

### SJA Activity

1. How many of the aforementioned recommended cyber hygiene practices do you follow?
2. Navigate to the FCC Smartphone Security Checker website using the URL provided in the "Resources" section. Use the tool for smartphone users to secure their phones. Select your mobile device operating system, then click on the "Generate Your Checker" button. What do you find?

### Resources

Express VPN. (n.d.). Four ways to get smart about *smartwatch security*. https://www.expressvpn.com/blog/smartwatch-security/

Endpoint Security. (n.d.). *Phone security: 20 ways to secure your mobile phone*. https://preyproject.com/blog/phone-security-20-ways-to-secure-your-mobile-phone

FCC. (n.d.). *Smartphone Security Checker*. https://www.fcc.gov/smartphone-security

FTC. (n.d.). *How to protect your privacy on apps*. https://consumer.ftc.gov/articles/how-protect-your-privacy-apps

### Digital Divide

All the benefits of telehealth and wearables underscore how important it is to ensure their equitable access adoption in underserved communities. The HINTS survey, for instance, found that Whites are more likely to rate their healthcare quality as excellent (34%) than other minority groups (26%–28%) and less likely to rate it as fair or poor (Health Information National Trends Survey (HINTS), 2019). This disparity can stem from a range of systemic exclusionary practices, often stemming from implicit bias made evident in the lag in telehealth utilization and the conveniences it offers. For instance, while 65% of White patients say that their providers have offered them online access to their electronic medical records (EMRs), fewer Black (57%), Hispanic (46%), and Asian (53%) patients report having received such offers (HINTS, 2019). Populations who are vulnerable such as seniors, people with economic or social disadvantages, individuals who are disabled, and those living in rural areas experience low telehealth use and report higher rates of chronic disease and premature death.

*Review* **Textbox 9.9** *for a look at the WPHC context of how one university-based project, Project ECHO, is driving global change in health, education, and climate change domains in an innovative manner.*

**Textbox 9.9    Project ECHO**

**Mini-Case Study**

*WPHC Context*

**Project ECHO** describes itself as a knowledge-sharing, distance-based telehealth network model for implementing best practices in disease management. It began in 2003 by aiding rural physicians in evaluating their patients' using telehealth conferencing with clinicians at the University of New Mexico, UNM).

Led by Sanjeev Arora, MD, a UNM professor of medicine, Project ECHO integrates technology in training law enforcement officers to work with individuals with mental health issues in encounters during patrols (e.g., using videoconferences with psychiatrists to train police officers in topics such as bipolar disorder, substance abuse disorder, post-traumatic stress disorder, and autism).

Studies have shown that the care delivered by ECHO-trained providers was equivalent to UNM specialists in domains such as hepatitis C case management. The ECHO model engages participants in a virtual community with their peers where they share support, guidance, and feedback. They focus on a collective understanding of disseminating and implementing best practices across diverse disciplines to continually improve the current knowledge of participants. Active learning, mentoring, and peer support make ECHO promote knowledge-sharing and dynamic engagement by bringing together specialists from multiple disciplines for a robust, holistic approach.

*SJA Prompt*

• The potential of the wearable industry to both deepen and bridge the digital divide in healthcare disparities is immense. What is one innovative way you can envision a wearable device addressing the challenges posed to the environment and the related racial health disparities in communities of color?

**Resource**

Project ECHO. (n.d.). University of New Mexico Health Sciences. https://hsc.unm.edu/echo/

*Digital Divide and SDoH*

Despite the promise of telehealth initiatives, the disparities in health outcomes stemming from disparities in telehealth use are closely connected. In fact, without consideration of the inequities stemming from SDoH and their integration in policy guiding telehealth initiatives, the disadvantages characterizing marginalized populations would only increase. As previous chapters have illustrated, SDoH attributes such as poverty, access to healthy food, safe places for physical activity, transportation, and employment opportunities are often more impactful than the provision of healthcare and clinical interventions in determining health outcomes.

*Read the **Scholar Interview** with **Dr. Sahar Khamis** to gain insight into the digital health disparities in women's global health. How can the work of communication scholars like Dr. Khamis impact the lives of women in their communities?*

## TEXTBOX 9.10    Gendered Health Disparities in the Digital Age: Ethnographic Studies in the Global South

**Dr. Sahar Khamis**
*University of Maryland*

Exploring women's health communication patterns and access to health information from an ethnographic standpoint has always been one of my main research interests. This dates back more than two decades ago, when I conducted my doctoral dissertation research on the women of the village of Kafr Masoud in rural Egypt and how and why they received health messages, including family planning messages, differently, based on a plethora of factors, including their socioeconomic status, level of education, generation, and media consumption patterns. One of the key findings was the gap between the younger more educated women, who had access to more diverse sources of health information from a variety of sources including the media, and the older uneducated women who relied mostly on interpersonal face-to-face communication and advice from trusted others (Khamis, 2000).

When I visited the same village again ten years later, I witnessed firsthand the huge impact which the introduction of new technologies had on these women's lives and their access to health information. With the introduction of satellite television and the internet, health-related information, whether regarding vaccinations, family planning, maternal health, childcare, or other issues, became much more accessible and available for a broader segment of women. The fact that, surprisingly enough, even some of the poorest homes in the village can now afford to watch not only television but the satellite dish too, in addition to the possibility of browsing the internet, created new avenues for more women to gain new information, including health information. However, it would be inaccurate to assume that this wider access to health information erased all disparities between different groups of women in this rural Egyptian village or in the Global South, more broadly. The fact remains that younger, more technologically savvy, more educated, and employed women had better access to new technologies and, consequently, better access to health information (Khamis, 2010).

This digital divide between the technological haves and have-nots widened even more amid the COVID-19 pandemic, with all the economic, social, and health implications it caused worldwide. This pandemic widened the gap even more between different groups of people, based on a myriad of geographical, educational, social, and economic factors. The gender factor, however, should not be overlooked since women, especially those in less fortunate communities in the Global South, lagged behind in terms of not only accessing healthcare services and vaccinations but also accessing much-needed health information, contributing to a wider "gender digital divide" between men and women, on one hand, and between various categories of women, on the other hand (Khamis & Campbell, 2020).

Even within the same country, as my latest coauthored study on women's access to maternal healthcare information in Ghana amid COVID-19 reveals, there are significant disparities between women in urban and rural areas when it comes to accessing much-needed health information, in general, and maternal health information, in particular, especially amid the COVID-19 pandemic. This study exposed how the pandemic exacerbated many of the already existing barriers to accessing maternal health information by limiting interpersonal communication with healthcare providers and escalating the need for relying on digital technologies to gain such information, despite the rarity and difficulty of accessing such technologies, especially in less developed countries in the Global South, and more so in less developed regions within these countries, such as rural areas (Khamis & Agboada, 2023).

Moving forward, it is imperative to conduct more research that tackles many of these gaps and the complexities and nuances of these disparities both globally and locally using a gender-sensitive lens that takes into consideration women's multiple invisibilities and the myriad barriers confronting them, economically, socially, and technologically.

## Resources

Khamis, S. (2000). Egyptian Rural Women and Television's Public Awareness Programmes. Unpublished PhD dissertation in Mass Media and Cultural Studies, Department of Sociology, University of Manchester, United Kingdom.

Khamis, S. (2010). New media and social change in rural Egypt. *Arab Media & Society*, issue 11, winter 2010. Available at: https://www.arabmediasociety.com/new-media-and-social-change-in-rural-egypt/

Khamis, S. & Campbell, E. (2020). Info-deficiency in an infodemic: The gender digital gap, Arab women, and the COVID-19 pandemic. *Arab Media & Society*, September 27, 2020. Available at: https://www.arabmediasociety.com/info-deficiency-in-an-infodemic-the-gender-digital-gap-arab-women-and-the-covid-19-pandemic/

Khamis, S. & Agboada, D. (2023). Maternal health information disparities and the gender digital gap in Ghana amid COVID-19, *Media and Communication*, volume 11, issue 1(in press).

### SDoH and Barriers to Telehealth Adoption

Because of its seminal role in supporting all facets of health and well-being, internet use is now recognized as a super SDoH. Thus, it becomes even more important to eliminate SDoH that relate to digital barriers to telehealth, particularly in rural and urban communities to reduce the health disparities faced by disadvantaged populations. While it is easy to see how a reliable broadband connection is essential for telehealth, it is equally important to realize that a lack of broadband and digital skills are even more significant barriers to telehealth adoption. Where we live makes a difference to our health status. Thus, it is not surprising that national statistics on internet access point to gaps especially in rural areas and for seniors. However, by itself, this data hides the variability and relationships that characterize low-income status at the intersection of the race and rural divide. For example, in the United States, 82.7% of all households had broadband internet subscriptions as of the 2019 American Community Survey five-year census data. But when the data is examined across smaller areas, disparities emerge. Cleveland, Ohio, was ranked by the National Digital Inclusion Alliance as the Worst Connected City in 2019. In Cuyahoga County, Ohio, home to Cleveland, at least about one-fifth of the county's neighborhoods, fewer than one-half of households have a broadband subscription. Equally significantly, many of the neighborhoods with low broadband subscription rates also have the lowest levels of smartphone ownership (about 37% and 68% of households).

*Review* **Textbox 9.11** *for a Discussion Question and Thought Scenario for Reflection in the domain of racial disparities, implicit bias, and negative health outcomes associated with health inequities and disparities.*

---

**Textbox 9.11   Discussion Question/Thought Scenario for Reflection**

**WPHC Thought Scenario**

Recent research findings provide ample evidence of how sociodemographic characteristics differ by race. Consider the following findings reported in a study by Cunningham and colleagues in 2015:

1. Blacks under 65 years of age were more likely to have no health insurance than Whites.
2. Blacks were more likely than Whites to have <12 years of education, be unemployed, live below the poverty level, and be less likely to live in a household where the head of household owned the home.
3. Blacks were more likely than Whites to report not being able to see a doctor in the past year because of cost.
4. Blacks aged 18–34 years were less likely to have a personal doctor or healthcare provider than Whites.
5. Blacks were more likely than Whites to report frequent mental distress and frequent physical distress at age ≥50 years.
6. Blacks had 40% higher death rates than Whites for all-cause mortality in all age groups <65 years.
7. The National Bureau of Economic Research (NBER) found that Black men seen by Black doctors agreed to more preventive services than those seen by non-Black doctors.

**SJA Discussion Question**

1. What efforts can wearable device manufacturers and telehealth platforms undertake to address implicit bias?
2. Can you design a training exercise that will help providers reduce disparate outcomes for minority patients in underserved communities?

**Resource**

Cunningham, T. J., Croft, J. B., Liu, Y., Lu, H., Eke, P. I., & Giles, W. H. (2017, May 5). Vital signs: Racial disparities in age-specific mortality among Blacks or African Americans–United States, 1999–2015. *MMWR*, 66(17), 444–456. https://www.ncbi.nlm.nih.gov/pmc/articles/PMC 5687082/

## Digitally Disconnected Neighborhoods

Digitally disconnected neighborhoods are also identified in national data as being the most racially segregated. In the most digitally disconnected neighborhoods, 84% of the residents are Black, whereas in neighborhoods that are the least digitally disconnected, about 3% or fewer residents are Black. This disconnect continues to be reflected in the rural and urban divide. About 80% or more residents in more privileged suburban neighborhoods have broadband subscriptions and/or smartphones. Although policy exists to bridge these disparities, its effective implementation poses challenges.

*Review **Textbox 9.12** for one example of the WPHC context of a policy initiative Connect2 Health addressing the challenges facing digitally disconnected neighborhoods. Respond to the SJA prompt. How does it help achieve the goals of health equity?*

---

### Textbox 9.12   Connect2Health (C2H): Broadband Connectivity as an SDoH

#### WPHC Context

The FCC's C2H Task Force emphasized the following considerations for broadband access and adoption in all communities toward achieving digital health equity (Connect2HealthFCC, n.d.):

- Implementing broadband-enabled health technologies (e.g., home hospitals)
- Supporting the transformation of healthcare through emerging technologies and innovations
- Supporting integrated care, e.g., between
  - Patients and caregivers
  - Health systems and clinicians
  - Social service agencies
  - Community health centers
  - Wellness providers (e.g., grocery stores, fitness centers)
- Empowering consumers for greater engagement

#### Vision

Everyone connected to the people, services, and information they need to get well and stay healthy.

#### SJA Prompt

- What are some challenges facing the digitally disconnected neighborhoods in your city? Speak to some community members and journal your experiences.
- How can some elements of the FCC's C2H Task Force recommendations be integrated to bridge digital health divide disparities in your neighborhood?
- Craft a vision and mission statement of digital health connectivity for your community.

---

**Resource**

Connect2HealthFCC. (n.d.). *Mission and vision.* https://www.fcc.gov/general/connect2healthfcc-mission-and-vision

---

### Connect2Health

By now you can see that so much of the benefits of technology in healthcare are dependent on the use of the internet. The C2H Task Force of the FCC posits broadband should be recognized as a "super" determinant of health. SDoH reflect the fact that health begins where we live, learn, work, and play; that these nonmedical factors (including education, income, and employment) affect health or can serve as a predictor of one's health status. Thus, recognizing them as super SDoH can help them receive greater attention in national broadband policies, population health, and government-wide efforts to address health inequities. Not surprisingly, achieving digital health equity through improving broadband access and adoption is an FCC priority.

Telehealth, telemedicine, and mhealth solutions to healthcare provide an opportunity for individuals to get personalized WPHC care to support continuity of care in a nonclinical environment. The COVID-19 pandemic spurred a leap in the integration of healthcare information technology in the delivery of healthcare in clinical and community settings. Such inroads promise a more equitable healthcare landscape. Evidence shows that telehealth approaches have gained in popularity for rural, underserved, and disadvantaged populations. As the value-based model of care (**Chapter 6**) underpinning the WPHC approach advances, telehealth will be increasingly integrated into settings, including primary care and mental healthcare.

From the lens of a WPHC SJA framework, the structural barriers facing the adoption of telehealth remain. These stem from a lack of clarity in reimbursement mechanisms, persistence of slower internet bandwidth speeds in rural areas, and regulatory and legislative barriers. Individual-level factors such as slower adoption of technology, particularly among older adults and challenges faced by the socially disadvantaged continue to serve as barriers to the widespread adoption of telehealth in marginalized and minority populations.

In conclusion, as discussed in **Chapter 9**, **Health Communication and Technology**, the promise of the wearable industry, telehealth, telemedicine, telecare, and mhealth can only be accomplished when the concerns and challenges related to health inequity and disparities are addressed. This chapter has examined the structural and contextual factors underscoring health inequity and disparities for marginalized and vulnerable populations. It has encouraged critical thought toward conceptualizing alternative ways for achieving better health for all in line with shared goals for societal and technological progress.

*Read **Textbox 9.13** and share your thoughts on the SJA prompt that follows.*

**Textbox 9.13    Present Challenges and Future Directions Exercise**

## WPHC Context

As technological innovations have advanced, many applications of telehealth are being explored to provide training and support in healthcare services in a variety of contexts. The Albuquerque Police Department (APD) became the first law enforcement agency in the United States to train its officers through videoconferencing with psychiatrists under the Project ECHO learning model (Stark, n.d.) Albuquerque police officers received mental health and crisis intervention team training. Using videoconference with UNM School of Medicine clinicians, APD officers examined the 2064 crisis intervention-related incidents that occurred from January through November 2016. They referred about 78% of the individuals examined for mental health evaluation and follow-up care instead of making an arrest.

## SJA Prompt

In several states, the law requires healthcare practitioners to attest that they have completed an implicit bias training program on their license renewal application (e.g., Maryland). However, findings suggest that there are still gaps in how it has changed what police officers do on their job, although it makes some difference in the reflection on unconscious associations that may affect decisions and actions (NPR, 2020). For the SJA Future Directions prompts that follow, you may consult the "Resources" provided in this textbox.

## SJA Future Directions

1. In what ways can the use of technology such as telehealth initiatives and wearables advance initiatives to address implicit bias and promote awareness in police agencies?
2. In what ways can the limitations and gaps in telehealth and wearables development hinder the initiatives to address implicit bias and awareness in police agencies?
3. Can you design a telehealth initiative that can support training in mental health awareness that explicitly addresses the representation and exclusion of minority and low-income populations?

## Resources

*Implicit bias training required for 2022 license renewal.* Retrieved December 31, 2022, from https://health.maryland.gov/boardsahs/Documents/implicitb.pdf

NPR. (2020, September 10). N*YPD study: Implicit bias training changes minds, not necessarily behavior.* Retrieved December 31, 2022, from https://www.npr.org/2020/09/10/909380525/nypd-study-implicit-bias-training-changes-minds-not-necessarily-behavior

Stark, J. (n.d.). Addressing implicit bias in policing. *Police Chief Magazine.* Retrieved December 31, 2022, from https://www.policechiefmagazine.org/addressing-implicit-bias-in-policing/

# References

American College of Sports Medicine. (2021, December 30). *Wearable tech named top fitness trend for 2022*. Retrieved December 31, 2022, from https://www.acsm.org/news-detail/2021/12/30/wearable-tech-named-top-fitness-trend-for-2022

Bent, B., Goldstein, B. A., Kibbe, W. A., & Dunn, J. P. (2020). Investigating sources of inaccuracy in wearable optical heart rate sensors. *NPJ Digital Medicine, 3*, 18. https://doi.org/10.1038/s41746-020-0226-6

Blanton, N. (2021, November 10). What is the future of wearable technology in healthcare? *Baylor College of Medicine*. Retrieved December 31, 2022, from https://blogs.bcm.edu/2021/11/10/what-is-the-future-of-wearable-technology-in-healthcare/

California Consumer Privacy Act (CCPA). Retrieved December 31, 2022, from https://oag.ca.gov/privacy/ccpa

Cilliers, L. (2020). Wearable devices in healthcare: Privacy and information security issues. *Health Information Management, 49*(2–3), 150–156. https://doi.org/10.1177/1833358319851684

Colvonen, P. J. (2021). Response to: Investigating sources of inaccuracy in wearable optical heart rate sensors. *NPJ Digital Medicine, 4*(38). https://doi.org/10.1038/s41746-021-00408-5

Deloitte (2021, December 1). *Wearable technology in healthcare: Getting better all the time*. Retrieved December 31, 2022 from https://www2.deloitte.com/us/en/insights/industry/technology/technology-media-and-telecom-predictions/2022/wearable-technology-healthcare.html

Department of Justice (2021, November 1). *Justice Department secures agreement with Rite Aid Corporation to make its online COVID-19 vaccine registration portal accessible to individuals with disabilities*. https://www.justice.gov/opa/pr/justice-department-secures-agreement-rite-aid-corporation-make-its-online-covid-19-vaccine#:~:text=The%20Justice%20Department%20and%20the,book%20their%20vaccination%20appointments%20online

Department of Justice. (2022, June 7). *Julian Vargas and American Council of the Blind v. Quest Diagnostics Clinical Laboratories Inc. et al*. https://www.justice.gov/crt/case/julian-vargas-and-american-council-blind-v-quest-diagnostics-clinical-laboratories-inc-et

Department of Homeland Security. *Securing Consumer Mobile Healthcare Devices: 2021 public-private analytic exchange program. Vulnerabilities in healthcare information technology systems*. Retrieved December 31, 2022, from https://www.dhs.gov/sites/default/files/publications/phase_iii_-_securing_consumer_mobile_healthcare_devices.pdf

eVisit. (2022). *What is telecare*. https://evisit.com/resources/what-is-telecare

FCC. (2022). *What we do*. Retrieved December 31, 2022, from https://www.fcc.gov/about-fcc/what-we-do

Federal Trade Commission (FTC). *Take action*. Retrieved December 31, 2022, from https://www.ftc.gov/

Ford, C., Xie, C. X., Low, A., et al. (2022). Comparison of 2 smart watch algorithms for detection of atrial fibrillation and the benefit of clinician interpretation: SMART WARS study. *JACC Clinical Electrophysiology, 8*, 782–791. https://doi.org/10.1016/j.jacep.2022.02.013

Gao, W., Emaminejad, S., Nyein, H. Y., Challa, S., Chen, K., Peck, A. et al. (2016). Fully integrated wearable sensor arrays for multiplexed in situ perspiration analysis. *Nature, 529*(7587), 509–514. https://doi.org/10.1038/nature16521

Haghi, M., Thurow, K., Habil, J., Stoll, R., & Habil, M. (2014). Wearable devices in medical internet of Things: Scientific research and commercially available devices. *Healthcare Information Research, 23*(1), 4–15. https://doi.org/10.4258/hir.2017.23.1.4

Health Resources & Services Administration. (HRSA). (2023). Office for the Advancement of Telehealth. What is telehealth? Retrieved on July 29, 2023 from https://www.hrsa.gov/telehealth/what-is-telehealth

HealthIT.gov. *Breaches of unsecured protected health information: Number of individuals affected by protected health information breaches: 2010–2015*. Retrieved December 31, 2022, from https://www.healthit.gov/data/quickstats/breaches-unsecured-protected-health-information

Iezzoni, L. I., Rao, S. R., Ressalam, J., Bolcic-Jankovic, D., Agaronnik, N. D., Lagu, T., Pendo, E., & Campbell, E. G. (2022). US Physicians' knowledge about the Americans with Disabilities Act and accommodation of patients with disability. *Health Affairs*, *41*(1). https://doi.org/10.1377/hlthaff.2021.01136

James, T. G., Argenyi, M. S., Guardino, D. L., McKee, M. M., Wilson, J. A. B., Sullivan, M. K., Schwartzman, E. G., & Anderson, M. L. (2022). Communication access in mental health and substance use treatment facilities for deaf American Sign Language users. *Health Affairs*, *41*(10), https://doi.org/10.1377/hlthaff.2022.00408

Jiang, D., & Shi, G. (2021). Research on data security and privacy protection of wearable equipment in healthcare. *Journal of Healthcare Engineering*, 6656204. https://doi.org/10.1155/2021/6656204

Kopf, M. (2022, March 15). The difference between telehealth vs. telemedicine. k health. Retrieved from https://khealth.com/learn/healthcare/telehealth-vs-telemedicine/

Lamensch, M. (2021, August 11). Putting our bodies online: The privacy risks of tech wearables. Retrieved December 31, 2022, from https://www.cigionline.org/articles/putting-our-bodies-online-the-privacy-risks-of-tech-wearables/

LeHong, H., & Velosa, A.(2014). *A hype cycle for the internet of Things*. Gartner Inc. Retrieved December 31, 2022 from https://www.gartner.com/en/documents/2804217

McCarthy, J. (2019). One in five U.S. adults use health apps, wearable trackers. Retrieved December 31, 2022 from https://news.gallup.com/poll/269096/one-five-adults-health-apps-wearable-trackers.aspx

Office of the National Coordinator for Health Information Technology. (2016, February). *Breaches of unsecured protected health information.* Health IT Quick-Stat # 53. https://www.healthit.gov/data/quickstats/breaches-unsecured-protected-health-information

US National Library of Medicine. (2020). *Apple Heart Study: Assessment of wristwatch-based photoplethysmography to identify cardiac arrhythmias*. Retrieved December 31, 2022, from https://clinicaltrials.gov/ct2/show/NCT03335800

Weber, Lauren (2022, March 14). Pandemic medical innovations leave behind people with disabilities. *Kaiser Health News.* Retrieved from https://www.orlandomedicalnews.com/article/5561/pandemic-medical-innovations-leave-behind-people-with-disabilities

Zinzuwadia, A., & Singh, J. P. (2022). Wearable devices–addressing bias and inequity. *The Lancet: Digital Health*, *7*(12), E856–E857. https://doi.org/10.1016/S2589-7500(22)00194-7

## Additional Resources

Agarwal, V., & Buzzanell, P.M. (2008). Trialectics of migrant and global representation: Real, imaginary, and online spaces of empowerment in Cyber*mohalla*. *Western Journal of Communication*, *72*, 331–348. https://doi.org/10.1080/10570310802445975

FCC. (n.d.). Broadband health imperative. https://www.fcc.gov/health/broadbandhealthimperative

*Telehealth: What to know for your family.* https://www.cms.gov/files/document/c2c-telehealth-patient-toolkitdigital508c.pdf

Chapter 10

# Health, Religion, and Spirituality

## Chapter Learning Outcomes

Upon completion of **Chapter 10, Health, Religion, and Spirituality**, the reader should be able to employ the **WPHC SJA framework** to:

1. Articulate how religion and spirituality are similar and distinct conceptually and specifically in relationship with the goals of medicine.
2. Identify the diversity of traditions that have shaped the medical-religious partnership from ancient times through their present-day contexts.
3. Apply culturally sensitive healthcare principles for individuals from all religious and spiritual backgrounds.
4. Provide ethically grounded recommendations for the integration of religion and spirituality in healthcare settings.
5. Identify the unique challenges and considerations of integrating religion and spirituality in diverse healthcare settings such as palliative care, hospice care, end-of-life care, and chronic care self-management.
6. Provide communicative recommendations that address religious differences from the perspective of bias and discrimination.
7. Understand the relevance of medico-religious partnerships and professions in the contemporary landscape in terms of their contribution to value-based care, quality of life, and social support through communities of faith.
8. Understand the contribution of religion and spirituality in compassionate, just, and transformative care through professional training such as clinical pastoral education.
9. Explain the relationship of religion, spirituality, and health behaviors in organizational and healthcare institutional settings.
10. Situate religion and spirituality in patient-centered care for religious minorities and vulnerable populations.
11. Apply the models for integrating spirituality into medicine to help bridge the gap in medicine with spirituality and religion through constructing inclusive and culturally sensitive communicative practices.

DOI: 10.4324/9781003214472-13

**Consider the following personal experiences shared by physicians:**

I start my day walking to mass at six in the morning. It's a way to make sure everything I do for the day is done for the right reason, as an offering to God. I aim to imitate Jesus Christ. He sowed healing, physically and spiritually. Medicine is one of the professions in which you can follow him and imitate him most closely.

(Jose Florez, MD, PhD, chief, Endocrine Division and Diabetes Unit, Massachusetts General Hospital, Boston, as quoted in Boyle, 2022)

Mental health "requires that we learn to grow muscles where our injuries were. In the words of the Eighty-fourth Psalm, that man is blessed 'who, going through the vale of misery, uses it for a well.' One thing we have learned is that a full discussion of mental health requires a rich bilingualism. It requires both the poetic and prophetic metaphors of religion and the precise, hard grammar of science."

(Allport, 1963, p. 187)

I have cared for babies who I was sure were not going to live through the night and they waited for their parents to arrive, to almost give them permission to die. I remember once, this baby had been dying all day. I was sitting by the baby holding hands with one of the nurses. Then the dad came and held the baby, and suddenly all the vital signs were completely stable. For that half an hour that the dad held the baby, the baby looked the best the baby had looked. Then baby went back into the bed, the dad left, the baby died. I can't explain that.

(Andrea Weintraub, MD, attending neonatologist, as quoted in Boyle, 2022)

I practice my religion and pray for my three children every day. Sometimes I pray for patients—the ones where my instinct tells me they need an extra boost. I come back to my office and pray for them and wish they can go back to their families and have a wonderful life.

(Roopa Kohli-Seth, MD, Director, Critical Care Institute, Mount Sinai Health System, New York, as quoted in Boyle, 2022)

I fast and I pray as much as I can. Sometimes when I walk in the patient's room, and I feel like it's a difficult case, I breathe in and ask God for help, to give me the strength. Because in the end, no matter what we do as physicians, there is always some kind of higher power that has control over the destiny of people.

(Heval Mohamed Kelli, MD, Cardiologist, Northside Hospital Cardiovascular Institute, Lawrence, Georgia)

The WPHC SJA perspective is central to providing socially just and ethical care in an equitable and accessible manner that ensures adverse effects (e.g., provider moral distress or negative patient outcomes) are avoided. From a WPHC SJA perspective, such everyday scenarios evoke profound yet challenging questions such as, To what extent should providers bring their faith into their practice? And how should providers acknowledge their patients' faith in the process of their care? Research shows that connecting medical care and spirituality helps healthcare providers deliver patient-centered care and find purpose in their professional life, a key tenet of the WPHC approach. At the same time, these scenarios also raise ethical dilemmas about navigating what constitutes the right way of providing care and doing good.

Religion and spirituality in medicine are important to patients and to healthcare providers alike (Zaidi, 2018). Religion and spirituality serve to bring purpose and meaning to healthcare settings in ways that help individuals feel whole and complete. At the same time, as the instances at the outset of the chapter indicate, their intersection in healthcare domains raises important ethical dilemmas. To illustrate these quandaries, two cases from a recent issue of religion and spirituality in medicine are provided Textbox 10.1 (Zaidi, 2018). Each illustrates an all-too-common quandary in healthcare settings and poses an ethical challenge for the healthcare provider.

*Read **Textbox 10.1** to see how the authors respond to these cases and to share your thoughts. Respond to the SJA prompt that follows.*

---

### Textbox 10.1   Ethics in WPHC

#### WPHC Context

The following cases are abstracted from the resources that are cited under them. Respond to the SJA prompt after reviewing them.

#### Case 1

A patient tells his physician that he doesn't want pain medication after a cholecystectomy because "God wants [him] to be in pain." Should the clinical team comply? [Abstracted from Frush et al., 2018]

> Yes, as long as the patient's bodily integrity and health isn't threatened. [75%]
> No [13%]
> Undecided [11%]

#### SJA Prompt

* Read the full case and its discussion in the *AMA Journal of Ethics* article titled "What should physicians and chaplains do when a patient believes God wants him to suffer?" What are your thoughts?

---

## Resource

Frush, B. W., Brewer, J., Eberly, J. B., & Curlin, F. A. (2018, July). What should physicians and chaplains do when a patient believes God wants him to suffer? *AMA Journal of Ethics*. Retrieved January 4, 2023, from https://journalofethics.ama-assn.org/article/what-should-physicians-and-chaplains-do-when-patient-believes-god-wants-him-suffer/2018-07

## Case 2

The night before a scheduled bypass surgery, a patient asks her surgeon to pray with her. How should he respond? [Abstracted from Christensen et al., 2018].

Say yes, but only if he shares her religion [10%]
Say yes, even if he does not identify with her religion [56%]
Say no and call the chaplain [6%]
Say no but offer to remain with the patient while she prays [25%]
Say no and do nothing else

## SJA Prompt

Read the full case and its discussion in the AMA Journal of Ethics article titled "How should clinicians respond to requests by patients to participate in prayer?" What are your thoughts?

## Resource

Christensen, A. R., Cook, T. E., & Arnold, R. M. (2018, July). How should clinicians respond to requests from patients to participate in prayer? *AMA Journal of Ethics*. Retrieved January 4, 2023 from https://journalofethics.ama-assn.org/article/how-should-clinicians-respond-requests-patients-participate-prayer/2018-07

Patients, providers, and caregivers often face such quandaries in healthcare settings. To help construct care that is ethical and meaningful for both the patient and the provider, many hospitals have turned to the role of the hospital chaplain. In situations where spiritual and religious values create conflict or provider moral distress, the medical chaplain can use their professional training to respond to the needs of the patient, as opposed to drawing upon their own interpretation of religion and spirituality. By serving as an intermediary between patients' families and physicians, the clinical hospital chaplain can help both discuss the goals of care and coordinate clinically effective and culturally sensitive religious and spiritual strategies for patient care (Zaidi, 2018). They also underscore that for many patients, religion and spirituality are important aspects of healthcare where healing includes feeling whole, and medicine, in its goal of treating patients, should treat them as whole persons, not simply their diseases (Koenig, 2000).

## Chapter Organization

**Chapter 10, Health, Religion, and Spirituality**, presents the relationship between health, religion, and spirituality and is laid out in a comprehensive and multidimensional manner to bring out the centrality of ethics in WPHC. The chapter keeps the SJA approach front and foremost and invites the reader to consider how religion and spirituality can help achieve the goals of medicine in an impactful and purposeful manner. **Chapter 10** is laid out as follows: **First**, the concepts of religion and spirituality are defined and from their historical role in medicine and faith-based initiatives to their dimensions and their relevance to culturally sensitive WPHC for individuals, particularly from minority populations. **Second**, the chapter covers the intersections of medicine and WPHC with religion and spirituality in different contexts, such as during times of stress, death, and dying. **Third**, the chapter addresses religious differences from the perspective of bias and discrimination and situates medical-religious partnerships and their role in integrating religion, spirituality, and quality of life in communities of faith. **Fourth**, the chapter covers religion and spirituality in compassionate, just, and transformative WPHC, including current contexts such as clinical pastoral education. **Fifth**, the chapter outlines the relationship of religion, spirituality, and health behaviors, while situating it within organizational and WPHC institutional settings. **Sixth**, the chapter offers avenues to think about, including religion and spirituality in WPHC-based patient-centered care, and considers its implications for vulnerable populations. **Seventh**, and in conclusion, the chapter provides models for integrating spirituality into medicine along with avenues for students to think about how medicine can bridge the gap between spirituality and religion, centering considerations of cultural diversity in WPHC contexts.

Along the way, students are provided multiple contexts for reflection, ranging from discussion questions to present challenges and future scenarios, opportunities to engage with the SJA actions to help advance the ethical goals of religion and spirituality in WPHC, implicit bias, cultural competence, inclusion, and respect in WPHC institutional settings and in interpersonal physician-patient contexts. Communication scholars Dr. Sarah Amira de la Garza and Drs. Kandi Walker, Madeline Tomlinson, and Joy Hart share their thoughts on religion and spirituality in WPHC from the perspective of mindful heresy and student action, respectively.

## Religion, Medicine, and WPHC Meaning Making

People often turn to prayer in times of distress. Religion and spirituality become especially important in times of challenging healthcare diagnosis and prognosis. Religion and

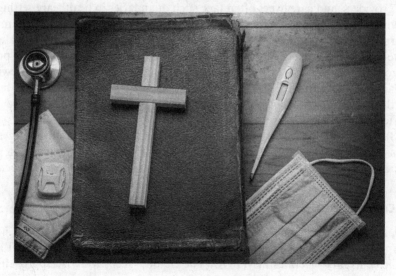

*Figure 10.1* Religion and Spirituality are Important Components of Culturally Sensitive Healthcare.

spirituality are reported to help cancer patients find meaning in their illness, provide comfort in the face of existential fears, and receive support from a community of like-minded individuals (Alcorn et al., 2010; Park, 2013; Preau et al., 2013). The National Health Interviews Survey found that 69% of cancer patients reported praying for their health compared to 45% of the general US population (Ross et al., 2008). This section covers the conceptual description of religion and spirituality, along with its dimensions, and provides a context for considering culturally sensitive care that can bridge the gap in meeting the needs of minority populations.

### Religion and Spirituality

Religion has been understood as "a system of beliefs and practices observed by a community, supported by rituals that acknowledge, worship, communicate with, or approach the Sacred, the Divine, God (in Western cultures), or Ultimate Truth, Reality, or nirvana (in Eastern cultures)" (Koenig, 2008, p. 11). Religion has provided individuals solace during serious illness through the ages (Koenig et al., 2000). Spirituality has been defined as "the way individuals seek and express meaning and purpose, and experience connectedness to self, others, the significant or sacred" (Puchalski et al., 2014). Others have emphasized that spirituality is referenced in a connection with a source larger than oneself and with feelings of transcendence whereas religion is referenced with practices such as religious affiliation and service attendance. Spirituality is conceptually related to but not like religion. People who describe themselves as spiritual may not necessarily see themselves as religious.

Review **Textbox 10.2** to see the four dimensions of religion and spirituality and their definitions.

---

**Textbox 10.2   Dimensions of Religion and Spirituality**

**WPHC Context**

**Affective dimension**:
Defined as the subjective emotional experience of religion and spirituality, such as a sense of transcendence, meaning, purpose, and connection to a source larger than oneself as well as struggling with or feeling anger toward God.

**Behavioral dimension**:
Defined as the use of religious or spiritual practices or behaviors to manage stress and life events such as those related to cancer and its treatment including meditation, prayer, pursuing a connection with God, attending religious services, and strengthening connections with religious persons, activities, or groups.

**Cognitive dimension**:
Defined as statements that an individual believes to be true about religion and spirituality, such as causal attributions, spiritual post-traumatic growth, religious fatalism, and intrinsic religious or spiritual beliefs.

**Physical dimension**:
Defined as comprising physical well-being (i.e., an ability to perform activities of daily living ranging from basic self-care to more strenuous physical activities), functional well-being (i.e., perceived difficulties in fulfilling roles at home, at work, or in the

community due to physical health), and self-reported physical symptoms (i.e., fatigue, pain, sleep, cognition, and other physical symptoms) [Jim et al., 2016].

**SJA Prompt:**

- Have you or someone close to you faced a healthcare challenge? Did you or your loved one turn to religion or spirituality as a way of making sense of the challenge?
- Would you prefer that your healthcare provider cared about your religious and spiritual beliefs in the delivery of care?
- In situations where delivery of care settings conflict with the religious and spiritual beliefs of patients (e.g., prayer time or type of food and medication prescribed), how should providers and healthcare institutions respond?

### Resource

Jim et al. (2016). Religion, spirituality, and physical health in cancer patients: A meta-analysis. *Cancer*, *121*(21), 3760–3768. https://doi.org/10.1002/cncr.29353

## Culturally Sensitive Religious and Spiritual WPHC

From a WPHC SJA framework, it becomes important to see that everyone, no matter what their religious or spiritual beliefs, receives culturally sensitive care that helps them achieve better health outcomes in alignment with their deepest beliefs. However, research shows that minority populations have been found to receive lower quality WPHC stemming from inadequate training and knowledge of WPHC providers in cultural sensitivity and inadequate assessment of culturally informed WPHC needs. For instance, the seven million American Muslims comprise an ethnically and racially diverse population that shares religiously informed WPHC values. These individuals can comprise individuals from African American, Arab American, and South Asian American ethnicities and nationalities. The diversity of values under this umbrella reflects a range of cultural beliefs surrounding gender (e.g., modesty), nutrition (e.g., *halal* food), and prayer (e.g., *namaz* time; *azaan*). Such values are of importance in the WPHC SJA perspective because they deeply influence the expectations of care and the ethics of being well individuals bring to WPHC.

### History of the Relationship of Medicine and Faith

The relationship of medicine with faith is not new. In fact, medicine has a rich history of partnership with faith-based initiatives. Ancient cultures ranging from ancient Egypt to China and the Mesopotamian civilizations through the Middle Ages with the Renaissance have interwoven the goals of health and healing with faith and the practice of spirituality. In fact, the traditions of medicine and religion separated as distinct fields only in recent history during the past 200–300 years in the Age of Enlightenment.

*Read **Textbox 10.3** for a glimpse of the wide range of how religion and health beliefs are interwoven in some of the major religious worldviews today. To what extent should patient hopes for a medical miracle shape provider expectations and delivery of care?*

## Textbox 10.3   Medical Miracle: Faith, Religion, and Spirituality

### WPHC Context

Medicine and religion have been intertwined throughout history in an intimate and complex relationship.

During times of serious illness, Trevor Bibler, a **clinical ethicist** (Bibler, 2019), says patients often ask, "Why is this happening to me?" And the question facing WPHC providers often is, "How should medicine respond to patients and families who hope for a miracle?"

A key struggle Bibler observes is in understanding how best to respect the religious and spiritual beliefs of patients and families, understanding what they mean by a **medical miracle**, and how WPHC professionals should approach the conversation. The challenge often lies in resolving the impasse when the hope for a miracle appears to conflict with a WPHC professional's idea of what good medicine looks like. Such questions call into focus the relationships between life, death, medicine, and the Divine. Each religion approaches these questions from its own unique perspective. Their intersection with medicine opens the door to a vast new landscape, one filled with hope, coping, and resilience but also ethical issues relating to the practice of science, medicine, and the intersection of different faiths (on the occasion when the provider and the patient subscribe to different religious and/or spiritual belief systems).

In the **Bible**, Jesus called his twelve disciples to him and gave them the authority to cast out evil spirits and to heal every kind of disease and sickness (Matthew 10:1).

In **Judaism**, the verses in the Torah quote: "And He said: 'If you will diligently harken to the voice of the Lord, your God, and will do that which is right in His sight, and will give ear to His commandments, and keep all His statutes, I will put none of these diseases upon you which I put on the Egyptians; for I am the Lord, your healer'" (Exodus 15:26) (Hakohen & Schwartz, n.d.).

In the **Qu'ran**, Abu Sa'id al-Khudri r.a. reported that the Prophet said, "Whenever a Muslim is afflicted with a hardship, sickness, sadness, worry, harm, or depression—even a thorn's prick, Allah expiates his sins because of it."

The **Bhagavad Gita** states (in Sanskrit), "The one who is not depressed in adversity or disturbed by pleasure and pain, and is devoid of attachment, fear and anger—he is indeed a steadfast one" (Gita II – 56).

**Buddhist** biographies of illness and disease and practice encourage finding spiritual meaning in illness (Chaudhury, 2017), such as "illness can motivate you to pursue your spiritual practice; illness can introduce you to the path of liberation; illness can intensi[fy] and enrich your training ... therefore the wise carry illness onto the path" (Longchenpa, 2).

### SJA Discussion Prompt

Given the diversity of religious views and practices, and the centrality of religion in sickness and illness, consider the following SJA questions:

- How do religious beliefs shape the expectations patients bring to WPHC?
- What role might religion and spirituality play in helping providers and patients achieve their goals of WPHC-centered outcomes?

- To what extent can and should religion and spirituality be accommodated in WPHC contexts?
- How should providers respond to a patient's hope for a medical miracle in times of a challenging diagnosis?

### Resources

Bibler, T. (2019, April 5). Exploring the role of faith in medicine. *Center for Medical Ethics and Health Policy*. Retrieved on January 4, 2023, from https://blogs.bcm.edu/2019/04/05/exploring-the-role-of-faith-in-medicine/

Chaudhury, K. (2017). Health and sickness: A Buddhist view and implications for social marketing. *Journal of Nonprofit & Public Sector Marketing, 29*(4), 450–464. https://doi.org/10.1080/10495142.2017.1326357

Hakohen, Y. B. S., & Schwartz, R. H. (n.d.). *Prevention: Torah perspectives on preserving health*. Retrieved on January 4, 2023, from https://www.jewishveg.org/schwartz/health.html

Seshadri, T. R. (1997). *The curative powers of the Holy Gita*. Full Circle.

*Sickness according to Qur'an and Sunnah*. Retrieved January 4, 2023, from https://www.missionislam.com/health/sickness.html

Although everyone has deeply personal views of religion and spirituality and their place in WPHC, the questions posed by Textbox 10.3 are not easy to answer. In their quest to deliver patient-centered care, today, many hospitals and faith-based service groups benefit from the support of religious communities. Religion and spirituality also influence patient care at individual and community levels, particularly when the needs and beliefs of a diverse community population must be considered. Research supports the imperative to provide religious and spiritual support. Spiritual support has been helpful in the cancer journeys of those diagnosed with cancer. For instance, researcher Andrea Meluch (2018) finds that spiritual support can help patients with meaning making and finding purpose in their diagnoses, fostering a connection with shared beliefs related to spirit and faith, and aiding well-being by providing feelings of centeredness.

Religion and spirituality are central to peoples' lives. As such, their role is intimately tied up with a view of what adequate WPHC should look like.

Look at **Textbox 10.4**. *Try your hand at responding to the discussion questions examining the challenges faced by WPHC providers and patients alike. What advice and recommendations would you give?*

### Textbox 10.4  Discussion Question/Thought Scenario for Reflection

#### Spirituality and WPHC: What Can Practitioners Do?

##### WPHC Context

The Gallup Poll measures Americans' views on God and religion as part of its *Values and Beliefs* poll in its Gallup Poll social Series. Gallup measured US adults' belief in God in three different ways in recent years. Interestingly, each different way of asking the question provided varying results through the years. In 2022, Gallup found 81% of Americans expressing belief when asked the simple question, "Do you believe in God?," down from 87% in 2017. In 1944, 96% believed in God.

## SJA Discussion Questions

Polls and surveys have consistently highlighted how religious and spiritual beliefs and practices are important in the lives of patients (e.g., Saad & Hrynowski, 2022). Given this data, medical students, residents, and physicians are often uncertain about whether, when, or how, to address spiritual or religious issues with their patients in healthcare settings. Think through some of the considerations regarding religion and spirituality in WPHC that have been discussed in the chapter from a WPHC SJA perspective (Spirituality and Medicine, 2014).

Write down your thoughts on the following questions:

- Is it important to attend to spirituality in medicine? Why?
- How would you advise a WPHC professional to take a "spiritual history" in a culturally sensitive manner?
- What would respect for persons from a spiritual perspective look like in WPHC-centered WPHC settings?
- What role should hospital chaplains play? How can they meet the gaps in diverse religious and spiritual perspectives?
- What role should your own personal beliefs play in your physician-patient relationship?
- What religious and spiritual beliefs and expectations do you bring to your meeting with your WPHC provider?
- What challenges can you identify in integrating discussions of spirituality with patients? What are some appropriate avenues for integrating these concerns?
- How can training for integrating spirituality in medicine be designed with physicians-in-training? What would such training include?

## WPHC Reflection Prompt

- How would you prefer your physician to approach religious or spiritual content with you?
- Will your response differ from a well visit to a visit before a serious surgery? If so, what expectations of religion and healthcare do you bring to your visit with your physician in each instance?

## Resources

Saad, L., & Hrynowski, Z. (2022, June 24). *The Gallup Poll. How many Americans believe in God?* Retrieved January 4, 2023, from https://news.gallup.com/poll/268205/americans-believe-god.aspx

Spirituality and medicine. (April 2014). *Ethics in medicine.* Retrieved on January 4, 2023, from https://depts.washington.edu/bhdept/ethics-medicine/bioethics-topics/detail/79

### Religion and Spirituality in Health Messages and Clinical Settings

Religion and medicine have deep historical roots. In health communication research, understanding how religion, spirituality, and health meaning making shape health behaviors is particularly important for understanding their relationship with health promotion and disease prevention (Parrott, 2004). For instance, Peterson explores the support experiences of coping with HIV and AIDS to argue that the connection between spirituality, communication, and social support can prove helpful in improving health outcomes (Peterson, 2011). Communication researchers Egbert et al. (2004) find evidence supporting how understanding communication within a religious group is an important facet for understanding the individual's self-concept regarding health. They also emphasize how religion and spirituality are important components in understanding one's willingness to disclose health-related information to a WPHC provider.

Patient disclosure of health-related information to their WPHC providers is an important component of trust in the WPHC relationship. Such research underscores the centrality of religion and spirituality in building a trusting and open WPHC relationship. Research also demonstrates the value of religion and spirituality in clinical health communication settings. In communicating health messages, religious and spirituality components including dimensions such as religious coping, decision-making, and spiritual well-being can be helpful in promoting self-efficacy, or an individual's feeling that they can perform a desired response or behavior (Witte, 1994). Increasing self-efficacy can be an important factor for individuals coping with chronic conditions or challenging health diagnoses that require substantial self-management. Questions posed by Egbert and other health communication researchers identify challenges around how religious commitment can be used in constructing persuasive health messages and to what extent it may be appropriate to do so. Additional questions include considering how a relationship with God can affect social support networks in times of health-related stress. Such research is even more relevant today when religion and politics are at the center of health-related decisions in many contexts ranging from reproductive health rights to end-of-life decision-making and vaccination. The intersection of health, religion and spirituality, and control and autonomy of the human body has never been more central in recent times.

*Examine the concerns raised by communication professors **Kandi Walker**, **Madeline Tomlinson**, and **Joy Hart** in **Textbox 10.5**, **Scholar Interview**, and share your thoughts on the SJA questions they raise.*

---

### TEXTBOX 10.5   Scholar Interview

**Dr. Kandi L. Walker, Dr. Madeline M. Tomlinson and Dr. Joy L. Hart**
*University of Louisville*

#### Religion, Politics, and Public Health

If scientists and governments deem a practice important for public health, should individuals be allowed exceptions? If so, what type of exceptions are acceptable? For example, should the government intervene when family members or guardians don't take children to receive biomedical care due to religious beliefs?

Most states allow religious exemptions to seeking medical treatment. An online search will reveal many news articles about cases where parents/guardians did not take their child for medical treatment, including some articles where the death of a child occurred. As you read through examples, think about questions like the following: When should the government step in, or should it step in at all, if parents/guardians do not seek medical attention for their child due to religious beliefs? Does your opinion change if the treatment is regarded as necessary to save or prolong life? How should the rights of the child, the parents/guardians, and the state (as well as public health interests) be weighed?

Would your opinions on the previous questions change if others might be harmed? For example, vaccines have been a point of discussion recently, with heightened interest in required school vaccines. For context, all 50 states require a child to have certain vaccines to attend public school. Most states allow religious exemptions to this mandate; however, states such as California, New York, Maine, Mississippi, and West Virginia allow exemptions only for medical reasons. What is the student vaccination requirement in your state? Does your state allow religious exemptions? For required vaccinations to attend public school, what arguments can be made in favor of limiting exemptions to medical reasons? Conversely, what arguments can be made in favor of allowing religious exemptions?

If separation of church and state is a fundamental tenet in the United States, what factors should be considered in potential health-related exemptions due to religion?

### Palliative Care, End-of-Life Decision-Making, and Chronic Conditions

The connections of medicine and WPHC with religion and spirituality evoked by the scholar interview with Drs. Walker, Tomlinson, and Hart become even more central during times of great stress. Consider the context of religion and spirituality during palliative care, hospice care, and in end-of-life decision-making. Palliative care is care given to people living with a serious illness (e.g., cancer) and can include end-of-life care. Religion and spirituality are key sources of support in palliative care contexts that help family members, caregivers, and WPHC providers navigate and make sense of health at the intersection of what it means to live a purposeful and meaningful life. An appropriate understanding of the intersection of health, religion, and spirituality is valuable for structuring communication in the sense-making involved in final communications with the terminally ill. An analysis of messages shared during final conversations by communication researchers highlights how they center religious faith and spirituality and can help guide provider-patient communication in palliative and end-of-life contexts.

#### Final Communication Messages

Researcher Maureen Keeley finds that final conversation messages reveal three "rules of conduct" that address areas such as (a) coping with life challenges after the death of a loved one, (b) being involved in the death and dying process, and (c) enacting religion and spirituality during death and dying (Keeley, 2004). In the context of chronic disease management, communication researchers have examined spirituality for designing health promotion messages. Spirituality has undergirded the communication strategy for HIV/AIDS prevention and education programs in global contexts. In Brazil, the unique features of the Afro-Brazilian religion were considered in the establishment of the Odo-Ya Project, which sought to provide spiritually based HIV education (Da Silva & Guimaraes, 2000). Organizationally, the integration of religion and spirituality in WPHC institutions has proved to be a valuable resource in structuring meaningful and culturally sensitive care for the sick.

*Examine* **Textbox 10.6** *to learn more about how one organization, the Bikur Cholim, has honored the mitzvah to help patients with their well-being in WPHC settings. Try your hand at the SJA prompt, examining how such care has been integrated into WPHC institutions.*

---

**Textbox 10.6**    *Bikur Cholim*: **Organizational Integration of Religion and Spirituality in WPHC Institutions**

**WPHC Context**

Learn more about how Bikur Cholim has honored the *mitzvah* to visit and extend aid to the sick. https://www.bikurcholimcleveland.org/

**SJA Prompt**

• Examine Bikur Cholim Baltimore's page on Johns Hopkins Hospital. How have different hospital systems exemplified religious inclusion and respect?

**Resource**

Bikur Cholim, Baltimore. Retrieved on January 4, 2023, from https://baltimorebikurcholim.org/hospitals/johns-hopkins-hospital/

---

*Delineating Religion and Spirituality*

Given their centrality in healthcare, the contexts in which religion and spirituality are enacted in WPHC bear careful understanding and interpretation for context, values, and outcomes. Understanding religion and spirituality in WPHC contexts starts from the understanding that being spiritual does not mean the same as being religious. For some individuals, religious rituals, and practices such as going to church or praying may hold special value during times of WPHC stress. For others, seeking meaning and purpose in connections with nature or the universe at an abstract level may hold greater value and be a source of support and wellness. Most discussions, however, place religion and spirituality in the same basket to structure discussions around their contribution.

Communication researchers have sought to delineate spirituality from religion in understanding the value of spirituality during serious illness. One of the challenges in separating spirituality from religion in providing guidance to WPHC workers is that there is very little evidence base to do so. McGrath examines how individuals construct spirituality in the face of life-threatening illness and the need to use such understandings to develop a language that is reflective of the commonalities of human experience (2005). She finds that for individuals who approach spirituality from a nonreligious framework, there is a lack of a shared language that can be used to communicate their insights and experience with serious illness.

## Religion, Spirituality, and Quality of Life

Providing culturally appropriate WPHC that acknowledges the religious and spiritual beliefs of the patients while attending to their physical well-being and health outcomes throws up several challenges. Currently, the most appropriate modes of conceptualization and delivery of care that are empathetic and patient-centered, while meeting the ethics of including religious and spiritual conversations in WPHC, are still very much under deliberation.

### Pastors and Communities of Support

Although there is much uncertainty in how to negotiate religion and spirituality in WPHC, there are some shared bonds and concerns among the two vastly different, yet similar professions of the clergy and the WPHC provider. WPHC providers and pastors are similar in that they have a shared common bond of trust with their patients and congregations. Medical-religious partnerships have significant value because of the established and trusting relationships they draw upon. Research has found that religious beliefs and practices may help people to cope better with stressful life circumstances, give meaning and hope, and surround depressed persons with a supportive community (Bonelli et al., 2012). Studies on cancer outcomes in patients show that religion and spirituality are associated with better patient-reported physical health, and patients' religious and spiritual needs should be attended to as part of comprehensive cancer care (Jim et al., 2016). Yet, what is unclear is how such spiritual and religious care should be provided in ethical and culturally respectful ways in WPHC contexts.

*How can WPHC providers be sensitive to the different religious and spiritual beliefs of their patients? Examine* **Textbox 10.7** *to understand some communication strategies that can guide the provision of culturally sensitive WPHC. Consider the WPHC implications of the recommendations and try your hand at the SJA prompt that might help guide your decisions.*

---

**Textbox 10.7   Addressing Religious Bias in WPHC**

Religious differences can give rise to bias and discrimination in the practice of WPHC. Here are some recommendations Swihart et al. (2022) provide for WPHC providers to gain knowledge and understanding of the backgrounds and beliefs of their culturally diverse or religious patients.

**WHPC Recommendations**

The recommendations are helpful in providing **culturally sensitive WPHC**:

Apologize for cultural mistakes.
Ask the patient and family how you can help make their experience more comfortable.
Avoid being judgmental.
Avoid making assumptions and be patient.
Avoid employees serving as interpreters for other employees.
Be aware of the uniqueness of their religion and their special needs.

---

Be respectful.
Observe body and facial language.
Recognize how values, behaviors, and beliefs may affect others.
Train staff about cultural competence.
Use medically competent and fluent interpreters with training in cultural competence.

Strategies for improving **cultural competence** in individuals and systems:

Encouraging family to participate in WPHC decision-making.
Incorporating culture-specific values into health promotion.
Providing cultural awareness training.
Providing an environment that allows traditional healers.
Providing interpreter services.
Recruiting minority staff.

### SJA Prompt

- Should religious and spiritually appropriate care only be provided in specific circumstances such as palliative care or hospice care?
- If so, what criteria would you recommend be applied to the determination of such circumstances?
- What ethical bases would you provide to support your recommendation?

### Resource

Swihart, D. L., Naga, S., Yarrarapu, S., & Martin, R. L. (2022). Cultural religious competence in clinical practice. *National Library of Medicine: National Center for Biotechnology Information*. Retrieved January 4, 2023, from https://www.ncbi.nlm.nih.gov/books/NBK493216/

### Compassionate, Just, and Transformative WPHC

The recent integration of religion and spirituality in WPHC has moved toward the goal of providing compassionate, just, and transformative care. Increasing recognition that WPHC is a human right rather than an economic and social privilege was sharpened through the disparities in health outcomes revealed by the COVID-19 pandemic. Exemplifying this shift, organizations such as the Association for Clinical Pastoral Education (ACPE) that are now recognized by the Department of Education, seek to provide contemporary standards for spiritual care and education. Clinical Pastoral Education (CPE) is characterized by a diverse membership that includes certified CPE educators, spiritually integrated psychotherapists, spiritual care professionals and practitioners, pastoral counselors, chaplains, faith communities, and seminaries. This diverse membership reflects ACPE's multidisciplinary, multifaith, multiracial ethic. Following the premise of WHPC, CPE training can help individuals further their spiritual health as part of achieving the goals of compassionate and transformative care. Compassionate and transformative care also seeks to achieve productive understandings of suffering and WPHC challenges that force individuals to re-examine their lifestyles and existing goals and priorities.

## Clinical Pastoral Education (CPE)

CPE has shifted toward emphasizing an experience that is responsive to cultural develop-ments in supporting pastoral growth. Many training institutions emphasize the heart of the CPE as "ministry with the sick, injured, and dying, and learning from that ministry" (Hopkins Medicine, 2022). The employment of reflection, discussion, and evaluation in a small group setting helps CPE trainees to become familiar with the WPHC environment, as well as behav-ioral sciences and theological reflection.

## Pastoral Care in Clinical Settings

CPEs seek to pay attention to the "spiritual needs and resources of each individual [by] par-ticipating in the comforting and loving activity of God in order to promote the restoration of health and wholeness" (Johns Hopkins Medicine, 2022). Parish nurses in faith-based organi-zations view themselves as promoters of health and employ a holistic approach to health combining emotional and spiritual dimensions in their delivery of WPHC (Anderson, 2004). In their study drawing upon Entman's framing perspective to study sermons given in the state of Connecticut after the Sandy Hook shootings, Olufowote and Matusitz find that clergy used "social support" and "social system" frames along with silence to delineate between the secu-lar and the spiritual and to mitigate and promote mental illness stigma (Olufowote & Matusitz, 2016).

## Medical Miracle

From the previous discussions, it is easy to see how religion and spirituality are important components of some patients' psychosocial framework when faced with an illness diagnosis or during chronic illness management. During times of great stress, many patients and their caregivers look toward their WPHC providers in the hope of a medical miracle. Other patients have reported improved outcomes when religion and spirituality are included in their WPHC conversations, whether this is through a wellness journey or when facing a frightening diagno-sis. At the same time, physicians, when faced with conversations from their patients about religion, are often unsure of how to respond and negotiate such requests for sharing personal information. To understand how physicians can respond to patient requests for religious dis-closure, Canzona and colleagues employ Petronio's Communication Privacy Management (CPM) Theory (Canzona et al. 2015).

## Constructing Religious and Spiritual Privacy Boundaries

Through the lens of the CPM, they examine how family medicine physicians construct and communicate privacy boundaries in response to patient requests for religious disclosure (Petronio, 2002). The CPM Theory provides a framework to help understand how individuals make decisions related to the disclosure of private information. It assumes that individuals believe they own their private information and will prefer to reveal information to others through a process that involves a negotiation of tensions between sharing and concealing information. Decisions regarding disclosure, the process by which information is given or received, are made because of the potential of such information to increase or decrease risk. For example, an individual will weigh whether disclosing a medical diagnosis, such as that of

HIV/AIDs or cancer, will cause greater concern or worry to their loved ones in making the decision on whether, when, and how to disclose such private information. The CPM is useful, for instance, in cases when quandaries arise in instances when patients inquire about their provider's religion to receive care congruent with their religious beliefs.

## Religion, Spirituality, and Health Behaviors

Spiritual care in health settings has also focused its attention on empowering individuals to utilize the spiritual resources of their own faith and traditions to heal. WPHC emphasizes achieving positive WPHC outcomes by helping individuals find a way of making meaning of suffering and pain. Such considerations are especially important in conditions that require lifelong management, such as chronic conditions.

### Chronic Condition Self-Management

An aging population and a growing concern with the chronic disease epidemic have spurred the need to consider religious and spiritual community-based approaches toward preventive care and lifestyle self-management for chronic diseases. The role of medical professionals in the management of chronic diseases and their acute exacerbations is well recognized. However, the responsibility for the day-to-day management of chronic conditions is placed largely on the individuals. There is increasing recognition that religious and spiritual care that is culturally sensitive can support health literacy at a community level effectively. This management could involve using medications correctly and on time, implementing lifestyle changes, sustaining preventive and desirable behaviors, and monitoring one's overall health (Galiatsatos et al., 2020).

### Preventive Care and Faith

To support individuals in their self-management of chronic conditions and to support preventive care in those at-risk, WPHC organizations have increasingly sought to find ways to reach out with pastoral care information and timely support when the use of medical services is required. WPHC organizations offering clinical pastoral services emphasize their ecumenical and interfaith basis. Care is also taken to respect everyone's religious and spiritual preferences and offer patients the right to accept or decline services.

*Look at **Textbox 10.8** for an overview of how organizations and WPHC institutions offer religious and spiritual services to achieve WPHC outcomes. Respond to the SJA prompt provided. What additional questions should be asked in this context that are currently not being asked?*

---

**Textbox 10.8   Religion, Spirituality, and WPHC**

**WPHC Context**

Organization, Mission, and Vision
Association for Clinical Pastoral Education (ACPE)

### Mission and Vision

ACPE's mission is to positively affect people's lives by nurturing connections to the sacred through experiential education and spiritual care. Its vision is to create measurable and appreciable improvement in spiritual health that transforms people and communities in the United States and across the globe.

## Johns Hopkins Medicine Department of Spiritual Care and Chaplaincy

### Mission and Vision

The spiritual care and chaplaincy mission of the Johns Hopkins Medicine Spiritual Care and Chaplaincy Program is to (a) provide excellent and effective spiritual care and chaplaincy support, which attends to the spiritual needs of the patients, their families, staff, and personnel; (b) provide opportunities for the discussion of the religious, spiritual, and ethical dimensions of WPHC for clergy, WPHC professionals, and interested laity; and (c) engage in partnership with the religious community [to] promote health and wholeness.

## Telehealth Equity Coalition (TEC)

### Mission and Vision

Focused on equity, inclusion, representation, accountability, collaboration, and innovation, the mission of TEC is to improve access to quality and affordable WPHC by increasing the adoption of telehealth, especially among those communities that have been left out or left behind. TEC seeks to offer a unique voice to optimize equitable telehealth delivery and utilization by taking a data-driven approach to identifying opportunities, advocating to improve telehealth policy, developing a first-of-its-kind open-source telehealth data dashboard and maps, and building a coalition of academics and supporters to advocate for greater access to telehealth.

## Trusted Connectivity Alliance (TCA)

### Mission and Vision

TCA's vision is to drive the sustained growth of a connected society through trusted connectivity that protects assets, end-user privacy, and networks.

Mission: To collectively define requirements and provide deliverables of a strategic, technical, and marketing nature, that enable all stakeholders in our connected society to benefit from the most stringent secure connectivity solutions that leverage our members' expertise in tamper-proof, end-to-end security.

## SJA Prompt

- What values did you identify in the previous mission and vision statements that demonstrate respect for persons?
- How do organizations enact socially just religious and spiritual communication?

- Could you identify any gaps for vulnerable and minority populations whose religious and spiritual care needs may not be adequately addressed?
- What recommendations would you provide to the aforementioned organizations to be more religiously and spiritually inclusive in an interfaith and diverse manner?

### Resources

ACPE. (2020). *About us*. Retrieved January 1, 2023, from https://acpe.edu/about-acpe. Telehealth Equity Coalition. https://www.telehealthequitycoalition.org/index.html
Johns Hopkins Medicine. (n.d.). *Our spiritual care and Chaplaincy mission*. Retrieved January 1, 2023, from https://www.hopkinsmedicine.org/spiritualcare/history-vision-mission.html

*Local Religious Organizations and Health Education Programs*

A key facet of WPHC SJA is collaboration and integration. As the overview of WPHC organizations and their mission and vision statements in Textbox 10.6 suggests, the role of **local religious organizations** in supporting **health education programs** for their **congregations** and communities has gained prominence.

#### MEDICO-RELIGIOUS PARTNERSHIPS

To illustrate, Johns Hopkins Medicine has partnerships with more than 500 individuals from local congregations to help their congregants manage chronic conditions. Although these **medical-religious partnerships** are important in the daily efforts to provide patient-centered WPHC, these partnerships are also valuable in times of crisis, such as when the COVID-19 pandemic struck (Adhikari et al., 2020).

#### FAITH LEADERS AS OPINION LEADERS

This education took the form of discussing COVID-19 health-related recommendations in actionable manners, such as, for example, in promoting masking behaviors and good hygiene. They also provided a valuable platform for individuals to share their struggles and successes and support their mental health challenges. Johns Hopkins Hospital held twice-weekly calls with community leaders with introductions, COVID-19 updates by physicians, and other updates and issues, with the final five minutes being reserved for a closing meditation. These meditations were designed to be inclusive of all faith traditions and nonsectarian. Specific religious observances of meditations, such as during Passover, Good Friday, or Ramadan, were also offered as appropriate. Such meditations helped community faith leaders gain support for their own spiritual nurturance while supporting resilience using spiritual tools for their congregants.

*Gaps in Furthering the Spiritual Health-Identity Connection*

The previous discussion indicates the significance of integrating religious and spiritual care with WPHC to achieve the goals of WPHC. With increasing evidence suggesting a strong relationship between religion, spirituality, and health there is a need to further understand how the terms are understood, practiced, and the processes by which they shape health outcomes (Miller & Thoresen, 2003). Communication researchers have examined how communication facilitates the spirituality-health connection. For instance, Kline finds that affirmation of a conception of God and spiritual law, of one's spiritual identity, and attaining a spiritual-based understanding of health helped testifiers and Christian Science practitioners enlisted to pray with testifiers to restore their health (Kline, 2011). The findings from this study suggest that for healthy individuals, the risk of mortality from cardiovascular disease is reduced for church/service attenders, largely through the healthy lifestyle it encourages (Powell et al., 2003). Yet, the landscape of aligning religious beliefs and workplace practices can be fraught for patients and providers alike at many levels. One instance in which the provider or employee's religious beliefs can come into conflict in the line of duty and its implications for those it serves is illustrated in Textbox 10.9.

*As you read through this thought scenario, consider the discussion questions given in **Textbox 10.9** for reflection and provide your recommendations.*

---

**Textbox 10.9   Discussion Question/Thought Scenario for Reflection**

**Religious Accommodations in Law Enforcement and Implicit Bias Training**

*WPHC Thought Scenario*

Law enforcement, religion and spirituality, and community health are central facets of WPHC. In several states, the law requires WPHC practitioners to attest that they have completed an implicit bias training program on their license renewal application (e.g., Maryland.gov 2022). However, findings suggest that there are still gaps in how it has changed what police officers do on their job, although it makes some difference in the reflection on unconscious associations that may affect decisions and actions (NPR, 2020). On the other hand, sometimes the demands of law enforcement conflict with freedom of religion. On such occasions, police officers' religious observances can sometimes feel discriminated against.

Lynn Grunloh writes about a devout Baptist police officer in Indiana who was forbidden by his religious beliefs from gambling and aiding others in their gambling efforts. These values came into conflict with his professional duties when he was assigned by the police force to a full-time position as a Gaming Commission agent at a casino in Indiana. Based on the definition of "employer," "person," "employee," and "religion," there are limited protections from religious discrimination while on duty. However, Title VII provides for an exemption that limits the breadth of such protection. Under Title VII, employers are required to reasonably accommodate employees' religious observances and preferences (Grunloh, n.d.; Department of Justice, 2023).

Grunloh explains that religious discrimination is prohibited "unless an employer demonstrates that he is unable to reasonably accommodate an employee's, or prospective employee's, religious observance or practice without undue hardship on the conduct of the employer's business." However, an accommodation of a religious observance or practice is not required if doing so would impose an undue hardship on the employer. Therefore, religious discrimination is not entirely prohibited under Title VII.

## WPHC Prompt

1. Look at the Community Resource Center (CRC) web page on the Department of Justice's website (https://www.justice.gov/crs/our-focus/religion). It provides some examples of how CRC supports communities experiencing tension based on religion through initiatives such as:

   - Facilitating dialogue between law enforcement and religious community members
   - Providing training to law enforcement awareness of civil rights issues impacting Muslim and Sikh Americans
   - Conducting programs with schools
   - Holding public "protecting places of worship" community forums and gatherings

2. Consider the case of the Tree of Life synagogue shooting in October 2018. In response, a daylong event was coordinated by federal agencies, the city of Pittsburgh, and a local university. CRC led the interagency initiative to increase the federal agencies' capacity to present and respond to hate crimes in Pittsburgh by forming a working group comprising local federal employees.

3. Considering the increased hate crimes against minority communities during the COVID-19 pandemic, many Asian Americans, Native Hawaiians, and Pacific Islanders were afraid to leave their homes (DOJ, n.d.). Their worry about contracting the virus was in addition to their fear for their physical safety. Review the press release dated May 20, 2022, titled "DOJ, Joined by the Department of Health and Human Services (HHS), Announce New Initiatives to Address and Prevent Hate Crimes and Hate Initiatives" (URL: https://www.hhs.gov/about/news/2022/05/20/justice-department-announces-new-initiatives-address-prevent-hate-crimes-hate-incidents.html).

## SJA Discussion Questions

Utilizing the resources provided in this discussion prompt, reflect upon some of the key concerns, conflicts, and tensions you might have begun to identify. As the *Police1* article included in the "Resources" tab in this textbox notes, law enforcement, as a profession, is extremely stressful, with officers responding to stresses from responding to calls for service, leadership within the department, society's expectations, spouses and family members, finances, or even from within, as officers tend to hold their actions and behaviors to very high standards (select URL from the "Resources" tab; *Police1*, 2017; Stark, n.d.).

- How do you see the role of religion and spirituality in policing?
- What are some challenges you can identify? For law enforcement officers? For community members? For minority and vulnerable populations?
- Based on your discussion and review of the resources provided, what are some initiatives that can help address the challenges that you've identified?

## Resources

Maryland.gov. (2022). *Implicit bias training required for 2022 license renewal.* Retrieved December 31, 2022, from https://health.maryland.gov/boardsahs/Documents/implicitb.pdf

National Public Radio (NPR). (2020, September 10). *NYPD study: Implicit bias training changes minds, not necessarily behavior.* Retrieved December 31, 2022, from https://www.npr.org/2020/09/10/909380525/nypd-study-implicit-bias-training-changes-minds-not-necessarily-behavior

Stark, J. (n.d.). Addressing implicit bias in policing. *Police Chief Magazine.* Retrieved December 31, 2022, from https://www.policechiefmagazine.org/addressing-implicit-bias-in-policing/

Grunloh, L. A. (n.d.). Religious accommodations for police officers: A comparative analysis of religious accommodation law in the United States, Canada, and the United Kingdom. Retrieved January 5, 2023, from https://mckinneylaw.iu.edu/iiclr/pdf/vol16p183.pdf

Department of Justice (DOJ). *Community Resource Center. Religion.* Retrieved January 5, 2023, from https://www.justice.gov/crs/crs-resource-center

DOJ. *Special report: Raising awareness of hate crimes and hate incidents during the COVID-19 pandemic.* Retrieved from https://www.justice.gov/hatecrimes/addressing-hate-crimes-against-AAPI

Police1. (2017, April 13). What is the role of religion and spirituality in policing. Retrieved on January 5, 2023, from https://www.police1.com/police-products/training/services/articles/what-is-the-role-of-religion-and-spirituality-in-policing-7iOZFuT5auxwr2eS/

## Including Religion and Spirituality into WPHC Contexts

### Patient-Centered Care

As the paradigm of patient-centered care advances, the practice of medicine has begun to attend to ways for including spirituality and religion in patient care. Recommendations advanced for integrating the body-mind-soul divisions in WPHC have further advanced the need to integrate religious and spiritual care with medical care. Given this interest, religious and spiritual preferences are increasingly at the intersection of the debate on how to provide care to patients in a manner that is meaningful to them. Several interesting challenges and quandaries have been raised by patients from different religious backgrounds and with varying expectations of what constitutes ethical and appropriate care. Such concerns are particularly impactful for minorities and those in vulnerable religious and spiritual communities of faith.

*Browse through some of the **Present Challenges and Future Directions** instances reflecting the concerns related to the American Muslim community and unrepresented patients in **Textbox 10.10**. How would you respond to the call for future action in these instances and others like this?*

**Textbox 10.10   Present Challenges and Future Directions Exercise**

**WPHC Accommodations for Minorities and Vulnerable Populations**

*WPHC Context*

*American Muslim Community*

Researchers Padela and colleagues include the following American Muslim participants' quotes in their study:

> "I look for females for (me and) my daughters, so the gender issue is really high on my list. It is not necessary that my doctor(s) … be … Muslim, but they do have to be female."
> "I would not even walk into a clinic (in which) I didn't have a choice of gender."
> "I've heard it from patients. I've heard it from families … when you don't eat because of (not having) halal food, it's definitely going to affect (your health)."
>
> "A prayer room is a form of healing on its own"… "I said, ok, before … they have to hook up the wires on (me) … I must do my last prayer. They gave me (only) three seconds … and start(ed) interfering." "So, we were praying but … nurses and … security (came) and asked if everything was ok. … Doctors were (thereafter) … hesitant to come back in the room and … everybody came by after that and kind of looked in the door (gawking)." "It's just like, you know, if they see a nun walking through the hospital, they say … hi sister, but they see a Muslim woman in a hijab … they might be thinking they need to keep security on hand."
>
> (Padela et al., 2012)

*Unrepresented Patients:*

*Adult patients who lack both decision-making capacity and any available surrogate decision-maker* are referred to as **unrepresented patients**. They are also referred to as **"unbefriended," "incapacitated patient without advocate."** About 16% of patients admitted to an intensive care unit (ICU) were **unrepresented**. Five percent of patients who died in an ICU were unrepresented. Fifty percent of critical care clinicians and hospitalists report seeing at least one unrepresented patient per month. In an ICU setting, they can face overtreatment, undertreatment, or otherwise be treated in a way that is not representative of their values (Pope et al., 2020; White et al., 2006). Their numbers are increasing particularly among the elderly, homeless, and mentally disabled.

SJA FUTURE ACTION

For each of the aforementioned instances, what recommendations would you make to provide culturally appropriate care that is mindful of the patient's religious beliefs? Consider the "Resources" section for recommendations made and their strengths and weaknesses.

**Resources**

*American Muslim Community*

Padela et al. (2012). https://www.ncbi.nlm.nih.gov/pmc/articles/PMC3358400/

## Team-Based Collaborations and Ethical Construction of WPHC

Several models have been proposed to help provide clinicians with a way to ethically construct spiritual care and to approach their patients with more empathy and trust. Ultimately, they offer an avenue for providers in WPHC settings to strengthen team-based collaborations between clinicians and chaplains (Zaidi, 2018). These models allow providers a systematic mechanism to assess spirituality in the medical encounter and discuss spiritual issues with their patients. By integrating the delivery of spiritual and religious care in medical contexts, the argument is that how patients experience illness can be better aligned with the medical facet of their treatment and aid patient-centered decision-making. The implications of such integrated decision-making are illustrated most explicitly in end-of-life decisions for patients, their families, and the WPHC system.

*Look at **Textbox 10.11** titled **Models for Integrating Spirituality into Medicine** for an overview of the HOPE model, the SPIRIT model, and the FICA Spirituality Tool.*

---

**Textbox 10.11   Models for Integrating Spirituality into Medicine**

**WPHC Context**

The Association for American Medical Colleges (AAMC) recommends the following three models of **HOPE, SPIRIT, and FICA** for approaching the topics of spirituality and religion in patient interviews (AAMC, 2023).

I.  The **HOPE model** for a formal spiritual assessment in a medical interview:

    H: Sources of hope, meaning, comfort, strength, peace, love, and connection
    O: Organized religion
    P: Personal spirituality and practices
    E: Effects on medical care and end-of-life issues

II.  The **SPIRIT model**:

    S: Spiritual belief system
    P: Personal spirituality
    I: Integration and involvement in a spiritual community
    R: Ritualized practices and restrictions
    I: Implications for medical care
    T: Terminal events planning (advance directives)

III. **FICA spiritual history** tool:

F: Faith and belief
Do you consider yourself spiritual or religious? Do you have spiritual beliefs that help you cope with stress? What gives your life meaning?

I: Importance
What importance does your faith or belief have in your life? Have your beliefs influenced how you take care of yourself in this illness? What role do your beliefs play in regaining your health?

C: Community
Are you part of a spiritual or religious community? Is this of support to you and how? Is there a group of people you really love or who are important to you? Churches, temples, mosques, or close friends are all examples of communities of support.

A: Address in care
How would you like me, your WPHC provider, to address these issues in your WPHC?

## SJA Prompt

Reflect upon your own religious and/or spiritual beliefs.

- How would you employ the aforementioned models to construct questions that WPHC providers can ask their patients?
- What would you advise WPHC providers **not** to do? Why?
- WPHC providers are often stretched for time. Would you consider it important to include the questions on religion and spirituality in the WPHC encounter?
- If so, at what stage of the WPHC relationship would questions pertaining to religion and spirituality be relevant?

## Resource

*Association of American Medical Colleges*. AAMC.org. Understanding the role of spirituality in medicine–A resource for medical students. Retrieved January 1, 2023, from https://www.aamc.org/media/24831/download

Ethical construction of WPHC centers the premise of honoring the dignity of everyone. Spirituality is oftentimes a key component of patients' and providers' WPHC and well-being. Communication scholar Dr. Sarah Amira de la Garza expands the notion of spirituality in social justice, wholeness, and communication while keeping in mind the ethics of planetary sustainability. Spirituality can help deliver care that is centered on the whole person and focuses not just on the disease indicators and its clinical treatment. As spirituality often goes beyond religion to include meaning making through family, nature, environment, and planetary relationships, it encourages a consideration of how we think about nature and its elements (e.g., wildlife, oceans, forests, sand, or rivers) in conceptualizing WPHC.

*Read **Textbox 10.12**, **Scholar Interview** to understand the notion of mindful heresy as proposed by **Dr. de la Garza** and its application in socially just WPHC.*

### TEXTBOX 10.12   Scholar Interview

**Dr. Sarah Amira de la Garza**
*Southwest Borderlands Scholar*
*Hugh Downs School of Human Communication*
*Arizona State University*

From the very beginning of my work looking at health communication, I have been driven by variations of the same question, one rooted in an awareness that our well-being is linked to our wholeness and spiritual nature as humans. Spirituality, as I have studied it and learned, is a dimension of human experience—often associated with religion, but not rooted in religion—rather in our capacity to see the interconnected wonder and wholeness of how we exist. Health and wholeness are very much related—it's not just about the body, but our experience of our health, as well. This continues to be what drives my commitment to social justice *and* contributing to the capacity for persons to live whole, healthy, and integrated lives. And our capacity to be conscious and to contribute to the well-being of our own bodies, as well as our communities and planet, is linked to our ability to share what we sense is needed for restoration and maintenance of healthy wholeness.

As humans, I believe a uniquely human conundrum is that of developing habits in service of avoiding discomfort, and it is paradoxically the biggest challenge we face to living a spiritually integrated pursuit of wholeness. My earliest work as a graduate student interested in health communication involved my curiosity around a patient's reticence and silence in exchanges with their doctors about critical aspects of their health. Whether it be out of respect for physicians, the power dynamics of the interaction, or cultural norms for interaction, I was fascinated, and disturbed, by the tendency to avoid asking questions, to leave out details that were "embarrassing," to fail to respond with detailed accounts of their symptoms, and such. The literature added to this challenge, providing evidence that patients who were considered "difficult," (pushy, insistent, asking many questions) tended to get better care. I was a student of conversation and human interaction, and my interest in health has always also been inherently an interest in justice—and what I observed was that the rules for ordinary conversation and "cooperation" in discourse were often obstacles to the pursuit of justice and access to WPHC. It remains so and is very much related to why I pursue work in what I have coined as *"mindful heresy."*

To pursue a healthy wholeness in our worlds requires that we not be mindlessly disciplined into silence when we have vital information, curiosity, concerns, and questions to share. **Mindful heresy** addresses the reality that sometimes, the only way to get justice, to feel the sense that a whole is being recognized and addressed, is to violate the orthodox norms of a group or setting. Many of the persons throughout history who later came to be recognized as great spiritual leaders, saints, and wise ones—during their lives were considered troublemakers, heretics, greatly challenging norms and religious doctrine of the day. Teaching people how to embody their commitment to justice in such a way that they can break the rules of propriety and politeness so that a message or cause can be heard, a response obtained, is an advanced spiritual practice that requires teaching our embodied minds to respond to certain discomforts as signs of pursuing justice and assuring we receive the care and attention that norms and customs may be denying us.

### Culturally Sensitive, Value-Driven, Religious, and Spiritual WPHC

The discussion of religion and spirituality illustrates the challenges in the provision of spiritual and religious care in culturally sensitive ways in WPHC settings and provides an overview of some models that can guide providers in their quest to be patient-centered in value-driven WPHC.

#### Bridging the Gap between Spirituality and Religion

Researchers Balboni and Balboni (2019) offer several recommendations for medicine to engage the gap between spirituality and religion: (a) clinicians, spiritual and religious experts, and funding organizations should partner to conduct research to better understand how spirituality in cultural and clinical contexts guides quality of life and medical decision-making; (b) training and socialization of clinicians in spiritual care. This follows research findings that physicians and nurses who were not religious themselves were more likely to provide spiritual care to seriously ill patients and overcome biases sustained through systemic silence; (c) establish a minimal standard of spiritual care provision for spiritual and religious collaboration and shared decision-making. Some guidelines here include asking each patient if and how spirituality and religion might be important to understandings of their illness and proceeding; accordingly, and (d) understanding the illness context as a hybrid of secular, sacred, and humanistic elements that are most effectively engaged when medical professionals and medical institutions partner with local religious communities and religious clergy. This partnership is deemed critical in WPHC of patients in a manner that addresses the patients' body, mind, and soul. Balboni and Balboni also argue for the integration of spiritual and religious community organizations in a humanistic and personal version of compassionate care that counterbalances the market-driven, technological, and bureaucratic pressures on the practice of medicine.

#### Inclusive Spiritual and Religious Care

The provision of religious and spiritually appropriate care that is inclusive of all patients' needs and diversity of beliefs is a central facet of a culturally sensitive and socially just WPHC landscape. Religious and spiritual beliefs can play out in the smallest of incidences and the most critical WPHC settings in ways that can cause distress to both providers and patients if they are not addressed appropriately.

Look at **Textbox 10.13**. Identify the elements of cultural diversity invoked in these instances.

---

**Textbox 10.13    Cultural Diversity in WPHC Contexts: Religious and Spiritual Beliefs**

**WPHC Context**

Consider the following contexts of religious and spiritual beliefs and the SJA recommendations provided under each. *What would you add to each context?* Then respond to the SJA prompt that follows.

- **Context of religious and spiritual beliefs**:
  Some religions have strict prayer times that may interfere with medical treatment. Consider inquiring about these and how they may affect the delivery of care.

**How WPHC providers can address cultural diversity in religious and spiritual beliefs**:

**SJA recommendation**: Provision of neutral prayer space. *What might be some organizational avenues for such initiatives? What evidence from WPHC outcomes could you employ to advocate for the designation of such spaces?*

- **Context of religious and spiritual beliefs**:
  Medicines based on animal products or that contain alcohol and caffeine. *How would you recommend WPHC providers take the composition of medication into consideration? If a patient inquires, what would be an appropriate manner for the WPHC provider to respond?*

**How WPHC providers can address cultural diversity in religious and spiritual beliefs**:

**SJA recommendation**:
Providing full disclosure and suggesting alternatives where possible. *Can you think of some possible scenarios based on your own faith (including atheism)? What communication practices can invite open disclosure from patients and providers alike? What would be some appropriate criteria for alternatives?*

- **Context of religious and spiritual beliefs**:

Diet and nutrition. *If a patient's diet and nutrition rules conflict with the ethic of care, how would you ethically best respond to this quandary?*

**How WPHC providers can address cultural diversity in religious and spiritual beliefs**:

**SJA recommendation**:
Find out when, whether, and how their patients are fasting. *What might be a first step in crafting culturally appropriate nutrition guidelines and nutrition therapy recommendations for a fasting regimen?*

- **Context of religious and spiritual beliefs**:

Modesty

**How WPHC providers can address cultural diversity in religious and spiritual beliefs**:

**SJA recommendation**:
Understanding privacy preferences in receiving care and the cultural meanings of modesty (i.e., receiving respect and caring). *How could you envisage WPHC providers communicating this religious and spiritual value through propriety in speech, dress, behavior, or lack of pretentiousness?*

- **Context of religious and spiritual beliefs**:

Preferred gender of WPHC providers. *In a situation where it may be challenging to accommodate such a preference, how might you respond in a patient-centered culturally sensitive manner?*

**How WPHC providers can address cultural diversity in religious and spiritual beliefs**:

**SJA recommendation**: Trying to accommodate to the fullest extent possible.

- **Context of religious and spiritual beliefs**:

Environment of care. Understanding how patients understand and prefer their environment of care. *What types of questions might WPHC providers ask to understand patient preferences for their environment of care? Why is environment of care important?*

**How WPHC providers can address cultural diversity in religious and spiritual beliefs**:

**SJA recommendation**:

Research the practices of one religion that you are not familiar with. *What are some of the forms that cultural diversity takes in WPHC settings?*

- **Context of religious and spiritual beliefs**:

Medical procedures. *What religious and spiritual considerations might underlie the performance of medical procedures? How can WPHC providers be sensitive to such considerations?*

**How WPHC providers can address cultural diversity in religious and spiritual beliefs**:

**SJA recommendation**:

Understand how their patients view the meaning and importance of the body and bodily integrity regarding medical procedures, including surgery and vaccination.

- **Context of religious and spiritual beliefs**:

Women's health and reproductive health

**How WPHC providers can address cultural diversity in religious and spiritual beliefs**:

**SJA recommendation**:

Understand laws and beliefs surrounding birth control, artificial insemination, abortion, menstruation, puberty, and menopause. *What communication principles might you follow based on the CPM Theory to structure conversations around reproductive and sexual beliefs?*

- **Context of religious and spiritual beliefs**:

Faith healing and prayers

**How WPHC providers can address cultural diversity in religious and spiritual beliefs**:

**SJA recommendation**:

Understand how patients feel about prayer in the WPHC setting. *How will you advise healthcare providers to communicate in a culturally sensitive and patient-centered manner with patients about their approach to prayer in the healthcare setting?*

- **Context of religious and spiritual beliefs**:

Alternative therapies

**How healthcare providers can address cultural diversity in religious and spiritual beliefs**:

**SJA recommendation**:

What communicative strategies can healthcare providers employ to be open to patients' communication of their preferences or decisions to try alternative therapies and share the current state of evidence-based knowledge on their decisions? *How can healthcare providers partner with their patients to keep them informed of the implications of their decisions and make a note of the therapies they have sought?*

## SJA Prompt

- Based on your understanding of the principles of social justice, what would you add to the recommendations for addressing cultural diversity in healthcare settings in the realm of religion and spirituality?

## Resource

Padela, A. I., Gunter, K., Killawi, A., & Heisler, M. (2012). Religious values and healthcare accommodations: Voices from the Muslim community. *Journal of General Internal Medicine*, *27*(6), 708–715, https://doi.org/10.1007/s11606-011-1965-5

## Challenges and Opportunities Ahead

In conclusion, **Chapter 10, Religion and Health**, has provided an overview of the historical evolution, the patient and provider landscape, the organizational landscape, and some of the ways that these intersect with the values and principles of WPHC and SJA. Ultimately, although there is agreement on the provision of compassionate care that is mindful of the patient's religious and spiritual beliefs, creating compassionate systems of care (Puchalski et al., 2014) is a challenging task. As has been illustrated in this chapter, all too often there is a need for constructing consensus on what spirituality means and how its parameters can be aligned with the vision and principles of medical practice. Further complicating the scenario is the fact that the standards and recommended strategies around inclusive, bias-free, and compassionate communicative norms surrounding religion and spirituality are still in the process of evolution. In addition, some healthcare contexts, more than others, such as palliative care settings, have been more sensitive to spirituality in the context of the practice of medicine, ethics, nursing, and social work.

Although the medical-religious partnerships are some of the oldest in the history of humankind, it is still a challenge to structure culturally sensitive care that centers patient religion and spirituality and communicates a caring, compassionate, and human-centered approach to healthcare that is also respectful and patient-centered. However, there is increasing recognition of the value of such integration and acknowledgment that the benefits of doing so are immense. Such care recognizes that the process of WPHC transforms not only the patients but also the healthcare provider, and thus may constitute a healing relationship, where both the patient and the provider can benefit.

Review **Textbox 10.14**. What WPHC quandaries do the mini-case study on religious concordance raise? How would you respond to the future challenges in the SJA Discussion Prompt?

---

### Textbox 10.14 Present Challenges and Future Directions Exercise-2

## Religious Concordance and WPHC

### WPHC Context

Consider the following case abstracted from an *AMA Journal of Ethics* "Case and Commentary" feature (Blythe & Curlin, 2019):

Ms. L is a 78-year-old woman who presents to a primary care clinic to establish care with a new physician, as she has recently moved. She is assigned to a newer physician on staff, Dr. O, who chats with her briefly and then begins to interview Ms. L. Within a few minutes of Dr. O's questions about her health history, Ms. L mentions her faith. "I found Jesus a long time ago," she says sincerely. "Do you believe in God?"

Dr. O is surprised but doesn't show it. "Yes, I do. Is it okay if we focus on your medical history for now?"

Ms. L pauses for a moment and goes on about her faith's importance. "An essential part of who I am is that I believe in God. I believe in Jesus. What God do you follow? Is it Jesus, Allah or another god?" Dr. O tries to focus on how to move on to obtain the rest of Ms. L's history, and replies, "I believe in Jesus and Allah, too." Ms. L straightens her spine and immediately replies, "No, you can't follow both."

Dr. O doesn't reply and moves on to her review of systems. "Do you know if there is a Christian doctor here?" Ms. L interrupts.

Dr. O replies, "I'm new to this clinic and don't really know the religious affiliations of my colleagues." Dr. O pauses and considers whether to continue examining Ms. L.

### WPHC Prompt-1

The concept of **cultural humility** requires that the healthcare provider "*incorporates a lifelong commitment to self-evaluation and critique, to redressing the physician-patient dynamic, and to power imbalances in developing mutually beneficial and non-paternalistic partnerships with communities on behalf of individuals and defined populations*" (Tervalon & Murray-García, 1998, p. 125).

### SJA Discussion Question-1

- Drawing on your understanding of religion and spirituality in healthcare, how would you advise the physician to respond? What is the rationale underlying your advice?

## WPHC Prompt-2

**Cultural competence** is defined as *"the ability of providers and organizations to effectively deliver healthcare services that meet the social, cultural, and linguistic needs of patients"* (Betancourt et al., 2002; Health Policy Institute).

## SJA Discussion Question-2

- How can you apply the principles of the concept of cultural humility and cultural competence in considering such requests?

## Resources

Betancourt, J. R., Green, A. R., & Carillo, J. E. (2002). *Cultural competence in healthcare: Emerging frameworks and practical approaches.* The Commonwealth Fund.

Blythe, J. A., & Curlin, F. A. (2019, June). How should physicians respond to patient requests for religious concordance? *AMA Journal of Ethics: Illuminating the Art of Medicine.* Retrieved on January 5, 2023, from https://journalofethics.ama-assn.org/article/how-should-physicians-respond-patient-requests-religious-concordance/2019-06

Health Policy Institute. *Cultural competence in healthcare: Is it important for people with chronic conditions?* Retrieved January 5, 2023, from https://hpi.georgetown.edu/cultural/

Tervalon, M., & Murray-García, J. (1998). Cultural humility versus cultural competence: A critical distinction in defining physician training outcomes in multicultural education. *Journal of Healthcare for the Poor and Underserved, 9*(2), 117–125. https://doi.org/10.1353/hpu.2010.0233

# References

Adhikari, S. P., Meng, S., Wu, Y. J., Mao, Y. P., Ye, R. X., Wang, Q. Z., et al. (2020). Epidemiology, causes, clinical manifestation and diagnosis, prevention, and control of coronavirus disease (COVID-19) during the early outbreak period: A scoping review. *Infectious Diseases of Poverty, 9*(1), 29. https://doi.org/10.1186/s40249-020-00646-x

Allport, G.W. (1963). Behavioral science, religion, and mental health. *Journal of Religion and Health, 2*(3), 187–197. https://www.jstor.org/stable/27504566

Alcorn, S. R., Balboni, M. J., Prigerson, H. G., et al. (2010). "If God wanted me yesterday, I wouldn't be here today": Religious and spiritual themes in patients' experiences of advanced cancer. *Journal of Palliative Medicine, 13*, 581–588. https://doi.org/10.1089/jpm.2009.0343

Anderson, C. M. (2004). The delivery of healthcare in faith-based organizations: Parish nurses as promoters of health. *Health Communication, 16*(1), 117–128. https://doi.org/10.1207/S15327027HC1601_8

Balboni, M., & Balboni, T. (2019, June 1). *Do spirituality and medicine go together?* Center for Bioethics. Harvard Medical School. News. Retrieved January 1, 2023, from https://bioethics.hms.harvard.edu/journal/spirituality-medicine#_edn1

Bonelli, R., Dew, R. E., Koenig, H. G., Rosmarin, D. H., & Vasegh, S. (2012). Religious and spiritual factors in depression: Review and integration of the research. *Depression Research and Treatment,* 962860. https://doi.org/10.1155/2012/962860

Boyle, P. (2022, March 15). A place for faith: Doctors bring spirituality to work. *AAMC news*. Retrieved January 1, 2023, from https://www.aamc.org/news-insights/place-faith-doctors-bring-spirituality-work

Canzona, M. R., Peterson, E. B., Villagran, M. M., & Seehusen, D. A. (2015). Constructing and communicating privacy boundaries: How family medicine physicians manage patient requests for religious disclosure in the clinical interaction. *Health Communication, 30*(10), 1001–1012. https://doi.org/10.1080/10410236.2014.913222

Da Silva, J. M., & Guimaraes, M. A. C. (2000). Odo-Ya Project: HIV/AIDS prevention in the context of Afro-Brazilian religion. *Journal of Health Communication, 5*, 119–123. https://doi.org/10.1080/10810730050019609

Egbert, N., Mickley, J., & Coeling, H. (2004). A review and application of social scientific measures of religiosity and spirituality: Assessing a missing component in health communication research. *Health Communication, 16*(1), 7–27. https://doi.org/10.1207/S15327027HC1601_2

Galiatsatos, P., Monson, K., Oluyinka, M. et al. (2020). Community calls: Lessons and insights gained from a medical–religious community engagement during the COVID-19 pandemic. *Journal of Religion and Health, 59*, 2256–2262. https://doi.org/10.1007/s10943-020-01057-w

*Hopkins Medicine*. (2022). Department of Spiritual Care and Chaplaincy. Retrieved from https://www.hopkinsmedicine.org/spiritual-care-and-chaplaincy/clinical-pastoral-education

Jim, H. S. L., Pustejovsky, J., Park, C. L., Danhauer, S. C.. Sherman, A. C., Fitchett, G. ... Salsman, J. M. (2016). Religion, spirituality, and physical health in cancer patients: A meta-analysis. *Cancer, 121*(21), 3760–3768. https://doi.org/10.1002/cncr.29353

Johns Hopkins Medicine. (2022). Department of Spiritual Care and Chaplaincy. Clinical Pastoral Education Program. *Clinical pastoral education at Johns Hopkins*. Retrieved January 1, 2023, from https://www.hopkinsmedicine.org/spiritualcare/education/

Keeley, M. P. (2004). Final conversations: Survivors' memorable messages concerning religious faith and spirituality. *Health Communication, 16*(1), 87–104. https://doi.org/10.1207/S15327027HC1601_6

Kline, S. L. (2011). Communicating spirituality in healthcare: A case study on the role of identity in religious health testimonies. *Journal of Applied Communication Research, 39*(4), 334–351. https://doi.org/10.1080/00909882.2011.608698

Koenig, H. (2008). Medicine, religion, and health. Book and media review. *JAMA, 300*(24), 2922–2927. https://doi.org/10.1001/jama.2008.871

Koenig, H. G., McCullough, M., & Larson, D. (2000). *Handbook for religion and health* (pp. 7–14). Oxford University Press

McGrath, P. (2005). Developing a language for nonreligious spirituality in relation to serious illness through research: Preliminary findings. *Health Communication, 18*(3), 217–235. https://doi.org/10.1207/s15327027hc1803_2

Meluch, A. L. (2018). Spiritual support experienced at a cancer wellness center. *Southern Communication Journal, 33*(3), 137–148. https://doi.org/10.1080/1041794X.2018.1459817

Miller, W. R., & Thoresen, C. E. (2003). Spirituality, religion, and health: An emerging research field. *American Psychologist, 58*(1), 24–35. https://doi.org/10.1037/0003-066x.58.1.24

Olufowote, J. O., & Matusitz, J. (2016). "How dark a world it is ... where mental health is poorly treated": Mental illness frames in sermons given after the Sandy Hook shootings. *Health Communication, 31*(12), 1539–1547. https://doi.org/10.1080/10410236.2015.1089458

Park, C. L., (2013). Spirituality and meaning making in cancer survivorship. In Markman, K., Proulx, T., & Lindberg, M. (Eds.), *The psychology of meaning* (pp. 257–277). American Psychological Association.

Parrott, R. (2004). "Collective amnesia": The absence of religious faith and spirituality in health communications research and practice. *Health Communication, 16*(1), 1–5. https://doi.org/10.1207/S15327027HC1601_1

Peterson, J. L. (2011). The case for connection: Spirituality and social support for women living with HIV/AIDS. *Journal of Applied Communication Research, 39*(4), 352–369. https://doi.org/10.1080/00909882.2011.608700

Petronio, S. (2002). *Boundaries of privacy: Dialectics of disclosure*. SUNY Press.

Powell, L. H., Shahabi, L., Thoresen, C. E. (2003). Religion and spirituality: Linkages to physical health. *American Psychologist*, *58*(1), 3652. https://doi.org/10.1037/0003-066x.58.1.36

Preau, M, Bouhnik, A. D., & Le Coroller Soriano, A. G. (2013). Two years after cancer diagnosis, what Is the relationship between health-related quality of life, coping strategies, and spirituality? *Psychology of Health and Medicine*, *18*, 375–386. https://doi.org/10.1080/13548506.2012.736622

Puchalski, C. M., Vitillo, R., Hull, S. K., & Reller, N. (2014). Improving the spiritual dimension of whole person care: Reaching national and international consensus. *Journal of Palliative Medicine*, *17*(6), 642–656. https://doi.org/10.1089/jpm.2014.9427

Ross, L. E., Hall, I. J., Fairley, T. L., Taylor, Y. J., & Howard, D. L. (2008).Prayer and self-reported Health among cancer survivors in the United States, National Health Interview Survey, 2002. *Journal of Alternative and Complementary Medicine*, *14*, 931–938 https://doi.org/10.1089/acm.2007.0788

Witte, K. (1994). Fear control and danger control: A test of the extended parallel process model (EPPM). *Communication Monographs*, *61*, 113–133.

Zaidi, D. (2018). From the editor. *AMA Journal of Ethics*, *20*(7), E609–612. https://doi.org/10.1001/amajethics.2018.609 Retrieved January 1, 2023, from https://journalofethics.ama-assn.org/article/influences-religion-and-spirituality-medicine/2018-07

## Additional Resources

Pope, T. M., Bennett, J., Carson, S. S., Cederquist, L., Cohen, A. B., DeMartino, E. S., Godfrey, D. M. ... Widera, E. W. (2020). Making medical treatment decisions for unrepresented patients in the ICU. *American Journal of Respiratory and Critical Care Medicine*, *201*(10), 1182–1192. Retrieved January 4, 2023, from https://www.atsjournals.org/doi/10.1164/rccm.202003-0512ST

White, D. B., Curtis, J. R., Lo, B., & Luce, J. M. (2006). Decisions to limit life-sustaining treatment for critically ill patients who lack both decision-making capacity and surrogate decision-makers. *Critical Care in Medicine*, *34*, 2053–2059. https://doi.org/10.1097/01.CCM.0000227654.38708.C1

# Chapter 11

# Global Health

DOI: 10.4324/9781003214472-14

messages from a mass media television series in South Africa. The researchers found that participation in the school-based program that used messages from another mass media platform was associated with a decrease in young women's HIV risk and impacted some key risky sexual behaviors.

Communication professor and social justice activist Dr. Dutta's work examines performance as a mode of organizing for social justice. Through his scholarship, Dr. Dutta aims to show how health communication can work in the service of the vulnerable and disadvantaged by connecting notions of justice and health (2011). Examining the work of an indigenous pediatrician, Dr. Binayak Sen with the marginalized populations in India, Dr. Dutta employs poetry to challenge structural forms of oppression.

The COVID-19 pandemic's impact affected everything ranging from people's health to their living conditions, livelihood, and community. The pandemic highlighted how global health concerns can impact everyone's life today, no matter where they live on the planet. Increasing world population and migration have increased the impact that global interrelationships and connections have on our daily lives. Terms like tropical medicine, which once seemed exotic, no longer seem as remote in the high-income regions of the world. On the other hand, the chronic conditions of obesity and diabetes mellitus that were once largely seen in high-income countries are now a challenge affecting developing countries as well. Such changing health patterns demonstrate the interconnected nature of global health. They also highlight the pervasiveness of its challenges ranging from environmental degradation, political instability, and war to genetic susceptibility (Houpt et al., 2007).

## Chapter Overview

Chapter 11, Global Health, will first cover the definitions of global health from a WPHC SJA perspective, laying out the differing foci of each and describing the concepts covered in global health. Second, it will outline its distinctions with international health and international public health campaigns to cover the SJA facets of health information seeking, social mobilization, public global health communication, collaborative partnerships in global health, and the different disciplinary domains that comprise the field of global health. Third, the chapter will discuss the challenges in constructing global health priorities that center health equity through the WPHC lens of structural and clinical priorities. Structural priorities will be covered through a comprehensive WPHC examination of the case of NTDs, highlighting the strengths and limitations of employing infrastructure, investment in global threat assessment, a global health security approach, and the need to design global cooperation as an integral part of multilateral support, coordination, and communication in global health security efforts. Clinical priorities will be covered through a WPHC-centered examination of NTDs through the SJA lens of health as a human right, global health risk communication, disease prevention, discriminatory laws, and stigma. Fourth, it will focus on how WPHC informs dialogic approaches to multisectoral partnerships in global health, centering multisectoral partnerships through the SJA lens of sustainability, agency, and empowerment in global health initiatives; technology and innovation; and resource mobilization. **Fifth**, it will focus on a WPHC SJA approach to giving voice to vulnerable populations and collaborative design, highlighting access and equity in global health, coproduction of solutions, accountability, and structural imbalances. Along the way, multiple engagement opportunities are provided ranging from an overview of the organizations in this arena to examining the CDC's work in global health. SJA exercises will guide the students to think through a range of vital examples thinking through subaltern communities and employing a WPHC SJA approach to examine NTDs, foundation support, the transnational nature of global health, and global health equity. The communication scholar interview with Dr. Uttaran Dutta will emphasize the need to keep marginalized populations, such as tribal communities, front, and center in the work of global health communication research.

## Definitions of Global Health

### Global Health

Global health emphasizes issues in health that cross-national borders. From a WPHC perspective, global health concerns highlight how the regions of the world are increasingly connected in extensive ways through travel, e-commerce, migration, and personal relationships. In an interconnected world, a health concern impacting one region of the planet will affect regions in another region of the planet as well. Addressing global health challenges emphasizes the importance of collaboration to achieve collective health goals. Seen through the lens of SJA, global health challenges emphasize the need to be attentive to concerns of equity in how health goals are achieved for differing development contexts.

### Definitions of Global Health

Several definitions of global health are in use today. Koplan and colleagues define global health as "an area for the study, research, and practice that places a priority on improving health and achieving health equity for all people worldwide" (2009). Others, such as Kickbush define global health as "those health issues that transcend national boundaries and governments and call for actions on the global forces that determine the health of people" (2006). These definitions have been critiqued for being too broad, not emphasizing collaborative effort enough, and not doing enough to emphasize an action-oriented approach needed to achieve the goals of equity (Beaglehole & Bonita, 2010).

### A RELATED TERM: INTERNATIONAL HEALTH

A related term, "international health," places greater emphasis on health issues in low-income countries such as infectious diseases and maternal and child health (2009). International health focuses on disease management across borders. For instance, international health contexts will focus on infectious diseases that spread with travel across national borders, necessitating communication about the disease and its risk factors in different national contexts.

*Examine* **Textbox 11.1** *to gain a deeper understanding of the major definitions of global health put forward by different researchers and organizations. Try your hand at the SJA activity that follows to critique the definitions.*

**Textbox 11.1   Definitions of Global Health**

**WPHC Prompt**

Examine the prominent definitions of global health provided here.

1. **Global health** is an area for study, research, and practice that places a priority on improving health and achieving equity in health for all people worldwide (Koplan et al. 2009).
   - Centers health research, practice, and equity.

2. **Global health** emphasizes transnational health issues, determinants, and solutions; involves many disciplines within and beyond the health sciences and promotes interdisciplinary collaboration; and is a synthesis of population-based prevention with individual-level clinical care (G20 Insights, 2021).
   a. Centers transnational nature, causes, and solutions and is more action oriented
   b. Centers interdisciplinary nature and collaboration
   c. Centers the relationship between public health and individual health solutions

3. **Global health** is a field of study, research, and practice that places a priority on achieving equity in health for all people. Global health is a discipline that advances efforts to improve the well-being of people and the planet (Keith Martin, CUGH, n.d.).

4. **Global health equity** is the mutually beneficial and power-balanced partnerships and processes leading to equitable human and environmental health outcomes on a global scale (August et al., 2022).

5. **Global health equity** is a world in which everyone can achieve the highest attainable level of health, and no one is disadvantaged from achieving this potential because of social position or any other socially, economically, demographically, or geographically defined circumstance or physical condition (CDC, 2022).

**SJA Activity**

- Compare and contrast the aforementioned definitions of global health to identify their strengths and weaknesses in designing socially just

  1. Bottom-up solutions
  2. Culturally sensitive initiatives
  3. Multisectoral partnerships
  4. Community-empowerment strategies

- Notice how the more recent definitions of global health lean into the notion of global health equity (McKinsey Institute, 2022). How does this emphasis help us address the challenges arising from income and resource disparity characterizing high- and low-income regions of the world and within populations in each region?

**Resources**

August, E., Tadesse, L., O'Neill, M. S., Eisenberg, J. N. S., Wong, R., Kolars, J. C., & Bekele, A. (2022). What is global health equity? A proposed definition. *Annals of Global Health, 88*(1), 50. http://doi.org/10.5334/aogh.3754

CDC. (2022). *Global health equity*. Retrieved from https://www.cdc.gov/globalhealth/equity/home.html#:~:text=CDC's%20vision%20for%20global%20health,defined%20circumstance%20or%20physical%20condition

Consortium of Universities for Global Health (CUGH). (n.d.). Retrieved from https://www.cugh.org/

G20 Insights. (2021). *Global equity for global health*. Retrieved from https://www.g20-insights.org/policy_briefs/global-equity-for-global-health/

Koplan, J. P., Bond, T. C., Merson, M. H., Reddy, K. S., Rodriguez, M. H., Sewnkambo, N. K., et al. (2009). Toward a common definition of global health. *Lancet, 373*(9679), 1993–1995. https://doi.org/10.1016/S1040–6736(09)60332-9

McKinsey Institute. (2022, July 21). *In sickness and in health: How health is perceived around the world*. Retrieved from https://www.mckinsey.com/mhi/our-insights/in-sickness-and-in-health-how-health-is-perceived-around-the-world

Although there are minor differences between the definitions of global health, what all definitions of global health have in common is a shared concern for improving the health of all populations and achieving equity in health for everyone. Health conditions like heart disease, stroke, TB, cancer, diabetes, and other noncommunicable diseases are prevalent globally. Global public health campaigns (e.g., immunization efforts) strive to address challenges ranging from obesity and SUDs to HIV/AIDS and mental health conditions.

## Global Public Health Campaigns

### Health Information Seeking

The success of global public health campaigns often depends on an accurate understanding of how health information is accessed and used in different parts of the world. Health information-seeking trends vary across global regions, populations, and cultures.

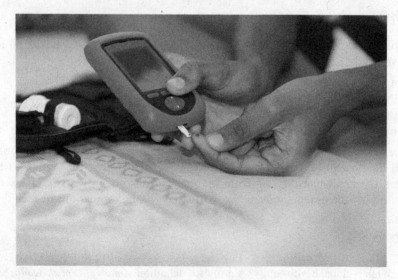

*Figure 11.1* Global Public Health Campaigns Benefit from an Accurate Understanding of How Health Information Is Accessed and Used in Different Parts of the World.

*Understanding Global Health Information Seeking*

Communication researchers Link et al. (2022) conduct a cross-country analysis of the challenges of how health information is provided and accessed using the US-based HINTS data administered by the NCI alongside the corresponding German research initiative called International Studies to Investigate Global Health Information Trends (INSIGHTS). They find that although the share of residents seeking health information is high in both the United States and Germany, there are subtle differences in how information is accessed in each country. They also find differences across the two countries in the primary sources used to seek health information. For instance, Germans will more often turn to health professionals as their primary source of health information, whereas US residents will turn to the internet as their primary source for gathering health information. Such research underscores how public health communication needs to be tailored in cross-national settings to address the health information-seeking preferences of individuals from different cultural and socioeconomic backgrounds.

*Examine **Textbox 11.2** for the definitions of the concepts associated with the field of global health and their location in a WPHC SJA context. Consider the implications of each conceptual domain for equitable and socially just global health efforts.*

---

**Textbox 11.2    Concepts Highlighted in Global Health**

- **Concept**
  Transnational health
     **Transnational health** emphasizes reaching across borders. Global health issues are transnational health issues that affect many countries and regions in the world.
     For example, infectious diseases such as the COVID-19 pandemic impacted almost all countries in the world.

- **Concept**
  SDoH
     Attending to SDoH helps public health professionals ask the question: How do the social, physical, and economic conditions in society impacting health affect those living in low-, middle-, and high-income countries differentially?
     Addressing SDoH emphasizes the need for building capacities and advocating for action to identify and eliminate disparities. It also involves providing support, building intersectoral partnerships, and uniform implementation of evidence-based policies.

- **Concept**
  Interdisciplinary collaboration
     Global health highlights interdisciplinary collaboration because it brings together knowledge from different domains.
     The domain of global health emphasizes transnational issues, determinants, and solutions. This approach is emphasized by the increasingly team-based training approach to global health.

- **Concept**
  Population-based prevention
  The term "population-based prevention" references the approach to healthcare interventions that emphasize the need to consider the entire population for achieving an equitable impact of reduction in disease risk factors.
  Population-based prevention approaches can be implemented at different scales. They can consider an entire population within a community, the structural systems that affect the health of those populations, and/or the individuals and families within those populations known to be at risk.

- **Concept**
  Individual-level clinical care
  Clinical care at the individual level understood in a global context highlights the need for caring humanely and expertly for patients; creating new knowledge through biomedical, behavioral, and health services research; and forging local, regional, national, and global partnerships that improve individual-level health outcomes.
  To promote individual health, physicians must promote public health by thinking globally and by valuing human rights, quality of life, social justice, and world peace.

- **Concept**
  Health equity
  Health equity in global health emphasizes that everyone, in every region in the world, should have the opportunity to live a healthy and vibrant life.

- **Concept**
  Intersectoral partnerships
  **Intersectoral collaboration and partnerships** are the coming together of different people, organizations, and sectors to work together to understand and solve complex issues.
  The push toward intersectoral collaboration assumes that cooperation among different social groups enables them to better solve common problems such as **public health crises** in a way that equitably addresses the needs and values of all sections of society.
  Such partnerships often bring together diverse organizations and people with different backgrounds and support the coordination of efforts of two or more sectors within the government.

## SJA Prompt

- Although the recent experience with the COVID-19 pandemic alerted the global health community to the interconnectivity of health risks, several challenges remain. What are some challenges that may prevent the global identification and spread of future infectious disease health risks?

## Social Mobilization

Communication researchers emphasize the necessity of trust-building and local, bottom-up social mobilization (SM) approaches. The SM approach advocates global democratization and collaboration in designing activist and pragmatic SM strategies to address differences and conflicts rooted in ethnicity, religion, and economics (Obregón & Waisbord, 2010). Examples illustrating the application of the SM strategy include CDC-supported polio, measles, and rubella campaigns collaborating with grassroots workers and drawing upon local community norms. In Vietnam, CDC partners implemented the Double X diagnostic strategy and tripled TB diagnoses, while improving access to TB treatment for people living with HIV (PLHIV). In Guinea, the CDC's Center for Global Health successfully scaled up interventions to eliminate parasitic diseases (Center for Global Health, 2022).

*Textbox 11.3 lists the different organizations working in the domain of global health. Probe the websites of these organizations and respond to the prompt given. What are some other examples of the CDC's Center of Global Health's efforts?*

---

**Textbox 11.3    Organizations Working in Global Health**

### WPHC Resources

Several organizations, both US-based, such as the CDC, and international, such as the WHO, work in the global health domain. The following list provides a few more resources to get you started on the path of learning about the many organizations that work in global health and their areas of focus

Global Health Organizations. https://globalhealth.washington.edu/sites/default/files/Global%20Health%20Internships%20%26%20Opportunities%20Resource%20List.pdf

World Health Organization. https://mphdegree.usc.edu/blog/world-health-organizations-guide/

Global Health and International Nonprofit Organization Websites. https://www.tephinet.org/global-health-and-international-nonprofit-organization-websites

Nongovernmental Organizations. https://www.who.int/emergencies/partners/non-governmental-organizations

Global Health Council. https://globalhealth.org/

Women in Global Health. https://womeningh.org/

Consortium of Universities for Global Health. https://www.cugh.org/

### SJA Activity

1. Critique the websites of the organizations listed to identify a conceptual area of global health that has been omitted.

   - What form of organization could you create to address that area? What mission statement and vision statement would it have?

- How would such a mission and vision meet the goals of a socially just organization?
- What forms of actions could global health organizations take that would help them further activism and action?
- Why is the area you have identified urgent and important?

2. Browse through the links provided under the preceding "WPHC Resources" section and pay attention to their areas of focus.

- Identify what is important about the SDoH area each of the organizations' website addresses.
- Are there emerging domains of interest that the organizations should be attending to in their work to avoid future disparities? What is an example of a gap in the mission of any one of the organizations?

## Public Health Communication

Public health communication focuses on communication efforts with populations in the larger public domain, such as through developing and sharing flyers, newsletters, or on websites and blogs and evaluating the effectiveness of various communication methods in protecting and advancing the health of key populations. International public health communication can facilitate collaboration between different countries and stakeholders as an important mechanism for sharing information. Researchers Dillard, Li, and Yang (2021) examined the relationship between information seeking and fear among women in the southern United States during the Zika-induced global health crisis. They conducted their study in the days just after the WHO declared Zika a global crisis. Their study finds that information seeking during times of disease crisis follows a complex pattern of proactive behaviors. Thus, public health communication agencies should plan their materials around this knowledge for maximum impact.

## Collaborative Partnerships in Global Health

Global health challenges increase in complexity with the overlap of global crises such as climate change, economic turmoil, and food and energy crises. Each of these crises has a connection with the health of the communities, families, and individuals living in those regions. No one organization or discipline or sector can fully address them on their own. Because global health problems span many different health concerns, regions, and conceptual domains, building collaborative partnerships across the different stakeholders becomes very important. Communication researchers Shankar et al. (2015) illustrate the impact of agency-based empowerment training on women entrepreneurs in Kenya. Women's involvement in clean cooking value chains globally has been minimal. These challenges constrain women's involvement in the energy sector. By employing an agency-based empowerment training model, the women were able to serve as active improved cookstove entrepreneurs in both urban and rural settings. Partnerships can help with the exchange of knowledge that exist among different countries and stakeholders. By including those who are affected by the problems, collaborative partnerships construct solutions that are equitable, sustainable, and empowering. Solutions constructed through equitable partnerships between all stakeholders are also more likely to be successful and long-lasting.

## Disciplines of Global Health

Building equitable partnerships and engagement in the domain of global health involves the collaborative efforts of interdisciplinary teams of specialists, researchers, and professionals working together in multiple fields. The disciplines of global health encompass the fields of medicine, health professions, natural sciences, social sciences, humanities, business, technology, and engineering. These include issues falling under the domain of infectious diseases or epidemiology to sanitation, economics, engineering and design, environment science, health behavior change, economics, sociology, political science, international policy, and international law, among others. Specialists from each of these different fields work together in the arena of global health. The problems addressed can range from stemming pandemics and infectious diseases; providing low-cost sanitation and clean water; administering immunization programs; providing vaccinations for preventive diseases; developing healthcare policies, such as that for anti-retroviral therapy; and management of local diseases. To involve local stakeholders and affected communities, a major aspect of global health should involve the coordination of interdisciplinary efforts that help ensure an effective, dialogic, and bottom-up response on an international scale. Thus, a challenge for these global centers is to emphasize and build equitable partnerships and empowering connections with local communities in the regions of their focus. Effective global health centers create strong links with low- and middle-income countries (LMIC) to give voice to locally defined priorities.

*Examine* **Textbox 11.4** *to understand the different disciplinary domains of global health from a WPHC SJA perspective. Read through the WPHC prompts under each domain to identify how the different domains might contribute. What do you notice? You may find that many educational, policy, and organizational centers of global health are in developed countries. Complete the SJA activity to examine the interconnected and interdependent nature of global health with climate change and consider its implications for global health and climate change communication.*

*In what ways is communication between the two interdisciplinary fields of global health and climate change interlinked? What are their shared concerns? How are they different? What communicative challenges are unique to each?*

---

### Textbox 11.4    One Health, Many Domains

| Domains Involved in Global Health | WPHC Foci: How Do the Different Domains Contribute? |
|---|---|
| Public Health | • **Public health professionals** work at the grassroots level within regional and national contexts.<br>• **Global health professionals** focus on healthcare problems, policy, and individual quality of life within communities at a global level.<br><br>**SJA Prompt**<br><br>• *Can you think of examples where public health and global health intersect today?* |

| | |
|---|---|
| Environmental Science | • **Pollution**, including chemical, water, and air pollution is closely associated with the rise of disease, and lower levels of physical activity, among other facets, contribute to the global epidemics of obesity, diabetes, and associated anabolic and metabolic diseases. |

**SJA Prompt**

• *How do you think the health of people living in developing countries may be affected by these concerns?*

| | |
|---|---|
| Biology | • The study of **global health biology** or biology of global health is gaining prominence across academic institutions (Drain, 2017). |
| | • The major in biology of global health focuses on global health issues at the local, national, and international levels, while combining the knowledge of basic science and disease research with work in interdisciplinary areas of policy, economics, ethics, law, and society. |

**SJA Prompt**

• *In what ways can different undergraduate majors complement the work of global health?*

| | |
|---|---|
| Economics | • A healthy population supports sustainable development and a strong **macroeconomy**. In turn, a strong economy will generate adequate resources for health systems. |
| | • The field of **health economics** focuses on how the economic behavior of stakeholders and recipients affects the quality and cost of medical care. It considers how health systems around the world can be restructured and improved (Benatar et al., 2011). |

**SJA Prompt**

• *In what ways do you think socially unjust and excessive patterns of consumption deplete and challenge global health?*

## WPHC Contexts and SJA Activities

1. The disciplines of geopolitical studies, population health, and healthcare economics consider different aspects, such as the interdependence of resources, equitable distribution of resources, and ethical prevention. How do these intersect across the different domains involved in global health?
2. Climate change is a global process with local and regional effects on communities. Most people will experience the effects of climate change at some point in their lives. Specific populations are more vulnerable to the effects of climate change than others. These effects can range from hurricanes, floods, wildfires, and mold exposure, to harmful algal blooms [National Institute of Environmental Health Sciences (NIEHS), 2022].

   a. What are some ways communication professionals can spread awareness of the relationship between health threats from climate change across the life span to build resilience in individuals, communities, and nations across the world?
   b. Who is at the highest risk?

c. How will you reach them?

d. Consider this fact sheet designed by NIEHS for the United States (https://www. niehs.nih.gov/health/materials/climate_and_human_health_508.pdf. What might such a fact sheet reveal about vulnerable regions globally?

## SJA Prompts

1. How might you imagine economic disparity across the world's population could affect access to healthcare and healthcare outcomes?
2. As you read through the textbook, the interconnection between society, health inequalities, and the need to provide adequate healthcare for all people may become clearer to you. Students in global health education address these concerns. What might be some essential communication skills required for work in the global health arena?
3. How can communication help in addressing some of the challenges of global health?
4. Can you conduct a similar exercise across the disciplines of cultural studies, political science, nursing, and sociology? What shared patterns do you notice?

## Resources

Benatar, S. R., Gill, S., & Bakker, I. (2011). Global health and the global economic crisis. *American Journal of Public Health, 101*(4). 646–653. https://doi.org/10.2105/AJPH.2009.188458

Drain, P. K. (2017). The emergence of undergraduate majors in global health. *American Journal of Tropical Medicine and Hygiene, 96*(1), 16–23. https://doi.org/10.4269/ajtmh.16-0687

National Institute of Environmental Health Sciences (NIEHS). (2022). *Climate change and human health*. Retrieved from https://www.niehs.nih.gov/research/programs/climatechange/index.cfm

## Constructing Global Health Priorities

In the complex global health landscape, it is key to understand not only how health can be defined but also how health-related priorities can be identified from a WPHC SJA perspective. It is important that global health practitioners ensure they conduct their work equitably and ethically by including local voices and supporting agencies. This section looks at the different priorities that fall under global health under the domain of structural and clinical priorities.

### Structural Priorities

Building research and public health communication infrastructure is critical for the successful detection of emerging infectious diseases, as well as for containing the impact of endemic diseases. Such public health communication efforts can make a significant difference in the management of outbreaks at a global level, particularly in disadvantaged global regions. Examples of public health efforts have that made a difference in stopping outbreaks include the polio outbreak in Mali, the yellow fever outbreak in Angola, and the avian flu outbreak in Cambodia (CDC, 2021). Structural priorities lay the foundation for global health efforts in improving health outcomes and doing so in a manner that achieves health equity for everyone, irrespective of where they are on the planet.

### Concerns

However, health communication researchers have highlighted the concern of misinformation circulating on the internet about global epidemics such as Ebola and global perception and response to the Ebola epidemic (Hai et al., 2017). The Ebola epidemic originated in West Africa. The authors analyzed English-language stories about the keyword "Ebola" from US and global sources to understand how social network theory and networked global public members shaped health communication efforts. Their findings highlight how public engagement on social media was primarily directed toward the risk of US domestic Ebola infections rather than Ebola infections in West Africa or on science-based information.

*Textbox 11.5 presents the WPHC domain of a few select NTDs, along with their causes, the affected vulnerable target populations, symptoms, and preventive public health measures (NIAID, 2015). Review these to complete the SJA activity below in designing a global health communication artifact.*

### Textbox 11.5    WPHC Domain—NTDs: An Overview

| NTD | Caused By | Who Does It Affect | Symptoms | How Is It Prevented |
|---|---|---|---|---|
| Dengue fever [European Center for Disease Prevention and Control (ECDC), 2014] | Carried by mosquitoes and caused by any of four dengue viruses | Those living in Asian, Pacific, and Latin American countries where it is a leading cause of death among children | Severe join and muscle pain; left untreated, hemorrhage and shock leading to death | Integrated vector management programs, dengue vaccine, reduction of mosquito breeding sites, personal protection measures |
| Leprosy (Hansen's Disease) (Cleveland Clinic, 2022) | Mycobacteria | Most cases detected in Asia and Africa | Permanent damage to skin, nerves, limbs, and eyes | Avoiding contact with infected people |
| Human African trypanosomiasis (sleeping sickness) [National Library of Medicine (NLM), 2022] | Parasite transmitted from tsetse flies | Rural and remote areas in sub-Saharan Africa | Headaches, fever, weakness, stiffness; if parasite migrates to central nervous system, it can cause seizures, psychiatric disorders, and death | Personal protection measures— avoid travel to endemic areas, avoid wearing dark contrasting colors |

## SJA Activity

Your task as a global health communication specialist is to employ communication messages and artifacts to increase evidence-based knowledge of the risk factors, disease prevention behaviors, and health promotion behaviors among the local community members.

1. Research any NTD listed in the table. Learn more about the cultural and social values that characterize the global region of their incidence.
2. In what ways might the affected populations be described as subaltern?
   a. What risk factors increase their vulnerability to NTDs?
   b. What forms of structural change are needed to envisage global health equity in the domain of NTDs?
3. Design a communication artifact that demonstrates the ethical principles of global health communication (equity, collaboration, partnership, cultural sensitivity, and empowerment) for the NTD.
   a. Try to use at least one visual in each artifact.
   b. Pay attention to your use of culturally appropriate symbols, colors, design elements, and music, if any.

## Resources

Cleveland Clinic. (2022, May 18). *Leprosy (Hansen's Disease)*. Retrieved from https://my.clevelandclinic.org/health/diseases/23043-leprosy-hansens-disease#:~:text=Who%20does%20leprosy%20affect%3F,bodies%20fight%20off%20the%20infection

European Center for Disease Prevention and Control (ECDC). (2014, August 12). *Factsheet about dengue*. Retrieved from https://www.ecdc.europa.eu/en/dengue-fever/facts

NIAID (2015, October 27). *Types of neglected tropical diseases*. Retrieved from https://www.niaid.nih.gov/research/neglected-tropical-diseases-types

National Library of Medicine (NLM). (2022, August 8). *African trypanosomiasis*. Retrieved from https://www.ncbi.nlm.nih.gov/books/NBK519580/

## Infrastructure, Investment, and Global Health Threat Assessment

International health communication can shape how local and national structural health priorities are addressed to allow LMICs to manage their resource, knowledge, and infrastructure needs to achieve health outcomes sustainably and efficiently, prioritizing those who are most vulnerable. The media can play an important role as a collaborator in emerging infectious disease reporting efforts and shaping how structural resources are directed by managing public opinion during global public health threats.

### Structural Priorities

For instance, communicating Water, Sanitation, and Hygiene (WASH) priorities can help provide opportunities for a hygienic environment for disadvantaged populations in the LMICs. Improving WASH infrastructure involves attending to structural priorities such as the provision of clean running water, sanitation facilities, and community health clinics. Establishing

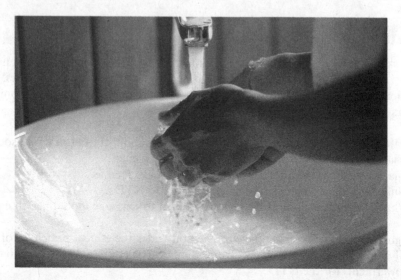

*Figure 11.2* WASH Priorities Can Help Provide Opportunities for a Hygienic Environment in LMICs.

infrastructure can involve investment in WASH facilities and education to end open defecation, wastewater treatment, safe reuse, increased water-use efficiency, ensuring freshwater supplies, and restoring water-related ecosystems (UN), Sustainable Development Goals, (SDGs) 3, 4, and 6, 2020).

### Potential for Negative Impact

Provision of clean water, sanitation, health clinics, power, and roads is one way of thinking about infrastructure. The potential for negative impact of international health communication regarding global epidemics is significant. Communication researchers Mason and Wright (2014) conduct a content analysis of domestic and international print news reports using vested interest theory examining how the crisis communication of the New Delhi Metallo-beta-lactamase-1 (NDM-1) virus in India and the severity of the threat were conveyed. Their analysis identified how the way the threat was communicated resulted in the negative outcome of India receiving an international communication warning and triggering false alarm systems regarding global health threats. Their findings corroborate the need for greater rigor in threat assessment protocols to ensure that a consistent voice is maintained in the messaging process and ensure that public trust in expert information sources. However, even with infrastructure elements in place, how decisions are made and how threats are communicated is important to understand their social impact.

### Social-Cultural Structure

Researchers Airhihenbuwa et al. (2014) interpret infrastructure as a social-cultural structure within which health decisions and communication may occur to understand how agency and identities give meaning to health behaviors and sociocultural practices. Airhihenbuwa (2007, 2005) defines social-cultural infrastructure as the "systems and mechanisms of culture that nurture social strengths by rendering them assets in containing epidemics" (p. 1). They recommend attending to complexity, plurality, and contradictions as centered in sociocultural frameworks for development in African contexts. SJA-centered global health communication attends to social and cultural values that are meaningful to community members and address the unique historical, social, economic, and political contexts in which the health challenges occur.

### Global Health Security

A second structural priority of global health is achieving global health security. A key global lesson from the COVID-19 pandemic was the need to protect the planet from global health threats. In 2022, the Global Health Council called for a new definition of global health security (Global Health Council, 2022). The revised definition of global health focuses on the multidisciplinary, multisectoral, and safety-focused orientation of the field. It addresses the holistic roots of global health and emphasizes the safety and security of all people. Structurally, factors such as existing prevention, detection, and response capabilities present at a national level in local programs, policies, laws, and initiatives inform global health security arrangements.

*Examine **Textbox 11.6** to understand the CDC's work in the international domain in the arena of global health security. Read the Guinea case study to prevent Ebola and attempt the discussion prompt activity that follows to support community collaboration and involvement.*

---

### Textbox 11.6    Mini-Case Study

#### CDC's Work in Global Health

#### *WPHC Context*

One of the CDC's efforts globally is in the direction of supporting the goal of achieving global health and health security for Americans. For instance, the CDC works to eradicate polio through the Polio Eradication Initiative and other vaccine-preventable diseases and keeps them from traveling to other countries (CDC, 2016).

The CDC's Global Health Security Agency (GHSA) is a global collaboration initiative. In this effort, CDC partners with 31 countries globally. The thrust of these efforts is to strengthen global public health capacity to prevent, detect, and respond to infectious disease threats. These countries range from Bangladesh, Burkina Faso, and Cameroon, to Ghana, Guinea, India, and Indonesia, and Pakistan, Peru, Senegal, Thailand, Ukraine, and Vietnam. Read on to see some of the objectives of the GHSA.

The GHSA seeks to

1. Prevent and reduce the likelihood of outbreaks—natural, accidental, or intentional.
   a. Promote national biosafety and biosecurity systems.
   b. Reduce infectious disease outbreaks.
   c. Prevent the emergence of antimicrobial drug-resistant organisms and zoonotic diseases.
   d. Strengthen international regulatory frameworks.

2. Detect threats early to save lives.
   a. Biosurveillance
   b. Rapid and transparent reporting and data sharing
   c. Novel diagnostics and laboratory systems
   d. Training of personnel

3. Respond rapidly and effectively using multisectoral, international coordination and communication.
   a. Interconnected network of Global Emergency Operations Centers and multisectoral response units
   b. Improve global access to countermeasures during health emergencies

## WPHC Guinea Case Study to Prevent Ebola

In 2015, Ebola spread from a remote area in Guinea to become the world's first epidemic of the virus. The CDC involved the community to stop the spread of infectious diseases by engaging in community outreach, building triage centers at healthcare facilities, and training healthcare workers (CDC, 2017). Through a five-year surveillance program called *Epi-détecte*, the CDC engaged with local health workers and the community to build trust and strengthen public health systems. Under this program, local community agents act as the surveillance system's eyes and ears on the ground and use mobile phone credits to contact their supervising health centers if they find a potential case or disease event. They also build trust and communication by getting to know families and sharing information on diseases, symptoms, and action steps.

## SJA Discussion Prompt for Supporting Community Collaboration and Involvement

1. Examine any one of the GHSA's goals presented earlier. How can local community priorities be centered on designing initiatives that prioritize their cultural and social values?
2. Balancing funding for resource allocation and regional priorities during global health epidemics can challenge effective coordination at global and local levels as a range of national priorities and cultural approaches collide. How can global health communication advocate for and create messaging that is inclusive, culturally responsive, and incorporate evidence-based public health knowledge in an equitable manner?
3. What challenges do you foresee global health communication practitioners facing?

## Resources

CDC. (2017, August 6). *Guinea module 1: Engaging communities to prevent disease outbreaks*. Retrieved from https://www.cdc.gov/globalhealth/security/stories/guinea-module-1-prevent-disease-outbreaks.html
CDC. (2016, January 16). *The Global Health Security Agenda*. Retrieved from https://www.cdc.gov/globalhealth/security/ghsagenda.htm

CRITIQUES OF GLOBAL HEALTH SECURITY

As a global health priority, global health security approaches have been critiqued for how health security risks are framed and prioritized. For instance, Ghebreyesus and Sands (2022) noted that although COVID-19 at its peak was killing people at the same rate as HIV, TB, and malaria combined, the death toll from these three diseases would have increased because of the lockdowns, resource-diversion, and interruption to lifesaving services imposed by the pandemic. The global health security framework has also been critiqued for its need to address the imperatives of where the LMICs' development and humanitarian issues pose as serious a concern as global health security threats pose to the industrialized and wealthy nations.

*Coordination and Communication*
To maximize effectiveness, public health considerations such as coordination and communication between different government agencies and sectors, political leadership, and engagement in global multilateral institutions are important considerations. In emphasizing the health security of all people on the planet, the revised definition seeks to highlight that global health security decisions involve a deep and fundamental discussion of human rights, equity, dignity, and sustainable development for all global regions. The notion of global health security has been critiqued by developing countries, which seek to understand the term as a public health concept removed from national security agendas. Trust-building initiatives in the use of shared health surveillance data, for example, need to emphasize that global cooperation will undergird policy in industrialized countries emphasizing the use of the term to reference the protection of their populations against external health threats such as those posed by pandemics and terrorism (Aldis, 2008).

*Program Design*
An important goal of global health security is designing programs to anticipate and protect people from the risk of dangerous pathogens and potential epidemics. The Division of Global Health Protection (DGHP) at CDC, for instance, leads global health security efforts by working with partner countries to build core public health capacities. These capacities help identify and contain outbreaks before they become epidemics. Public health considerations also emphasize the risk environment, accounting for the social, political, and environmental risks of emerging infectious diseases. From a public health perspective, analyzing the risk environment will include integrating the economic, regulatory, and political systems to coordinate data on global travel, migration, commerce, land use, climate, and geopolitical stability (Ravi et al., 2019).

*Building Multilateral Support*
A third, related priority of global health is constructing multilateral support. Multilateral support seeks to leverage the support of large donors such as the United States and donor agencies. Multilateral institutions are better able to protect the world against health threats. With collaborative partnerships, multilateral institutions can mobilize support, seek sustained financing from organizations such as the WHO, and work together as active participants in these efforts.

*Clinical Priorities*
International health communication scholar Professor Dutta has questioned the public health-centered behavior change approach to helping the disease and illness concerns of disadvantaged

global communities. The CCA emphasizes how larger factors like policy and infrastructure can be interlaid with social and cultural factors to help vulnerable individuals carve out their own space and voice. Through extensive immersive research on the marginalized tribal Santalis in India, Dutta argues how food, hunger, and the structural barriers posed by poverty emerge as central to the meaning of health and illness (Dutta, 2004). The WHO estimates that about 25% of the disease burden in the developing world is due to environmental factors (National Institute of Environmental Health Sciences, NIEHS, 2022). The negative health outcomes of poverty are closely related to the environment. In 2004, about 1.9 million individuals, primarily children, died from inadequate access to clean water and sanitation.

### Invitation for a Dialogic Approach

Communication researchers Clair and colleagues examined how health policies and programs related to open defecation (OD) in India could make an effective impact on the concern. Taking a dialogic and dialectical approach, the researchers find that, to be effective, health policy needs to be multipronged and poly-vocal and address social communication, gender, cultural, health, and work identity issues (2019). Two million people, mostly women and children, die each year from exposure to indoor air pollution from cooking with solid fuels such as wood, dung, and charcoal. Noncommunicable diseases (NCDs) such as heart disease, stroke, diabetes, cancer, and chronic respiratory conditions predominantly impact LMIC. About 80% of all deaths due to NCDs occur in the developing world. Moreover, people in the developing world die from NCDs at a younger age than people in the developed world. About 29% of all deaths from NCDs in the low-and middle-income countries occur in individuals under the age of 60. NCDs are particularly susceptible to environmental hazards, including air pollution, toxic chemics, and built environments that discourage physical activity. Disease and disability related to polluted environments take a toll on human suffering, add to the financial burden of affected countries, and decrease economic productivity (NIEHS, 2022).

### Neglected Tropical Diseases (NTDs)

The clinical priorities of global health span domains ranging from addressing tropical infectious diseases to the heightened emphasis on mental health and overall well-being. According to the WHO, NTDs comprise a group of about 20 distinct conditions prevalent mainly in tropical regions of the world (see Textbox 11.5). NTDs affect over 1.7 billion of the world's population. Their impact is the most severe among disadvantaged communities, women, and children in developing LMICs. In these regions, the NTDs are responsible for some of the most devastating health, social, and economic consequences to more than a billion people. They cost the affected communities the equivalent of billions of US dollars annually in direct health costs, loss of productivity, and reduced socioeconomic and educational attainment. Besides these impacts, NTDs are also responsible for consequences such as disability, stigmatization, social exclusion, and discrimination. A greater realization for increased public awareness around mental health concerns and greater political attention that will empower employer and local government involvement is needed to meet the gaps in mental health awareness, resources, and services.

*Review **Textbox 11.7** that centers on the WPHC SJA perspective of **health as a human right** in the context of NTDs. Try your hand at designing a culturally sensitive SJA-informed communication artifact following the instructions in the textbox.*

---

**Textbox 11.7    Health as a Human Right: The Case of NTDs**

**WPHC Context**

The WHO recognizes over 20 NTDs. All the NTDs are preventable and to a large extent, treatable. The NTDs are described in **Textbox 11.5**.

These NTDs affect over one billion people globally. Those affected tend to be some of the most disadvantaged individuals living in low-income countries. They especially highlight human rights challenges pertaining to inequity in access to preventative chemotherapy and morbidity management, stigma and discrimination, and patients' rights and nondiscrimination in healthcare settings.

**SJA Discussion Prompt**

The enjoyment of the highest attainable standard of health has been recognized in the WHO Constitution as a fundamental right of every human being.

1. Design a brochure that highlights the connection between the right to health and the need to address interventions for NTDs as a human rights issue.
2. What principles and facets of global health communication did you incorporate into your brochure?

**Resources**

Sun, N., & Amon, J. J. (2018). Addressing inequity. *Health and Human Rights*, *20*(1), 11–25. Retrieved from https://www.ncbi.nlm.nih.gov/pmc/articles/PMC6039727/

WHO. (2022). *Neglected tropical diseases*. Retrieved from https://www.who.int/health-topics/neglected-tropical-diseases#tab=tab_2

---

### Global Health Risk Communication

Addressing these constructs in risk communication of NTDs plays an important role in sharing information that is accurate, unbiased, and trust-worthy. Global health risk communication involves the exchange of information between experts and the public regarding a health threat to the survival, health, economic, or social well-being of a population. For example, understanding risk communication from the target audience's perspective can help health communication professionals. In this instance, health professionals might use social media and other channels of information to spread awareness of how the epidemiology of NTDs is closely intertwined with environmental conditions in complex ways through its effect on the geographic spread of vector-borne diseases and its effect on ecosystem habitats in which vectors and nonhuman hosts thrive. Communication of information on NTDs by health authorities can emphasize how such diseases can be prevented through controlling vectors by approaches such as mass spraying of insecticides in areas where vectors breed or gather to kill them before they become parasite carriers. Mass media can also spread awareness of newer ways of vector control including by genetically altering the vectors themselves so they cannot carry the parasite. When these genetically altered vectors are released into the population, they will breed and spread their genetic abnormalities to future generations.

NTDs are often vector-borne, i.e., are transmitted by the bite of an infected species such as mosquitoes, ticks, worms, flies, and fleas. Risk communication is central to the prevention and control of NTDs by impacting risk perception, increasing awareness, and bringing about behavior change. Mulderij-Jansen et al. (2020) look at how risk communication through the exchange of real-time information such as advice and opinions between experts and individuals can help prevent and control NTDs. Their study finds that television, radio, and newspapers were important mass media channels for information sharing regarding dengue and *chikungaya*, while interpersonal channels such as family, friends, and neighbors, also played an important role in information sharing. They also found that women were more likely than men to use the internet and that internet use decreased with age. Their study employed the Health Belief Model (HBM) and the Theory of Planned Behavior. They examined each of the constructs in the theory, including the essential role of cultural constructs and trust between the community and local health authorities.

### Disease Prevention

Public health measures such as vaccination campaigns are important during global health risk communication. Other global health domains, such as those of NTDs can be easily prevented even without vaccines. In such cases, knowledge gained through increasing awareness and health promotion behavior change can support positive global health outcomes. Clean water, sanitary food handling, and good hygiene can prevent diseases such as guinea-worm disease, schistosomiasis, soil-transmitted helminthiasis, and trachoma (NIAID, 2009). As NIAID notes, education of at-risk vulnerable populations is an important step in controlling the spread of NTDs. With proper awareness, people learn how to control environmental factors that invite NTDs and thus, learn to reduce their risk. A good example of education as an effective approach to controlling NTDs is malaria by increasing awareness of how eliminating areas of standing water will remove habitats for mosquitoes to breed and thus reduce the risk of mosquito-borne diseases. The provision of treated bed nets will also support such measures by reducing the risk of diseases carried by flies that circulate at night.

### Sustainable Development Goals (SDGs)

Even given these formidable impacts and challenges in mitigating the vectors and transmission modes of NTDs, these diseases have ranked very low historically from the global health agenda. In fact, NTDs were almost absent from the global health agenda until the 2015 SDGs, target 3.3. Their neglect has the downstream effect of exacerbating global health inequities and with it economic, social, intellectual, and personal attainment of a large part of the globe. The 2030 global target includes a 90 percent reduction in the number of people requiring treatment for NTDs, a 75% reduction in disability-adjusted life years (DALYs) related to NTDs, at least 100 countries eliminating at least one NTD, and the eradication of two diseases globally (dracunculiasis and yaws).

### Cross-Sectoral Nature

This neglect of NTDs has been attributed partly to their cross-sectoral nature. The widespread impact of NTDs intersects closely with many of the goals of the SDGs. According to the WHO, if interventions to tackle NTDs were to be made a global priority, it would also impact the accomplishment of progress in achieving all the SDGs. The WHO has sought to create integrated cross-cutting approaches to target NTDs. These approaches highlight the coordination and scaling-up of key interventions such as preventive chemotherapy, individualized case management, vector control, veterinary public health, and provision of WASH. Cross-sectoral approaches also include social and cultural change.

For example, from a public health perspective, eliminating leprosy includes minimizing rates of infection and disease but also the steps that need to be taken to address the stigma and discrimination of those infected. This involves clinical expertise (e.g., contact tracing for new cases and preventive chemotherapy), alongside vaccination initiatives. Equally important, it also involves garnering political commitment to ensure equity and access to resources for leprosy management, partnerships, and coalitions at a national level to engage all stakeholders; institutional collaboration to build capacity in the healthcare system; and monitoring of antimicrobial resistance and adverse drug reactions (WHO. 2022).

*Review **Textbox 11.8** to read through the WPHC thought scenario provided to illustrate global health disparities. Respond to the Discussion Questions that follow. How does the critical example provided help you employ SJA to understand the ethical challenges facing global health communicators?*

---

**Textbox 11.8   Discussion Questions/Thought Scenarios for Reflection**

**WPHC Thought Scenario**

Researchers Benatar et al. (2011) note

Modern advances in healthcare have benefited only about 20% of the world's population. In the 1990s, 89% of the annual world expenditure on healthcare was spent on 16% of the world's population, who bear only about 7% of the global burden of disease in DALYs.

- Annual per capita expenditure on healthcare ranges from more than $6,000 in the United States (17% of the gross domestic product, GDP) to less than $10 in the poorest countries in Africa (< 3% of GDP).
- Half of the world's population lives in countries that cannot afford annual per capital health expenditures of more than $15, and many people do not have access to even basic drugs.
- About 51%–60% of the world's population (3.2–3.8 billion people) live in miserable conditions, below what is defined as the "ethical poverty line" of living on $2.80 to $3.00 per person per day. This population has not benefited at all from the tremendous progress in science and medicine.

Consider the previous statistics when considering the following indicators:

Rapid economic growth or the real-world annual income, measured in purchasing power parities, increased from $25.096 trillion in 1990 to $71.845 trillion in 2009.

Unprecedented advances in science, technology, and medical care have brought us artificial intelligence algorithms that can read chest X-rays better than radiologists, inexpensive genomic sequencing that can guide personalized cancer treatments, and vast improvements in population health management through big data and analytics.

However, the humanitarian challenges to equitable access to healthcare and healthcare outcomes have only compounded as the COVID-19 pandemic revealed.

Such vast disconnects between progress and healthcare equity have led many researchers like Benatar to call for new ways of thinking that transcend national and institutional boundaries. They call for recognizing the **interdependence** of health and disease in a globalizing world with privilege and impoverishment. Such thinking foregrounds the need to see sustainable improvement in health and well-being as a necessity for all.

## SJA Discussion Questions

1. How would you understand what it means for people to flourish in different cultural, regional, and physical environments?
2. What would such a criterion for human flourishing involve (such as, for example, a condition in which essential life needs are met)?
3. Consider the fact that less than one-third of the world's population flourishes amid conditions of relative affluence and more than two-thirds do not have their essential needs met. What role should social justice play in producing caring social institutions to help all individuals achieve their full potential?

### Destigmatization

By supporting destigmatization, patient empowerment, and dialogue, communication researchers can utilize dialogue, interaction, participation, and engagement in different settings from the community to the family. International health communication can thus make an important contribution to controlling the spread and mitigating the severity of NTDs. Communication of these public health approaches and strategies is an important component of WPHC and the management of global health challenges such as leprosy. Krishnataray's (2010) experimental study examined the relative effectiveness of diffusion and participatory strategies in health communication campaigns in leprosy destigmatization in the state of Madhya Pradesh, India. He looked at the effect of cast on knowledge, perception of risk, and behavioral involvement. His study found that participatory strategies that promoted dialogue and interaction and incorporated people's knowledge and action factors had a greater impact on leprosy destigmatization through increasing knowledge, lowering perception of risk, and increasing behavioral involvement. By using a qualitative phenomenological approach, researchers Nasir and colleagues examine the life experience of leprosy families to support the healing of leprosy patients in Indonesia. Studying family communication provides insight into how leprosy sufferers who experience clinical, psychological, social, and behavioral impacts of the disease can find support in overcoming the severity of the disease. Their study finds that efforts in the family to understand, support, establish communication, and increase involvement by restoring self-confidence can help in the recovery of leprosy (2022).

## Dialogic Approaches to Multisectoral Partnerships in Global Health

In this section on dialogic approaches to multisectoral partnerships in global health, multisectoral partnerships are discussed through the SJA lens of an integrated approach highlighting facets like multisectoral coordination, sustainability, agency, and empowerment in global health initiatives, resource mobilization, and technology and innovation.

## Multisectoral Partnerships

Multisectoral partnerships can make a significant difference in the health of vulnerable global populations. In his editorial, scholar Scott Ratzan (2010) highlights how maternal and children's health problems associated with childbirth in developing countries can be positively impacted by UN initiatives that focus on maternal and children's health services. The United States invests almost $10.4 billion in global health annually (Kaiser Family Foundation, 2022). This represents an increase of approximately 96% since 2006. A large percentage of this investment is focused on protecting the health of US citizens and residents. Public health efforts in the international arena remain focused on areas such as tracking and preventing emerging infectious diseases to make the world a safer place.

### Actors and Stakeholders

A range of actors and stakeholders comprise the field of global health. These range from donors, multilateral international nongovernmental organizations, global health initiatives, and online networks of individuals. Hoffman and colleagues estimate that there may be more than 40 bilateral donors, 26 UN agencies, 20 global and regional funds, and 90 global health initiatives that comprise the global health landscape (The National Archives, 2007). A focus on integrated approaches, multisectoral coordination, universal health coverage, and country ownership can help speed up progress against NTDs.

*Review **Textbox 11.9** to understand the WPHC context of how foundation support can work to support and expand civil rights in the domain of global health. Respond to the SJA Discussion Prompt that follows.*

---

**Textbox 11.9   Multisectoral Partnerships in Foundation Funding and Health Equity**

### WPHC Context

A report on racial justice to the Rockefeller Foundation puts forward community solutions to achieve health equity. This report suggests that the following are needed to achieve the goals of **health equity** (The Rockefeller Foundation, 2023):

1. Foundation support should expand civil rights and racial justice to take on injustice and educate the public on the nature and causes of exclusion, race, ethnicity, and class.
2. Foundation support should explore creative approaches to sustain broad constituencies in areas such as health, education, and community revitalization.
3. Foundation support should allocate provision of funding to increase organizational capacity.
4. Foundation support should focus on strategic funding of national, regional, and local groups to design community solutions, connect with the broad national civil rights community, build partnerships, and speak in their own voice.

## SJA Discussion Prompt

One of the ways foundation support can integrate equity into their goals and objectives is through exploring creative ways of building local agency.

- How can foundation support empower marginalized communities to use local democracy to challenge structures that isolate and impoverish them?
- Civil rights have been understood as encompassing the domains of healthcare, education, employment, and housing. What forms of multisectoral partnerships can you envisage in these key domains to bring about effective change in the health outcomes of disadvantaged communities?

## Resources

The Rockefeller Foundation. (2023). *The Rockefeller Foundation and Digital Square at PATH commit to $5M to strengthening data-driven health systems & global immunizations.* Retrieved on February 21, 2023, from https://www.rockefellerfoundation.org/news/the-rockefeller-foundation-and-digital-square-at-path-commit-5m-to-strengthening-data-driven-health-systems-global-immunizations/

### Sustainable Partnerships

Creating sustainable partnerships across multiple stakeholders is essential for successful global health initiatives. Such stakeholders include organizations with a health mission, such as public health agencies, hospitals, or federally qualified health centers. They can also include community health organizations, faith-based organizations, businesses, education sectors, academia, philanthropy, housing, justice, planning and land use organizations, public safety, and transportation agencies, alongside collaborations with public- and private-sector agencies. At the heart of successful global health initiatives are communication strategies that make sustainable partnerships effective.

### EMPOWERMENT-CENTERED APPROACHES

Communication researchers Kraft et al. (2014) found that evidence-based behavior change interventions addressing gender dynamics are central to improving child health outcomes in low-and middle-income countries. Their study found that empowerment approaches that incorporated participatory action and shifted gender norms around communication and decision-making between spouses for maternal-child health increased educational and economic resources and modified norms to reduce child marriage were important in making a difference.

### COMMUNITY-BASED SOLUTIONS

Such broad-based alliances are crucial in increasing the capacity to deploy needed skills in a timely manner, provide resources, and fulfill a multitude of roles in designing community-based solutions. For example, a public health agency or a church congregation can serve as a convener of coalitions in data analysis involving the local hospital, university, or school district. They can also support fundraising and designing locally based creative solutions (Baciu & Sharfstein, 2016).

### Technology and Innovation
Employing technology and innovation is another approach to supporting multisectoral partnerships in global health.

### TECHNOLOGY

Precision public health is an evolving field where data and information come together to help envisage targeted solutions that address global health problems. Communication research that examines how to tailor messages informed by audience research data to a target audience can increase the effectiveness of public health messages. Lazarus and Wyka (2020) examined how COVID-19 vaccine acceptance varied by age, gender, and level of education globally. Such studies show how data and information coupled with cultural understandings can be effective in disseminating and promoting health-related information across different cultural contexts in global settings.

### INNOVATION

Several lifesaving products have been developed through cross-sectoral partnerships between corporations, public health organizations, and domestic governments that have focused on innovation as an approach to global health. For example, inhaled oxytocin was developed through the Saving Lives at Birth initiative, which was a collaboration between the healthcare company GlaxoSmithKline, Monash University, and other groups. This product stops maternal hemorrhaging by being placed in an asthma inhaler and thus does not require refrigeration or delivery by injection. Another example is Becton's Odon device, which is used for assisted vaginal delivery in delayed labor. This device is one of the first innovations in assisted vaginal delivery in over 200 years.

*Review* **Textbox 11.10** *to gain a deeper WPHC-centered contextual understanding of global health issues and their transnational nature. How is climate change communication similar? Respond to the SJA Discussion Prompt provided.*

---

**Textbox 11.10   The Transnational Nature of Global Health**

**WPHC Context of Transnational Health**

Global health issues, such as those involving infectious diseases, do not stay within the borders of one country but spread to multiple countries and regions of the world. HIV/AIDS, malaria, Zika, and TB are a few examples of diseases that affect countries across the world. Likewise, when we think about climate change, it impacts the health of people in different regions across the globe in different ways. Pollution from emissions or natural causes like wildfire smoke and volcano eruptions does not stay in the region it started in.

---

**SJA Discussion Prompt**

1. Can you think of additional health concerns not identified in the discussion that are not limited to any one country?
2. How can we understand the connections between the health of all people? Can you think of an example?
3. What forms of actions can people take where they live daily to support the health of all in our world? In what ways do these actions connect the local and the global?

---

### Resource Mobilization

Resource mobilization is a key facet for global health initiatives. Communication researchers Prio and Kaufmann (2010) examine the Global Polio Eradication Initiative (GPEI) that underestimated the difficulty and costs of the campaign. Coupled with funding shortfalls, the program faltered, emphasizing the necessity of engaging in advocacy for resource mobilization.

#### FOUNDATION SUPPORT

Foundation support has also been critical in supporting investment in communities of color and low-income communities, and advancing the civil rights movement for social justice through advocacy and organizing for structural change. The environmental justice movement has received valuable support toward organizational infrastructure building, community organizing, leadership development, and effective participation in policy and legal arenas (National Academies of Sciences, Engineering, and Medicine, 2017).

#### CORPORATE FUNDING

Corporate funding agencies such as the Warner Music Group Social Justice Fund (WMG BFF SJF) have also made a difference. The WMG BFF SJF has a mission to support global organizations that work to build just and equitable communities in the areas of education, arts and culture, and criminal justice reform. Their work is built on the philosophy that work in these areas can make a difference in dismantling structural racism and advancing equity and justice for all people (2022).

## Giving Voice to Vulnerable Populations and Collaborative Design

The section on giving voice to vulnerable populations and collaborative design centers SJA concerns of access and equity, coproduction of solutions and capacity, and accountability and structural imbalances.

### Subaltern Communities

Communities that are marginalized, "Othered," and displaced within post-colonial social structures are often referred to as subaltern communities. Centering an SJA lens, communication researchers Shastry and Dutta (2017), employ a CCA to critique the neglect of indigenous cultural practices in the public health management of Ebola, thus under-cutting the agency of local communities. The CCA looks at how structure (policies, infrastructure), culture, and individual agency can be brought together to help marginalized individuals, or subaltern communities, find their own voice. It emphasizes the co-creation of practices in a way that is transformative of the oppressive conditions to bring about positive health outcomes (Dutta, 2008). They note how the legitimacy of the indigenous practices was undermined as pathogenic in favor of highlighting the global risks. They present the CCA as a framework for integrating the relationship between indigenous cultural practices, structural determinants of WPHC, and the everyday agency of individuals of affected communities to develop authentic and ethical health communication messages.

*How will you think about what makes an ethical health communication message for indigenous global audiences? Read **Textbox 11.11, Scholar Interview**, to see what challenges one health communication researcher, **Dr. Uttaran Dutta**, faced in responding to the tribal communities he was researching during his fieldwork in India.*

---

### TEXTBOX 11.11    Scholar Interview

#### Dr. Uttaran Dutta
*Arizona State University*

My Field Research Experience ... More Than Just Data-Collection

In my early fieldwork attempts, as a student, I used to conduct in-depth interviews and observe participants in community settings to learn about the conditions of marginalization, and the underserved realities. In other words, I was trying to do field research as sincerely and as academically correct as possible. From the perspectives of many underprivileged communities, such a way of approaching action research was not fully convincing and/or meaningful. They essentially questioned the relevance and appropriateness of my kind of field research in the day-to-day context of their struggle and survival.

For instance—years ago, I went to various geographically-remote regions of eastern India—one of them was an indigenous Himalayan village, to conduct fieldwork. During research interactions, villagers asked me about the practical significance of my research in their day-to-day contexts. They essentially questioned my notion of just "learning about situated needs of underserved communities" without giving something back to the society. One senior resident of the village told me, "You said that you are interviewing us to collect data. That will fulfill your purpose of publishing and securing your career. Now tell us, what are you going to offer our community in return? What will be your contributions in developing or empowering the indigenous people in this village?". A young villager further added, "So many people like you visit our villages. Oftentimes, they give us assurances to develop our community. Then, as soon as they leave the village, they forget about their commitments." Villagers were annoyed of hearing void promises from the outsiders like me; essentially, they wanted to learn about my dedication and accountability in co-developing practical/useful solutions for their contextual needs.

In response, I made a public promise to the villages (as well as to myself)—while doing field research, I will try my best to arrange/organize resources and means so that we (communities and I) can co-create meaningful and sustainable changes at the margins. Following the oath, my later research activities yielded many community-centered and community-led outcomes—including, a mini-hospital, an indigenous library, a tribal museum, an indigenous craft center, a tribal audio-visual recording studio, among others.

### Access and Equity in Global Health

At the heart of justice is global health communication practices that focus on larger social and structural processes while giving voice to the lived experiences and narratives of stigmatized and vulnerable populations. Khan's (2020) study looks at stigma related to HIV/AIDS from the space of ethnographic field research. Arguing that behavioral research is inadequate for the goals of critiquing power, structure, domination, and control, Khan takes a CCA to sigma reduction interventions. Achieving health equity in global contexts means that everyone should have access to healthy environments and conditions in which to be able to live in a manner that sustains and promotes good health.

### Multisectoral Approach

A multisectoral approach involves coordination between different stakeholders and sectors to create a shared vision and approach and to work together to achieve a shared goal. Typically, such collaboration is between local, regional, and national organizations with donor organizations, funders, international nongovernmental organizations, or large research institutes. Achieving health equity implies addressing the factors that comprise the social determinants of global health, eliminating disparities in health systems, and ensuring equal healthcare access in every community, from those that are the closest to us, to those that are far away.

### Coproduction of Solutions

Coproduction of solutions and identification of challenges along with the communities that are affected helps create collaborative partnerships. Mulvale et al. (2019) share how participatory global health projects may unintentionally reinforce existing inequities through perpetuating power differentials. They suggest meaningful engagement, a focus on relationships, and flexibility to respond to the need of vulnerable populations through a focus on user-centered evaluations of co-designed public services. The focus of such partnerships is to create interconnections that link people, nations, and governments in ways that boost collective power to tackle global crises (Deloitte, 2022).

### COLLECTIVE ACTION

Such partnerships encompass the spectrum from health and other government agencies (e.g., education and transportation), collective action to address cross-border health risks, share data, information, and best practices across governments and climate change partnerships for mitigating risks, particularly in less-developed countries.

### PRIORITIZING EMPATHY

Communication researchers Muralidharan and Kim (2020) employ Social Cognitive Theory (SCT) to address the issue of domestic violence through a campaign heightening awareness of the issue through narrative health messages that would prompt bystanders to intervene. Their campaign asked bystanders to call a helpline number as a way of intervening when they encounter domestic violence. As domestic violence stems from deeply rooted patriarchal norms, the researchers found that narratives had a stronger impact on attitude toward the ad and reporting intention and that these effects were mediated by empathy, becoming even stronger when bystander efficacy was low.

## HUMAN-CENTERED DESIGN

Creative approaches such as human-centered design have increasingly sought to place communities and individuals at the center of the solution. Their emphasis is on achieving health equity through community engagement as a driver of solutions. Such place-based initiatives have sought to design solutions that help improve other social determinants of health. Active Living by Design (2016) is one such example. In these cases, collaboration helps to bring multisectoral partnerships and leverage new forums such as by combining professional education, joint conferences, new educational tracks, and new positions within universities to bring together a planner embedded in a public health department and health workers embedded in a planning department. Such partnerships push the envelope in designing solutions that help achieve health equity.

### Philanthropy

Likewise, with $46 billion spent annually on global health causes, philanthropy spends more on health-related causes than any other cause. With the COVID-19 pandemic, philanthropy provided critical funding for vaccine development, medical equipment, mutual aid, social welfare, and global health infrastructure. In addition, traditionally, the philanthropic sector has focused on providing support for leadership and capacity development and on providing a forum that brings together individuals and organizations in an inclusive manner across a broad landscape of community members to achieve a common goal. Such funding encourages the capacity of participants to fully engage by supporting the development of new leaders from within the communities. These pathways are essential for creating sustainable change going beyond the funding duration (National Academies of Sciences, Engineering, and Medicine, 2017).

### Accountability and Structural Imbalances

The benefits of such multisectoral partnerships are immense. However, there are cautions. Some scholars have warned against conflicts of interest in close global health philanthropy and institutional relationships. Basu and Dutta (2007) argue for co-constructing local meanings of health in marginalized tribal populations in India through structural capabilities and equitable negotiation of the tensions between tradition and modernization of health interventions. Stuckler et al. (2011) study the relationships between private foundations that are tax-exempt and for-profit corporations in their initiatives targeting global health. They find that many public health foundations have associations with private food and pharmaceutical corporations. In some instances, they note, the corporations directly benefit from the foundation grants, and the foundations are in turn invested in the success of the corporations. Further conflicts of interest arise when personnel move between food and drug industries and public health foundations. Such relationships can get complicated when foundation board members and decision-makers also sit on the boards of for-profit corporations that benefit from their grants.

## THE NEED FOR TRANSPARENCY

Oftentimes, the standard disclosure protocols for employees in such conflict-of-interest positions are unclear, leading to a lack of transparency. Others have noted the different emerging forms of accountability faced by private philanthropies in global health, such as the Bloomberg Initiative—that combine audit and epidemiology as a form of accountability (Reubi, 2018). Such questions center on where health funding is going versus where it is most needed, and who gets to decide (The Alliance Magazine, 2021).

## NEED TO ELIMINATE STRUCTURAL IMBALANCES

Structural imbalances can run the risk for philanthropy to perpetuate structural imbalances that give rise to health problems in the first place (Youde, 2018). One way to address this is by making reliable and credible healthcare information available to providers through mechanisms that ensure the integrity of the global healthcare knowledge system that embraces global health professionals, policymakers, researchers, publishers, librarians, and information specialists (Pakenham-Walsh, 2012). Effective global health communication, communication researchers have argued, centers advocacy with awareness and funding support for collective efforts in a manner that ensures collaboration between individual countries and the international community.

As we conclude **Chapter 11, Global Health**, consider all the ways that you have engaged with social justice and approaches during this book. Global health communication emphasizes the unity within the differences and disparities that characterize international WPHC contexts.

What role can global health communicators play in ensuring health as an equitable and fundamental right from a perspective? What challenges face global health communication practitioners and scholars in this goal?

*Textbox 11.12 encourages you to envision one way of designing an equitable global healthcare scenario that also meets the WPHC paradigm.*

---

### Textbox 11.12   Present Challenges and Future Directions Exercise

#### Global Health Equity

#### *WPHC Context of Global Health Equity*

Health equity is an ambitious goal for global health. It involves the coming together of many scientific disciplines, organizations, partnerships, and coalitions, toward the achievement of health, nutrition, and well-being goals of the world's most disadvantaged populations. This goal is made more challenging by the fact that health inequities and disparities are growing, not just globally but also nationally, regionally, and within communities everywhere. All the challenges make it seems as though health inequities are intractable, complex, and impossible to solve. Each stakeholder brings to the table their own values, and the conflicting values, explanations, priorities, and interventions often stymie meaningful progress.

## SJA Prompt

Design an equitable healthcare scenario for each of the following scenarios (abstracted from *Johns Hopkins Alliance for a Healthier World*)

1. An effort to enhance economic opportunity in a disadvantaged community also produces hazardous waste that damages air, water, and soil, and harms human health, particularly for marginalized populations.
2. A policy that incentivizes the development of medicines that provide benefits for those who can afford them at the expense of preventive measures and new drug development for conditions that primarily affect the poor.
3. A push to improve access to antimicrobials that has led to their widespread use in animals and humans that has improved food supplies and human health but has also contributed to antimicrobial resistance and its deadly consequences that have challenged the health of disadvantaged populations.

## Resource

Johns Hopkins. *Alliance for a Healthier World. Health equity: Defining a complex concept.* Retrieved December 27, 2022, from https://www.ahealthierworld.jhu.edu/understand-health-equity

## References

Airhihenbuwa, C. O. (2005). Theorizing cultural identity and behavior in social science research. *CODESRIA Bulletin*, Nos. 3–4, 17–19.

Airhihenbuwa, C. O. (2007). *Healing our differences: The crisis of global health and the politics of identity.* Lanham, MD: Rowman & Littlefield.

Airhihenbuwa, C. O., Makoni, S., Iwelunmor, J., & Munodawafa, D. (2014). Sociocultural infrastructure: Communicating identity and health in Africa. *Journal of Health Communication, 19*, 1–5. https://doi.org/10.1080/10810730.2013.868767

Aldis, W. (2008). Health security as a public health concept: A critical analysis. *Health Policy and Planning, 23*(6), 369–375. https://doi.org/10.1093/heapol/czn030

Baciu, A., & Sharfstein, J.M. (2016). Population health case reports: From clinic to community. *JAMA, 315*(24), 2663–2664.

Beaglehole, R., & Bonita, R. (2010). What is global health? *Global Health Action, 3*. https://doi.org/10.3402/gha.v3i0.5142

Basu, A., & Dutta, M. J. (2007). Centralizing context and culture in the co-construction of health: Localizing and vocalizing health meanings in rural India. *Health Communication, 21*(2), 187–196. https://doi.org/10.1080/10410230701305182

CDC. (2021, December 17). *Global health protection and security.* Retrieved from https://www.cdc.gov/globalhealth/healthprotection/ghs/about.html

Center for Global Health. (2022). *CDC's 75 years in public health. Making an impact through global partnerships.* Retrieved February 18, 2023, from https://www.cdc.gov/globalhealth/resources/reports/annual/2022/pdf/cgh_annualreport_2022.pdf

Clair, R. P., Rastogi, R., Lee, S., Clawson, R. A., Blatchley III, E. R., & Erdmann, C. (2019). A dialectical and dialogical approach to health policies and programs: The case of open defecation in India. *Health Communication, 34*(11), 1231–1241. https://doi.org/10.1080/10410236.2018.1473705

Deloitte. (2022). *Government trends 2022*. Retrieved from https://www2.deloitte.com/us/en/insights/industry/public-sector/government-trends/2022/global-health-partnerships-collaboration.html

Dillard, J. P., Li, R., & Yang, C. (2021). Fear of Zika: Information seeking as cause and consequence. *Health Communication, 36*(13), 1785–1795. https://doi.org/10.1080/10410236.2020.1794554

Dutta, M. J. (2004). Poverty, structural barriers, and health: A Santali narrative of health communication. *Qualitative Health Research, 14*(8), 1107–1122. https://doi.org/10.1177/1049732304267763

Dutta, M. J. (2008). *Communicating health: A culture-centered approach.* Cambridge, UK: Polity Press

Dutta, M. J. (2011). Health, human rights, and performance. *Health Communication, 26*(7), 679–682. https://doi.org/10.1080/10410236.2011.575542

Ghebreyesus, T.A., & Sands, P. (2022, September 21). Why the world can't afford to give HIV, TB, and malaria a chance to bounce back. *The Global Fund.* Retrieved on July 30, 2023 from https://www.theglobalfund.org/en/opinion/2022/2022-09-21-these-three-diseases-kill-half-as-many-people-now-as-they-did-20-years-ago/

Global Health Council. (2022, March 8). *GHC Priorities for 2022.* Retrieved from https://globalhealth.org/ghc-priorities-for-2022/

Hai, R., Seymour, B., Fish, S. A., II, Robinson, E., & Zuckerman, E. (2017). Digital health communication and global public influence: A study of the Ebola epidemic. *Journal of Health Communication, 22*(Sup1), 51–58. https://doi.org/10.1080/10810730.2016.1209598

Houpt, E. R., Pearson, R. D., & Hall, T. L. (2007). Three domains of competency in global health education: Recommendations for all medical students. *Global Health, 82*(3), 222–225. https://doi.org/10.1097/ACM.0b013e3180305c10

Johnson, S., Magni, S., Dube, Z., & Goldstein, S. (2018). Extracurricular school-based social change communication program associated with reduced HIV infection among young women in South Africa. *Journal of Health Communication, 23*(12), 1044–1050. https://doi.org/10.1080/10810730.2018.1544675

Kaiser Family Foundation. (2022, September). *The U.S. government and Global Health.* Retrieved from https://www.kff.org/global-health-policy/fact-sheet/the-u-s-government-and-global-health/

Khan, S. (2020). Examining HIV/AIDS-related stigma at play: Power, structure, and implications for HIV interventions. *Health Communication, 35*(12), 1509–1519. https://doi.org/10.1080/10410236.2019.1652386

Kickbush, I. (2006). The need for a European strategy on global health. *Scandinavian Journal of Public Health, 34*, 561–565. https://doi.org/10.1080/14034940600973059

Kraft, J. M., Wilkins, K. G., Morales, G. J., Widyono, M., & Middlestadt, S. E. (2014). An evidence review of gender-integrated interventions in reproductive and maternal child health. *Journal of Health Communication, 19*(S1), 122–1441. https://doi.org/10.1080/10810730.2014.918216

Krishnatray, P. K. (2010). Public communication campaigns in the destigmatization of leprosy: A comparative analysis of diffusion and participatory approaches. A case study in Gwalior, India. *Journal of Health Communication, International Perspectives, 3*(4), 327–344. https://doi.org/10.1080/108107398127148

Lazarus, J. V., & Wyka, K. (2020). Hesitant or not? The association of age, gender, and education with potential acceptance of a COVID-19 vaccine: A country-level analysis. *Journal of Health Communication, 25*(10), 799–807. https://doi.org/10.1080/10810730.2020.1868630

Link, E., Baumann, E., Kreps, G. L., Czerwinski, F., Rosset, M., & Suhr, R. (2022). Expanding the health information national trends survey research program internationally to examine global health communication trends: Comparing health information seeking behaviors in the U.S. and Germany. *Journal of Health Communication, 27*(8), 545–554. https://doi.org/10.1080/10810730.2022.2134522

Mason, A.M., & Wright, K.B. (2014). The life cycle of a virus: The infectious disease narrative of NDM-1. *Journal of Health Communication, 20*(1), 1–14. https://www.doi.org/10.1080/10810730.2014.901442

Mulderij-Jansen, V., Elsinga, J., Gerstenbluth, I., Duits, A., Tami, A., & Bailey, A. (2020). Understanding risk communication for prevention and control of vector-borne diseases: A mixed method study in Curaçao. *PLoS Neglected Tropical Diseases, 14*(4), Article e0008136. https://doi.org/10.1371/journal.pntd.0008136

Mulvale, G., Moll, S., Miatello, A., Robert, G., Larkin, M., Palmer, V. J., Powell, A., Gable, C., & Girlin, M. (2019). Codesigning health and other public services with vulnerable and disadvantaged populations: Insights from an international collaboration. *Health Expectations, 22*(3), 284–297. https://doi.org/10.1111/hex.12864

Muralidharan, S., & Kim, E. (2020). Can empathy offset low bystander efficacy? Effectiveness of domestic violence prevention narratives in India. *Health Communication, 35*(10), 1229–1238. https://doi.org/10.1080/10410236.2019.1623645

National Academies of Sciences, Engineering, and Medicine. (2017). Partners in promoting Health Equity in communities. In A. Baciu, Y. Negussie, A. Geller, et al. (Eds.), *Communities in action: Pathways to health equity.* Washington DC): National Academies Press. Retrieved from https://www.ncbi.nlm.nih.gov/books/NBK425859/

Nasir, A., Yusuf, A., Listiawan, M. Y., & Makhfudli, M. (2022). The life experience of leprosy families in maintaining interaction patterns in the family to support healing in leprosy patients in Indonesian society. A phenomenological-qualitative study. *PloS Neglected Tropical Diseases, 16*(2), e0010951. https://doi.org/10.1371/journal.pntd.0010264

National Academies of Sciences, Engineering, and Medicine. (2017). Health and medicine division, board on population health and public health practice, committee on community-based solutions to promote health equity in the United States. In A. Baciu, Y. Negussie, A. Geller, et al. (Eds.), *Communities in action: Pathways to health equity.* Washington (DC): National Academies Press (US); The Root Causes of Health Inequity. Retrieved from: https://www.ncbi.nlm.nih.gov/books/NBK425845/

National Institute of Allergy and Infectious Diseases (NIAID). (2009, February 5). *Neglected tropical diseases prevention.* Retrieved from https://www.niaid.nih.gov/research/neglected-tropical-diseases-prevention#:~:text=Vector%2Dborne%20NTDs%E2%80%94those%20that,before%20they%20become%20parasite%20carriers

National Institute of Environmental Health Sciences. (2022, December 8). *Global environmental health and sustainable development.* Retrieved from https://www.niehs.nih.gov/health/topics/population/global/index.cfm

Obregón, R., & Waisbord, S. (2010). The complexity of social mobilization in health communication: Top-down and bottom-up experiences in polio eradication. *Journal of Health Communication, 15*(S1), 25–47. https://doi.org/10.1080/10810731003695367

Pakenham-Walsh, N. (2012). Toward a collective understanding of the information needs of healthcare providers in low-income countries, and how to meet them. *Journal of Health Communication, 17*(S2), 9–17. https://doi.org/10.1080/10810730.2012.666627

Prio, G. A., & Kaufmann, J. (2010). Polio eradication is just over the horizon: The challenges of global resource mobilization. *Journal of Health Communication, 15*(S1), 22–83. https://doi.org/10.1080/10810731003695383

Ratzan, S. C. (2010). A call to action: The global effort on women's and children's health. *Journal of Health Communication, 15*(4), 355–357. https://doi.org/10.1080/10810730.2010.496299

Ravi, S. J., Meyer, D., Cameron, E., Nalabandian, M., Pervaiz, B., & Nuzzo, J. B. (2019). Establishing a theoretical foundation for measuring global health security: A scoping review. *BMC Public Health, 19*, 954. https://doi.org/10.1186/s12889-019-7216-0

Reubi, D. (2018) Epidemiological accountability: Philanthropists, global health, and the audit of saving lives. *Economy and Society, 47*(1), 83–110. https://doi.org/10.1080/03085147.2018.1433359

Shankar, A. V., Onyura, M. A., & Alderman, J. (2015). Agency-based empowerment training enhances sales capacity of female energy entrepreneurs in Kenya. *Journal of Health Communication, 20*(S1), 67–75. https://doi.org/10.1080/10810730.2014.1002959

Shastry, S., & Dutta, M. J. (2017). Health communication in the time of Ebola: A culture-centered interrogation. *Journal of Health Communication, 22*(S), 10–14. https://doi.org/10.1080/10810730.2016.1216205

Stuckler, D., Basu, S., & McKee, M. (2011) Global health philanthropy and institutional relationships: How should conflicts of interest be addressed? *PLoS Med.* 8(4), e1001020. https://doi.org/10.1371/journal.pmed.1001020

The Alliance Magazine. (2021). *Focus on global health*. Retrieved from https://www.alliancemagazine.org/global-health-philanthropy/

The National Archives. (2007, September 5). *The international health partnership launched today. Department for International Development*. Retrieved February 18, 2023, from https://webarchive.national archives.gov.uk/ukgwa/20071104143716/http://www.dfid.gov.uk/news/files/ihp/default.asp

United Nations (UN). (2020). *Sustainable development: Make the SDGs a reality*. UN Department of Economic and Social Affairs. Retrieved February 18, 2023, from https://sdgs.un.org/

Warner Music Group Social Justice Fund. (2022). Retrieved from https://www.wmg.com/fund

WHO. (2022, January 11). *Leprosy*. Retrieved from https://www.who.int/news-room/fact-sheets/detail/leprosy

WHO. (2022b). Leprosy. Retrieved from https://www.who.int/news-room/fact-sheets/detail/leprosy#:~:text=Leprosy%20is%20a%20curable%20disease,%2Ddrug%20therapy%20(MDT)

Youde, J. (2018). Philanthropy and global health. In C. McInnes, K. Lee, & J. Youde (Eds.), *The Oxford handbook of global health politics* (pp. 409–425). https://doi.org/10.1093/oxfordhb/9780190456818.013.24

# Index

Pages in **bold** refer to tables.

Printed in the United States
by Baker & Taylor Publisher Services